Progress in Pain Research and Management
Volume 6

Reflex Sympathetic Dystrophy: A Reappraisal

Mission Statement of IASP Press

The International Association for the Study of Pain (IASP) is a nonprofit, interdisciplinary organization devoted to understanding the mechanisms of pain and improving the care of patients with pain through research, education, and communication. The organization includes scientists and health care professionals dedicated to these goals. The IASP sponsors scientific meetings and publishes newsletters, technical bulletins, the journal *Pain,* and books.

The goal of IASP Press is to provide the IASP membership with timely, high-quality, attractive, low-cost publications relevant to the problem of pain. These publications are also intended to appeal to a wider audience of scientists and clinicians interested in the problem of pain.

Previous volumes in the series
Progress in Pain Research and Management

Pharmacological Approaches to the Treatment of Chronic Pain: New Concepts and Critical Issues, edited by Howard L. Fields and John C. Liebeskind

Proceedings of the 7th World Congress on Pain, edited by Gerald F. Gebhart, Donna L. Hammond, and Troels S. Jensen

Touch, Temperature, and Pain in Health and Disease: Mechanisms and Assessments, edited by Jörgen Boivie, Per Hansson, and Ulf Lindblom

Temporomandibular Disorders and Related Pain Conditions, edited by Barry J. Sessle, Patricia S. Bryant, and Raymond A. Dionne

Visceral Pain, edited by Gerald F. Gebhart

Progress in Pain Research and Management
Volume 6

Reflex Sympathetic Dystrophy: A Reappraisal

Editors

Wilfrid Jänig, Dr med

Physiologisches Institut
Christian-Albrechts-Universität zu Kiel
Kiel, Germany

Michael Stanton-Hicks, MB BS

Pain Management Center
Cleveland Clinic Foundation
Cleveland, Ohio, USA

IASP PRESS • SEATTLE

© 1996 IASP Press,
International Association for the Study of Pain

All rights reserved. No part of this publication may be reproduced, stored in a retrieval system, or transmitted, in any form or by any means, electronic, mechanical, photocopying, recording, or otherwise, without the prior written permission of the Publisher.

Timely topics in pain research and treatment have been selected for publication, but the information provided and opinions expressed have not involved any verification of the findings, conclusions, and opinions by IASP. Thus, opinions expressed in *Visceral Pain* do not necessarily reflect those of IASP or of the Officers and Councillors.

No responsibility is assumed by IASP for any injury and/or damage to persons or property as a matter of product liability, negligence, or from any use of any methods, products, instruction, or ideas contained in the material herein. Because of the rapid advances in the medical sciences, the publisher recommends that there should be independent verification of diagnoses and drug dosages.

Library of Congress Cataloging-in-Publication Data

Reflex sympathetic dystrophy : a reappraisal / editors, Wilfrid Jänig, Michael Stanton-Hicks.
    p.   cm. — (Progress in pain research and management; v. 6)
    Includes bibliographical references and index.
    ISBN 0-931092-13-2
    1. Reflex sympathetic dystrophy. I. Jänig, Wilfrid. II. Stanton-Hicks, Michael d'A. III. Series.
    [DNLM: 1. Reflex Sympathetic Dystrophy. 2. Pain—physiopathology.
W1 PR677BL v.6 1996]
RC422.R43R442 1996
616'.0472—dc20
DNLM/DLC
for Library of Congress   95–45160

Contents

	List of Contributing Authors	vii
	Preface	ix
1.	The Puzzle of "Reflex Sympathetic Dystrophy": Mechanisms, Hypotheses, Open Questions *Wilfrid Jänig*	1
2.	Clinical Characteristics of Patients with Complex Regional Pain Syndrome in Germany with Special Emphasis on Vasomotor Function *Ralf Baron, Helmut Blumberg, Wilfrid Jänig*	25
3.	Clinical Characteristics of Patients with Reflex Sympathetic Dystrophy (Sympathetically Maintained Pain) in the USA *Phillip A. Low, Peter R. Wilson, Paola Sandroni, Catherine L. Willner, Thomas C. Chelimsky*	49
4.	Reflex Sympathetic Dystrophy in Children and Adolescents: Differences from Adults *Robert T. Wilder*	67
5.	Complex Regional Pain Syndromes: Symptoms, Signs, and Differential Diagnosis *Robert A. Boas*	79
6.	Diagnostic Algorithm for Complex Regional Pain Syndromes *Peter R. Wilson, Phillip A. Low, Marshall D. Bedder, Edward C. Covington, Richard L. Rauck*	93
7.	Animal Models and Their Contribution to Our Understanding of Complex Regional Pain Syndromes I and II *Gary J. Bennett, William J. Roberts*	107

8. Afferent Mechanisms Mediating Pain and Hyperalgesias in Neuralgia
   Martin Koltzenburg 123

9. Quantitative Sensory Testing in Patients with Complex Regional Pain Syndrome (CRPS) I and II
   Richard H. Gracely, Donald D. Price, William J. Roberts, Gary J. Bennett 151

10. The Challenge and the Problem of Placebo in Assessment of Sympathetically Maintained Pain
    Donald D. Price, Robert H. Gracely, Gary J. Bennett 173

11. Psychological Issues in Reflex Sympathetic Dystrophy
    Edward C. Covington 191

12. Use of Regional Anesthetics for Diagnosis of Reflex Sympathetic Dystrophy and Sympathetically Maintained Pain: A Critical Evaluation
    Michael Stanton-Hicks, P. Prithvi Raj, Gabor B. Racz 217

Epilogue 239

Index 243

Contributing Authors

Ralf Baron, Dr med, PD *Klinik für Neurologie, Christian-Albrechts-Universität zu Kiel, Kiel, Germany*

Marshall D. Bedder, MD *Advanced Pain Management Group, Portland, Oregon, USA*

Gary J. Bennett, PhD *Neurobiology and Anesthesiology Branch, National Institute of Dental Research, National Institutes of Health, Bethesda, Maryland, USA*

Helmut Blumberg, Dr med, PD *Neurochirurgische Universitätsklinik, Klinikum der Albert-Ludwigs-Universität, Freiburg, Germany*

Robert A. Boas, MB BCh, FANZCA, FRCA *Pain Clinic, Auckland Hospital, Auckland, New Zealand*

Thomas C. Chelimsky, MD *Department of Neurology, Case Western Reserve University, Cleveland, Ohio, USA*

Edward C. Covington, MD *Chronic Pain Rehabilitation Program, The Cleveland Clinic Foundation, Cleveland, Ohio, USA*

Richard H. Gracely, PhD *Neurobiology and Anesthesiology Branch, National Institute of Dental Research, National Institutes of Health, Bethesda, Maryland, USA*

Wilfrid Jänig, Dr med, PD *Physiologisches Institut, Christian-Albrechts-Universität zu Kiel, Kiel, Germany*

Martin Koltzenburg, Dr med *Department of Neurology, University of Würzburg, Würzburg, Germany*

Phillip A. Low, MD *Autonomic Disorders Research Center, Department of Neurology, Mayo Clinic, Rochester, Minnesota, USA*

Donald D. Price, PhD *Anesthesiology Department, Medical College of Virginia, Richmond, Virginia, USA*

Gabor B. Racz, MD *Department of Anesthesiology, Texas Tech University Health Science Center, Lubbock, Texas, USA*

P. Prithvi Raj, MD *Pain Medicine Center, Los Angeles, California*

Richard L. Rauck, MD *Department of Anesthesiology, Bowman Gray School of Medicine, Winston-Salem, North Carolina, USA*

William J. Roberts, PhD *R.S. Dow Neurological Sciences Institute, Portland, Oregon, USA*

Paola Sandroni, MD *Autonomic Disorders Research Center, Department of Neurology, Mayo Clinic, Rochester, Minnesota, USA*

Michael Stanton-Hicks, MB BS, Dr med, FRCA, ABPM *Pain Management Center, The Cleveland Clinic Foundation, Cleveland, Ohio, USA*

Robert T. Wilder, MD, PhD *Department of Anesthesia, Children's Hospital, and Department of Anaesthesia, Harvard Medical School, Boston, Massachusetts, USA*

Catherine L. Willner, MD *Autonomic Disorders Research Center, Department of Neurology, Mayo Clinic, Rochester, Minnesota, USA*

Peter R. Wilson, MB BS, PhD *Pain Clinic, Mayo Clinic, Rochester, Minnesota, USA*

The following participants at the workshop in Orlando, Florida, contributed in the acquisition of the material that is described in this volume:

James N. Campbell, MD *Department of Neurosurgery, The Johns Hopkins Hospital, Baltimore, Maryland, USA*

J. David Haddox, DDS, MD *Center for Pain Medicine, The Emory Clinic; Department of Anesthesiology, Department of Psychiatry and Mental Health Sciences, Emory University School of Medicine, Atlanta, Georgia, USA*

Samuel J. Hassenbusch, MD, PhD *M.D. Anderson Cancer Center/ Neurosurgery, University of Texas, Houston, Texas, USA*

Nagy Mekhail, MD, PhD *Pain Management Center, The Cleveland Clinic Foundation, Cleveland, Ohio, USA*

Harold Merskey, DM *Department of Psychiatry, The University of Western Ontario, and Department of Research, London Psychiatric Hospital, Ontario, Canada*

Wen-Hsien Wu, MD *Pain Management Center, University of Medicine and Dentistry New Jersey, New Jersey Medical School, Newark, New Jersey, USA*

Preface

Interest in the sympathetic nervous system and pain has been reawakened in the last 15 years in clinical as well as in basic research (Basbaum and Besson 1991; Jänig and Schmidt 1992; Fields and Liebeskind 1994). This has led to an increase in knowledge and to interesting controversies that challenge old beliefs about the role of the (efferent) sympathetic nervous system in the generation of certain pain states seen in humans after trauma. It is commonly assumed that this system plays a key role in the generation of these pain states, mainly because sympathetic blocks appear to be rather successful in treating these pains. Clinical pain states treated in this way are often called "reflex sympathetic dystrophy" (RSD, Bonica 1990). This term expresses a philosophy and implies that the sympathetic nervous system is involved in the generation of this pain syndrome. There is, however, considerable argument about this hypothesis.

A conference held in Orlando, Florida, in November 1993 focused mainly on this issue. The immediate result of the conference was that, as an extension of a previously published consensus statement (Jänig et al. 1991), a consensus was reached about a redefinition of RSD without alluding to the sympathetic nervous system or to mechanisms. This led to the description of "complex regional pain syndrome" (CRPS), which is replacing the terms reflex sympathetic dystrophy (now largely identical with CRPS type I or CRPS I) and causalgia (now largely identical with CRPS type II or CRPS II). It was agreed that the term sympathetically maintained pain (SMP) is a symptom and should not be used to characterize a pain syndrome. The precise definition of CRPS I and II are described in the second edition of *Classification of Chronic Pain* (Merskey and Bogduk 1994) and elsewhere (Stanton-Hicks et al. 1995). The new classification is open to changes depending on future clinical and basic research.

The chapters of this volume are not the proceedings of the conference presentations. The topics were chosen during discussion after the conference and concentrate on clinical diagnosis (including quantitative assessment of sensory, autonomic, and motor disturbances) clinical research, and aspects of basic research for the understanding of the clinical phenomenology and psychological aspects, including the placebo problem. *Reflex Sympathetic Dystrophy* was chosen as title for this book because the participants were aware that it will take time to replace this deeply ingrained term. Editors and authors hope that this volume will trigger a more rational approach to diagnosis and treatment of CRPS and will initiate more basic and clinical research in this field.

REFERENCES

Basbaum, A.I. and Besson, J.M. (Eds.), Towards a New Pharmacotherapy of Pain, Dahlem Workshop Reports, John Wiley & Sons, Chichester, 1991.
Bonica, J.J., Causalgia and other reflex sympathetic dystrophies. In: J.J. Bonica (Ed.), The Management of Pain, 2nd ed., Lea & Febiger, Philadelphia, London, 1990, pp. 220–243.
Fields, H.L. and Liebeskind, J.C. (Eds.), Pharmacological Approaches to the Treatment of Chronic Pain: New Concepts and Critical Issues, Progress in Pain Research and Management, Vol. 1, IASP Press, Seattle, 1994.
Jänig, W. and Schmidt, F.R., Reflex Sympathetic Dystrophy: Pathophysiological Mechanisms and Clinical Implications, VCH Verlagsgesellschaft, Weinheim, 1992.
Jänig, W., Blumberg, H., Boas, R.A. and Campbell, J.A., The reflex sympathetic dystrophy syndrome: consensus statement and general recommendations for diagnosis and clinical research. In: M.R. Bond, J.E. Charlton and C.J. Woolf, (Eds.), Proceedings of the VIth World Congress on Pain, Pain Research and Clinical Management, Vol. 4, Elsevier, Amsterdam, 1991, pp. 372–375.
Merskey, H. and Bogduk, N. (Eds.), Classification of Chronic Pain: Descriptions of Chronic Pain Syndromes and Definition of Terms, 2nd ed., IASP Press, Seattle, 1994.
Stanton-Hicks, M., Jänig, W., Hassenbusch, S., Haddox, J.D., Boas, R. and Wilson, P., Reflex sympathetic dystrophy: changing concepts and taxonomy, Pain, 63 (1995) 127–133.

1

The Puzzle of "Reflex Sympathetic Dystrophy": Mechanisms, Hypotheses, Open Questions

Wilfrid Jänig

Physiologisches Institut, Christian-Albrechts-Universität zu Kiel, Kiel, Germany

The sympathetic nervous system regulates the function of all innervated tissues and organs throughout the vertebrate body with a few exceptions, such as the skeletal muscle fibers. In the periphery it forms the major efferent component of the peripheral nervous system. It contains integrative neuronal connections and complete reflex arcs. In the central nervous system (CNS) it has a high representation in spinal cord, brain, and hypothalamus. The various sympathetic functions include regulation of: blood flow to organs (cardiovascular system); digestion, transport, and absorption of food and fluid (gastrointestinal tract); evacuation of colon and urinary bladder; reproduction (genital organs); and constancy of body temperature (thermoregulation). These functions are essential for the preservation of the integrity and constancy of the inner milieu of the organism (homeostasis) at rest and during exposure to challenges from the environment (Cannon 1929, 1939). Many of these functions of the autonomic nervous system are closely linked to the functions of neuroendocrine systems.

The diversity of the effector organs of the sympathetic nervous system and the specificity and wide range of the effector responses during the ongoing regulations require an organization that is specific for the target organs. Thus, preganglionic and postganglionic sympathetic neurons constitute several functionally separate pathways to different target organs (Fig. 1). Each functional set of preganglionic neurons synapses with a particular set of postganglionic neurons. The activity of the postganglionic neurons is transmitted by discrete neuroeffector connections to the target organs (i.e., to blood vessels, glands, nonvascular smooth muscles, enteric neurons, cardiac muscles). Thus, many "private lines" exist between the thoracolumbar spinal cord and the autonomic target organs (Jänig and McLachlan 1992a,b). The paravertebral ganglia probably act primarily as pure relay stations, whereas some neurons in the prevertebral ganglia operate by integrating afferent input from the viscera. Each sympathetic motor path is associated with a distinct organization in spinal cord, brain stem, and hypothalamus (Jänig 1985a, 1988a, 1995a, in press; Jänig and McLachlan 1987). Whether there exist functional classes of sympathetic neurons that innervate and regulate unexpected target organs, such as immune competent cells or connective tissue, is unclear (Jänig 1995c),

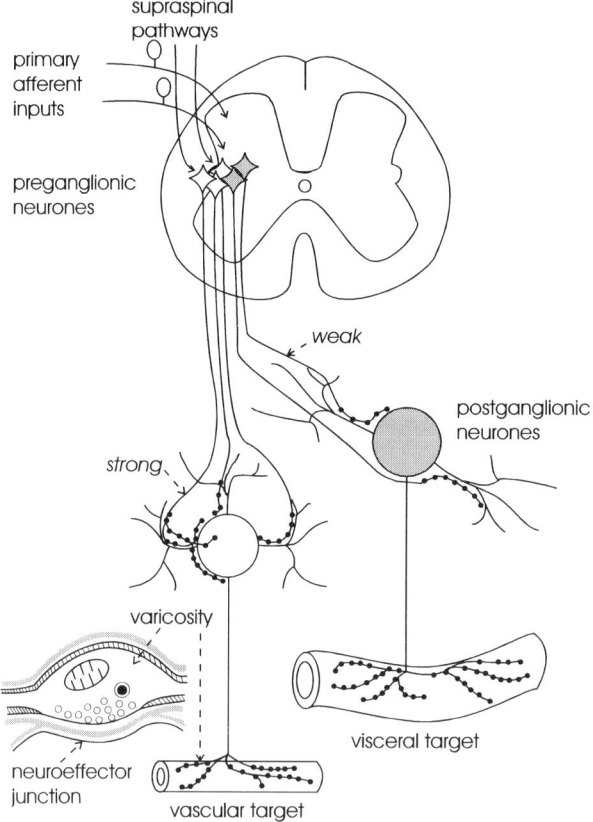

Fig. 1. Organization of the sympathetic nervous system in building blocks. Separate functional pathways exist from within the CNS to the effector organs. Preganglionic neurons located in the intermediate zone integrate signals decending from brain stem and hypothalamus and arising segmentally from primary afferent fibers. The preganglionic neurons project to peripheral ganglia and converge onto postganglionic neurons. Some preganglionic synaptic inputs to postganglionic neurons in paravertebral ganglia and to some postganglionic neurons in prevertebral ganglia are strong and are always suprathreshold. The postganglionic axons form multiple neuroeffector junctions with their target cells. (Jänig and McLachlan 1992a)

although histological investigations suggest that this occurs (for review see Ackerman et al. 1991; Felten and Felten 1991). Furthermore, it is possible that the sympathetic axon terminals are functioning as mediator elements in inflammatory processes, e.g., of the joint capsule, independent of their accepted function of transmitting centrally derived messages by release of transmitter substances to the target tissue (Miao et al., in press).

SYMPATHETIC NERVOUS SYSTEM AND PAIN

The sympathetic nervous system can be associated with pain in two ways (Fig. 2). *First,* it shows both generalized and specific localized reactions in response to noxious, tissue-damaging events. The generalized reactions are organized in the mesencephalon, hypothalamus, and suprahypothalamic brain structures and are best understood as components of the different patterns of *defense behavior*, such as *confrontational defense*, *flight*, and *quiescence* (Bandler and Shipley 1994, see references; Jänig 1995c). Confrontational defense and flight are represented in the dorsolateral periaqueductal gray of the mesencephalon, activated from the body surface and associated with endogenous nonopioid analgesia. Quiescence is represented in the ventrolateral periaqueductal gray, activated from the deep body domains and associated with an endogenous opioid analgesia. These stereotyped preprogrammed elementary behaviors and their association with the endogenous control of analgesia enable the organism to cope with dangerous situations that are always associated with pain or impending pain.

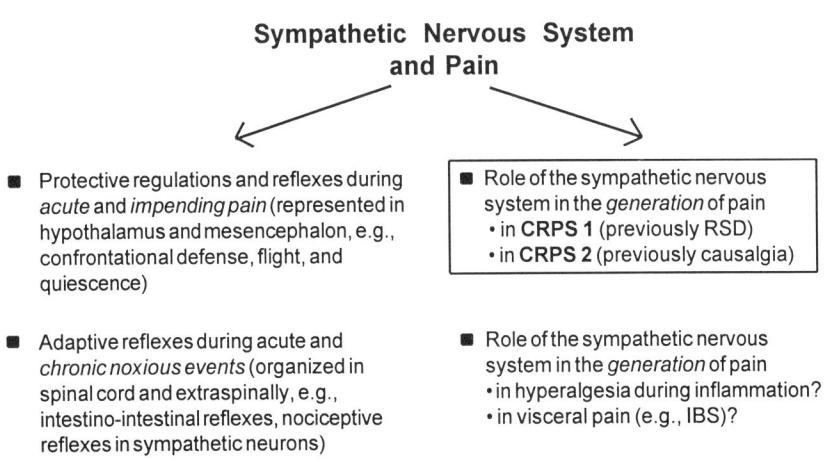

Fig. 2. Characteristics of the sympathetic nervous system and pain; CRPS, complex regional pain syndrome; IBS, irritable bowel syndrome.

More localized and selective reactions of the sympathetic nervous system are organized within the spinal cord and in the periphery, i.e., somatosympathetic, viscerosympathetic, and viscerovisceral reflexes. The hypothalamomesencephalic and the spinal levels of integration are presumably protective under normal biological conditions and are associated with activation of both the adrenocortical system by the hypothalamohypophyseal axis and the somatomotor system (Jänig 1985c; Jänig and Baron, in press).

Second, tissue damage in the extremities with and without any obvious nerve lesion is sometimes followed by diffuse burning pain and hyperalgesia, which can sometimes be relieved by blockade of the (efferent) sympathetic activity to the affected extremity. Spontaneous pain and hyperalgesia may be correlated with changes of blood flow and sweating, changes of posture and movements including an increase in physiological tremor, and trophic changes in skin, appendages of skin, subcutaneous tissues, fascia, and bone. These changes are thought to be, directly or indirectly, associated with the sympathetic nervous system. Like the pain, these changes may be alleviated by blockade of sympathetic activity, although this sometimes needs to be repeated several times to be successful (Bonica 1979, 1990). Pain syndromes of this type are called reflex sympathetic dystrophy (RSD) and sympathetically maintained pain (SMP), terms initially introduced by Evans (1946) and Roberts (1986), respectively. To avoid the mechanistic implications of such terminology, researchers have made recent efforts to define the clinical phenomenology in consensus statements that use purely descriptive terms such as complex regional pain syndrome (CRPS) (see pages 5–6; Jänig et al. 1991; Merskey and Bogduk 1994; Stanton-Hicks et al. 1995).*

The sympathetic nervous system may be causally involved in other pain states, such as hyperalgesia during inflammatory processes in tissues (Levine and Taiwo 1994) and possibly even visceral pain in functional diseases of visceral organs (e.g., irritable bowel syndrome, nonulcer dyspepsia, interstitial cystitis, angina pectoris; Jänig and Häbler 1985).

It is the contribution of the sympathetic nervous system to *pain after traumatic injury to the extremities* that has led to considerable confusion and speculation in regard to the underlying mechanisms and precise diagnostic criteria. Several well-documented clinical observations strongly argue that the sympathetic nervous system is involved in the generation of pain and the other associated changes in patients with RSD, SMP, and related disorders (Chapters 2–5, this volume; Jänig 1990a; Stanton-Hicks 1990; Jänig and Schmidt 1992; Blumberg and Jänig 1994):

---

* For practical reasons, the term reflex sympathetic dystrophy (RSD) will be used generically instead of RSD/SMP in this chapter. It is equivalent to CRPS type I and II.

- Pain is sometimes relieved following sympathetic blocks (by local anesthetics applied to paravertebral ganglia [Bonica 1990], or by other sympatholytic procedures such as regional application of guanethidine [Hannington-Kiff 1974], or intravenous phentolamine [Arnér 1991; Raja et al. 1991; Campbell et al. 1992]). Furthermore, placebo-controlled, double-blind regional sympatholytic block is analgesic in patients with presumed reflex sympathetic dystrophy (Hord et al. 1992).
- Pain can be rekindled or enhanced by an alpha-adrenoceptor agonist applied to the affected extremity (e.g., iontophoretically through the skin or injected into the skin in patients with superficial burning pain and hyperalgesia) (Wallin et al. 1976; Torebjörk 1990; Davis et al. 1991; Torebjörk et al. 1995; Wahren et al. 1995). Injection of epinephrine around chronic nerve-end neuromas can elicit or enhance pain in humans (Chabal et al. 1992).
- Guanethidine injected intravenously into the affected extremity initially elicits pain that is presumably generated by noradrenaline released from postganglionic terminals (Blumberg and Jänig 1994).
- Continuous electrical stimulation of decentralized thoracic sympathetic ganglia in conscious causalgic patients who had surgery reproducibly elicited the tingling and burning pain after latencies of 420 seconds (Walker and Nulsen 1948). White and Sweet (1969) confirmed this observation.

These observations made on some patients with pain after peripheral trauma strongly support the notion that the *efferent* sympathetic nervous activity can be involved in the generation of pain. However, these observations do not prove that the sympathetic nervous system is causally involved in the generation of pain and other phenomena in *all* patients with RSD. Furthermore, the vasomotor changes, the changes of sweating, and the trophic changes, which are commonly observed in many patients, cannot serve as an argument as to whether the sympathetic nervous system is *actively* involved in the generation of pain. Finally, these and other observations cannot be explained away by referring to the confusing clinical situation, to the commonly inaccurate and vague diagnosis of RSD (which leads to negative therapeutic consequences), or to the placebo effects of sympathetic blocks (Ochoa and Verdugo 1993; Ochoa et al. 1994; Chapter 10, this volume).

OPERATIONAL DEFINITION OF RSD

A descriptive and operational definition of RSD was adopted at the VIth World Congress on Pain (Jänig et al. 1991). This definition was a compromise and it was clear to the authors that the term RSD is inappropriate mainly because it may a priori imply, *first*, that the sympathetic nervous system is causally involved and, *second*, that the clinical phenomenology is the result of a reflex activation of sympathetic neurons. However, in many patients there is no proof that the sympathetic activity is elevated and there are indications that an indistinguishable clinical picture (including the pain!) can be generated by different mechanisms. The authors were also aware that it is almost impossible to replace the term RSD by another until more reliable quantitative clinical data are available and we have better ideas about the underlying pathophysiology.

As an extension and completion of this consensus statement, and to avoid ambiguities, a revised taxonomic system for RSD was recently presented (Merskey and Bogduk 1994; Stanton-Hicks et al. 1995). Disorders previously considered to be RSD and causalgia were classified under the neutral umbrella term *complex regional pain syndrome* (CRPS), which is based entirely on clinical criteria. The inclusion criteria under this overall CRPS syndrome are the presence of regional pain (spontaneous and evoked) and other sensory changes following a noxious event. The pain is associated with changes in skin color, skin temperature, abnormal sweating, edema, and sometimes motor abnormalities. Two types of CRPS have been recognized: CRPS type I, corresponding to RSD, and CRPS type II, corresponding to what was formerly considered as causalgia. CRPS I and II are open to further differentiation. The term sympathetically maintained pain (SMP) was not considered as a separate disorder but as a description of a type of pain that can be found in a variety of pain disorders, including CRPS I and II (Baron et al. and Wilson et al., this volume). Here I will use the term CRPS (dealing mainly with CRPS I) except when referring to the literature.

RSD AND THE PLACEBO PROBLEM

Ochoa has repeatedly stressed the problem that most diagnoses of RSD done on patients with trauma, with and without nerve injury, are not correct in respect to the active role of the sympathetic nervous system in the generation of pain (Ochoa 1992; Ochoa and Verdugo 1993; Ochoa et al. 1994). He emphasized that the "diagnosis is traditionally considered to be established medically when patients respond with subjective improvement to diagnostic sympathetic blocks of one kind or another" (Ochoa and Verdugo 1993) (e.g., diagnostic blocks with a local anesthetic applied to the sympathetic chain or with regional guanethidine; diagnostic block of the alpha-adrenoceptor-mediated coupling to primary afferent neurons by phentolamine injected i.v.). He insists that most sympathetic blocks are not placebo-controlled and implies that these patients are high placebo responders and may react positively (e.g., with relief of pain) to placebo blocks (Verdugo et al. 1994a,b). He questions whether the diagnosis of sympathetically maintained pain, as established by sympathetic blocks, exists at all in these patients. He maintains that the "concept of SMP is unfounded and stems from (1) neglect of proper placebo control when performing sympathetic blocks and (2) neglect of careful neurological evaluation in patients with chronic 'neuropathic' pain" (Verdugo et al. 1994b). Ochoa believes that "the unescapable conclusion is that an overall majority of patients qualifying for the purely descriptive 'diagnosis' of 'RSD' and 'SMP' carry a distinct, potentially treatable, neuropsychiatric cerebral disorder" (Ochoa 1992).

There is no question that, in a research setting, sympathetic blocks performed for diagnostic purposes should be placebo-controlled if possible to avoid inadequate treatment (Chapter 10, this volume). The relief of spontaneous pain and evoked pain (mechanical allodynia, cold allodynia, hyperalgesia) should be measured quantitatively by using the visual analogue scale or an equivalent scale. The effectiveness of the sympathetic blocks should be verified by using an objective parameter (e.g., increase of temperature of the tips of fingers or toes to greater than 35°C, Blumberg and Jänig 1994; Chapter 12, this volume). At least Arnér (1991) and Price et al. (1992) have done some placebo controls of their sympathetic blocks, although obviously not to the satisfaction of Ochoa.

It is certainly an unsettled issue whether the brain can influence (or even initiate?) symptoms of CRPS including the pain. In a literature review on psychological aspects of reflex sympathetic dystrophy, Mary Lynch concluded that the emotional and behavioral changes seen in patients with RSD are probably the result of pain, and that there is no worthwhile evidence supporting the hypothesis that psychological factors or certain personality traits predispose to RSD (Lynch 1992; Chapter 11, this volume).

Finally, the contributions of basic research do *not* consist of supplying animal models of CRPS as such, but in supplying working models (e.g., sensory, autonomic, motor) of components of CRPS to understand the mechanisms that lead to the clinical phenomenology and to gain a better approach to rational treatment that also includes the psychological components.

Although Ochoa has raised some important points, multiple independent lines of evidence reviewed below and elsewhere in this volume support the hypothesis that sympathetic activity contributes to pain in both animal models and the human clinical situation.

SOME CLINICAL CHARACTERISTICS OF CRPS

The key clinical symptoms that may be seen in CRPS are as follows (Blumberg 1988, 1992; Willner 1993; Blumberg et al. 1994; Blumberg and Jänig 1994; Chapters 2 and 3, this volume):

- Pain (spontaneous, hyperalgesia, allodynia)
- Abnormal regulation of blood flow and sweating
- Edema of skin and subcutaneous tissues
- Trophic changes of skin, appendages of skin, and subcutaneous tissues
- Active and passive movement disorders including an increased physiological tremor
- The disturbances are mostly restricted to one extremity, generally to its distal part. They generally are not restricted to the site of the trauma but are also present in nontraumatized parts of the affected extremity.
- The different symptoms are variable in their expression and combination.

The variability of symptoms in CRPS I is highlighted by published work about psychophysical measurements on patients with chronic CRPS. In small groups of patients various somatosensory abnormalities, largely associated with the skin, are observed: constant burning pain, touch-evoked allodynia, and cold allodynia (all three may be dependent on the sympathetic innervation); numbness, dysesthesia, paroxysmal pain, heat-evoked hyperalgesia and hypoalgesia (not dependent on the sympathetic innervation); and other sensory abnormalities. More than one of these sensory abnormalities may be present in the same patient (Price et al. 1989, 1992; Gracely et al. 1992; Bennett 1994; Wahren et al. 1995; Chapters 8 and 9, this volume). The diversity of these sensory abnormalities are related to the differentiation of the somatosensory system, in the periphery and in the CNS, into different sensory channels that have input from the different classes of sensory receptors (Willis and Coggeshall 1991; Chapter 8, this volume).

By the same token it is not farfetched to assume that the pathophysiological changes that are related to the efferent systems are also diverse, i.e., to the sympathetic nervous system (blood flow, sweating, swelling, possibly trophic changes) and to the somatomotor system (tremor, active and passive movement disorders). These efferent systems are, in the periphery and in the CNS, functionally as diverse as the afferent ones; therefore, we may expect distinct pathophysiological changes with distinct changes in the regulation of the effector organs.

The skin of the extremities is, for example, innervated by cutaneous vasoconstrictor and sudomotor neurons. Both types of neurons belong to two sympathetic pathways that are distinctly organized in the periphery and in the neuraxis. They are involved in the regulation of heat transfer through the skin, and of turgor and friction of skin; the latter two are probably important for improving sensory discrimination by hairless skin during manipulation. The regulation of the activity in both systems is always correlated. Depending on the thermal load of the body, the activity patterns are reciprocally organized, i.e., during body heating the cutaneous vasoconstrictor activity is low or absent and the sudomotor activity high; during environmental cooling the opposite is seen. These patterns are centrally preprogrammed. In other conditions, such as during emotional states, both systems may be simultaneously activated. In patients with CRPS I the activity relationship of these two sympathetic systems becomes abnormal.

POSSIBLE MECHANISMS THAT MAY INVOLVE THE SYMPATHETIC NERVOUS SYSTEM

The key question in basic and clinical research is: "How can the sympathetic nervous system become coupled in the periphery to primary afferent neurons to produce the different components of pain observed in these patients?" This coupling has to be postulated to explain the beneficial effects of sympathetic blocks, at least in some pathophysiological conditions. The type of coupling must be such that primary afferent neurons are excited or sensitized, the afferent activity enters the nociceptive pathways in the central nervous system, or sympathetically dependent activity in primary afferent nociceptive neurons generates changes (sensitization) of central neurons; otherwise it is almost impossible to explain the relatively prompt effects of sympathetic blocks or of "sympathetic" stimulation in some of the patients.

A further problem is addressed by the following question: "In which way is change of activity in the sympathetic neurons related to the generation of blood flow changes, sweating, swelling, somatomotor changes, and trophic changes?" These changes may not be causally related to the pains that are observed in the patients, yet they may be expressions of parallel processes in the central nervous system and in the periphery. It is unlikely that these changes occur simply as a consequence of a generalized increase or decrease of sympathetic activity.

Basic research is conducted on models developed from testable hypotheses. Whether a model (and also the therapeutic strategy that may be based on that model) might apply to a particular group of patients depends on the clinical diagnosis. Thus, consensus about criteria of clinical diagnosis is critical (Jänig et al. 1991; Stanton-Hicks et al. 1995; Chapters 2 and 3, this volume). Although several pathophysiological mechanisms may operate in parallel in CRPS and have been extensively discussed in the literature, animal models and human experimental models (Bauman et al. 1991; Koltzenburg et al. 1992; LaMotte et al. 1992; Torebjörk et al. 1992 and others) usually test only one component. This does not preclude the possibility of reducing a clinical entity to one mechanism (Campbell et al. 1992; Jänig 1992a). The results presented here are derived from model situations and help to understand the clinical situation (for reviews, Jänig 1990a, 1992b; Jänig and Schmidt 1992; Jänig and McLachlan 1994).

THE AFFERENT SYSTEM (Fig. 3, components 1 and 3)

Afferent neurons with small-diameter fibers that supply the affected territory, in particular the nociceptive ones, may be sensitized by the initial trauma. Damaged primary afferents generate ongoing activity and react with reduced threshold to mechanical, thermal, and chemical stimulation. Lesioned afferent axons may generate spontaneous and evoked ectopic impulses.

Both the decoding of nociceptive and nonnociceptive afferent information by neurons in the spinal cord (particularly in the dorsal horn), and the descending control of transmission of nociceptive information exerted by supraspinal systems, is changed. Neurons of the central nociceptive pathways can be sensitized by massive or continuous input in nociceptive afferents that supply the primary lesioned as well as the unlesioned tissues (Jänig 1988b; Cervero et al. 1989; see contributions in Bond et al. 1991; Jänig and Schmidt 1992; Willis 1992; Wall and Melzack 1994). Now nonnociceptive afferent inputs from the skin and the deep somatic domain may gain access to the nociceptive system (Woolf et al. 1992; Shortland and Woolf 1993), leading to pain elicited by stimulation of these afferents.

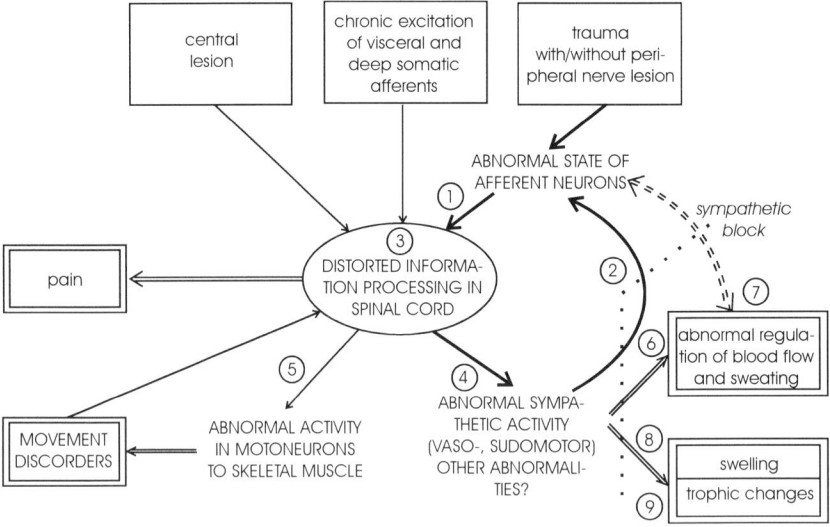

Fig. 3. General hypothesis about the neural mechanisms of generation of CRPS I and II following peripheral trauma with and without nerve lesions, chronic stimulation of visceral afferents (e.g., myocardial infarction) and deep somatic afferents and, rarely, central trauma. The clinical observations are double-framed. Note the vicious circle (arrows in bold black). An important component of this circle is the excitatory influence of postganglionic sympathetic axons on primary afferent fibers in the periphery. For details see text. Numbers 1–9 are the components referred to in the text. (Modified from Blumberg and Jänig 1983 and Jänig 1985b, 1990a)

In principle it is possible to correlate the different types of pain and abnormal sensations that are observed in the patients with distinct pathophysiological changes of the primary afferent neurons and of the spinal cord (Gracely et al. 1992; Chapter 8, this volume).

However, an intriguing problem remains that does not fit into this model situation and thus not in the general heuristic hypothesis displayed in Fig. 3. In many patients RSD develops after trauma that is comparatively minor and does not involve nerve damage or damages only small nerves. In these patients no ongoing activity may be initiated in nociceptive afferents at the site of trauma. They may have diffuse continuous pain inside the affected extremity combined with the other changes characteristic for RSD. Do nociceptive afferents of the deep somatic domain become spontaneously active in these patients or does low-rate ongoing activity, which is normally present in some deep somatic afferents but does not normally activate nonsensitized dorsal horn neurons (Schaible and Grubb 1993), become capable of activating the now sensitized dorsal horn neurons?

COUPLING BETWEEN SYMPATHETIC POSTGANGLIONIC NEURONS AND AFFERENT NEURONS (Fig. 3, component 2)

Noradrenergic postganglionic neurons are coupled in some abnormal way to the primary afferent neurons, leading to an abnormal afferent impulse traffic to the spinal cord that is initiated from the sympathetic nervous system. This coupling is the cornerstone of any hypothesis explaining CRPS in those patients in whom blockade of the sympathetic supply abolishes the pain. The coupling to both nociceptive afferent neurons as well as nonnociceptive afferent neurons may be important.

Several ways of coupling between sympathetic and afferent neurons have been proposed and recently tested in animal models (Jänig and Koltzenburg 1991a, 1992; Jänig and McLachlan 1994); some are supported by controlled investigations of patients with RSD in whom cutaneous sensations were investigated before and after interruption of sympathetic impulse traffic to the peripheral target tissue (Price et al. 1989, 1992; Gracely et al. 1992; Wahren et al. 1995). These include:

• Direct chemical (noradrenergic) coupling between the noradenergic terminal and the afferent terminal possibly via α_2-adrenoceptors (Perl 1992; Sato and Perl 1991; Chen et al., in press), leading to excitation or sensitization of the afferent fibers (Devor and Jänig 1981; Häbler et al. 1987; Jänig 1990b; Sato and Perl 1991; Perl 1992; Chen et al., in press)

• Coupling in the traumatized nerve, which is possible but has yet to be experimentally supported

• Coupling in the dorsal root ganglion to afferent neurons with large-diameter fibers and possibly unmyelinated fibers (McLachlan et al. 1993; Devor et al. 1994; Michaelis et al., in press)

• Indirect coupling via the microvascular bed or nonneural cells close to afferent receptors. These proposed indirect mechanisms are still hypothetical.

• Indirect coupling in which the postganglionic noradrenergic axon terminal serves as mediator element in the sensitization of nociceptive afferents (Levine et al. 1986, 1993; Levine and Taiwo 1994). This hypothetical way of indirect coupling involves noradrenaline or other compounds (e.g., prostaglandin E_2) released from the noradrenergic terminal. This idea is based largely on results from experiments in which evoked pain behavior of rats was quantitatively measured and changed by various pharmacological interventions. This peripheral mechanism of sensitization most likely operates during inflammation.

• Ephaptic coupling between sympathetic and afferent fibers. This coupling has been described between lesioned afferent axons, i.e., in experimental neuromas, but not between sympathetic and afferent fibers (Blumberg and Jänig 1982).

The activation of afferent fibers via these types of coupling seems to require activity in sympathetic neurons, yet not the sensitization of the afferent neurons. It is not necessary that the activity in the sympathetic neurons be increased or otherwise changed. Furthermore, the afferent neurons must express adrenoceptors, at least for the direct chemical coupling. The mechanism by which functional adrenoceptors appear in the membranes of the afferent neurons (upregulation of existing adrenoceptors, novel appearance of adrenoceptor mRNA, novel translation or transcription of mRNA leading to synthesis of adrenoceptors, uncovering of "hidden" adrenoceptors) and the signals that induce these changes are unknown (Jänig and McLachlan 1994).

ACTIVITY IN SYMPATHETIC NEURONS (Fig. 3, component 4)

The discharge pattern in the neurons of the sympathetic outflow to the affected extremity may change following trauma affecting peripheral nerve lesion. The idea is that the change of dorsal horn neurons, generated by continuous discharge of nociceptive afferents induced by the trauma (central sensitization) is reflected in altered sympathetic discharge (Blumberg and Jänig 1983, 1985; Jänig and Koltzenburg 1991b,c). This possible change in sympathetic activity is not necessarily causally related to the generation of nociceptive impulse activity and of pain. Thus, a change of activity in sympathetic neurons is certainly not a condition for the pain in CRPS to develop, yet it may aggravate the sensory abnormalities indirectly via the vasomotor changes. Altered sympathetic activity may be important to explain the other changes (vasomotor changes, changes of sweating, swelling, trophic changes) seen in patients with CRPS, which are not restricted to the territories of the lesioned nerves or the trauma. However, we have no idea about the role of sympathetic activity in generation of the edema and the trophic changes.

SYMPATHETIC TARGET ORGANS (Fig. 3, components 6 and 7)

In the case of nerve lesions (but possibly also under other conditions that do not change the micromilieu of the blood vessels) the regulation of small blood vessels by noradrenergic (vasoconstrictor) neurons (neurovascular transmission) may be changed following regeneration of lesioned postganglionic axons. Furthermore, blood vessels may develop hyperreactivity to circulating catecholamines and other compounds and to impulses in vasoconstrictor neurons. The mechanisms of this process are poorly understood (Jänig and Koltzenburg 1991b; Jobling et al. 1992; Koltzenburg et al. 1995).

Blood vessels in skin and deep somatic tissues (e.g., joint capsule) are also under afferent control. Activation of polymodal nociceptors generates precapillary vasodilatation and (in hairy skin and deep somatic tissues) postcapillary plasma extravasation. Both may be enhanced or reduced following trauma (Jänig and Koltzenburg 1991b; see contributions in Jänig and Schmidt 1992).

THE SOMATOMOTOR SYSTEM (Fig. 3, component 5)

The discharge pattern in alpha and gamma motoneurons may also be changed as a consequence of the sensitization of spinal neurons leading to reduction of active range of motion and muscular strength and to increase of physiological tremor (Schwartzman and Kerrigan 1990; Deuschl et al. 1991). Mechanisms leading to these changes are unexplored.

TISSUE CHANGES (Fig. 3, components 8 and 9)

Whether and how the nervous system is involved in the generation of the swelling (edema) and trophic changes in CRPS is most controversial. Many clinicians almost take it for granted that both changes are associated with the sympathetic nervous system. And, indeed, the swelling disappears after sympathetic blocks (Blumberg et al. 1994), and the trophic changes may disappear after sympathetic blocks, provided they are not irreversible. It could well be that it is afferent neurons with unmyelinated fibers (Fig. 3, component 7) that are primarily involved and that the sympathetic neurons act indirectly via the abnormal regulation of the blood flow through the affected territory of the extremity. The mechanisms by which the trophic changes are generated are therefore unclear.

A GENERAL EXPLANATORY HYPOTHESIS

Fig. 3 outlines a general hypothesis that explains several phenomena observed in patients with CRPS (Blumberg and Jänig 1983; Jänig 1985b, 1990a). The main clinical observations are double-framed; the initiating events are at the top, the most important one being trauma with and without nerve lesions. This heuristic hypothesis consists of several components (numbers in Fig. 3 and see above). Each component is fully or partially supported by experiments on animals and some by experimental investigations on humans.

Although heuristic, this hypothesis must be broken into parts to be tested. The prevalence of the different components varies for the generation of CRPS I and II, which may help to explain the different clinical phenomenologies. For example, in CRPS type 1, which may develop after trauma without nerve lesion, chemical sympathetic afferent coupling may not be important.

Under physiological conditions, peripheral sympathetic pathways are distinct with respect to their target organs (Fig. 1) and somatosensory pathways are functionally distinct with respect to the peripheral receptors and the corresponding sensations (Chapters 8 and 9, this volume). In CRPS the situation may radically change. The sympathetic (efferent) and sensory channels may no longer be separated. Activity in sympathetic neurons may lead to continuous activity in afferent nociceptive neurons. This putative continuous nociceptive activity could generate spontaneous pain and sensitize dorsal horn neurons, resulting in allodynia and hyperalgesia (Price et al. 1989, 1992; Bennett 1994; Chapters 7 and 8, this volume). Sensitized central neurons in the spinal cord could then be activated by stimulation of low-threshold mechanoreceptive afferents. This could be the spinal substrate of dynamic mechanical allodynia (e.g., particularly in patients with CRPS II). Any type of sympathetic-afferent coupling is compatible with this model. If the sympathetic neurons were also coupled to the low-threshold mechanoreceptors, it is theoretically even possible that the pain is maintained in part via this pathway provided the central nociceptive pathways are sensitized.

This vicious circle does not require, for the generation of pain, that the sympathetic activity be increased or changed in its pattern. It is also compatible with decreased activity in sympathetic neurons. To emphasize, there is no proof that activity in sympathetic neurons is increased in patients with CRPS (Blumberg 1988; Torebjörk 1990; Drummond et al. 1991). However, any change of the pattern of activity in the sympathetic neurons supplying the affected extremity could aggravate pain and the associated phenomena.

CRPS IS A NEUROLOGICAL DISEASE

The possible pathophysiological mechanisms of CRPS and the involvement of the peripheral and central nervous system (somatosensory system, somatomotor system, sympathetic nervous system) provide strong arguments that CRPS is a *neurological* disease. The neurological nature of CRPS has not been emphasized in the past for two major reasons:

First, most patients developing CRPS I are seen by anesthesiologists (in particular those running pain ambulances and pain clinics), surgeons, and orthopedic surgeons, and only a minority by neurologists.

Second, classically the autonomic nervous system does not appear to belong to the central nervous system and thus not to the domain of the neurosciences. By the same token, the pathophysiology of this system does not appear to belong to neurology (but see Bannister and Mathias 1992; Low 1993). In Continental Europe the autonomic nervous system still has the name "vegetative nervous system" and as such it is considered to be involved in the regulation of "vegetative functions" of the body in contrast to the functions of the central nervous system (previously subsumed under the so-called "Animalische Physiologie," from "anima" meaning soul). This old (Aristotelian) dichotomy between "vegetative" and "animal" physiology is today obsolete, yet may still influence our thinking.

That CRPS is a neurological disease is amply supported by the material presented here (Fig. 3, Table I). Provocatively it may be asked, is CRPS:
- a neurological disease involving the spinal cord?
- a neurological disease involving primarily the sympathetic nervous system?
- a peripheral α-adrenoceptor disease of the primary afferent neuron?
- a peripheral neurovascular disease?
- a neuropathic pain syndrome with sympathetic involvement?

LACK OF EXPLANATION FOR MANY CLINICAL OBSERVATIONS

The clinical phenomenology of CRPS I and II raises several questions that can just barely be answered satisfactorily based on known pathophysiological mechanisms. There may be several reasons for this: (1) the focus on the pain and other sensory phenomena is one-sided; (2) the conceptual basis of the organization of the sympathetic nervous system, which forms the basis for clinical investigations, is obsolete (Jänig 1995b); (3) the knowledge about the regulation of the micromilieu of the nociceptors in the superficial and deep somatic domains is incomplete; (4) and probably most important, we still lack sufficient quantitative clinical data that address the changes occurring in the

Table I

Characteristics arguing that reflex sympathetic dystrophy is a neurological disease

Clinical Phenomena	Neural Systems Involved	Pathophysiological Mechanisms
PAIN: spontaneous, hyperalgesia, allodynia (mechanical, cold, warm); hyperpathia; other paraesthesias	*Periphery:* nociceptive, afferent neurons silent afferent neurons non-nociceptive afferent neurons (cutaneous, deep, somatic, visceral)	change of receptive properties and impulse pattern; sensitization and recruitment of silent afferents; activation/sensitization of afferent neurons by sympathetic postganglionic neurons
	Dorsal horn, supraspinal control: nociceptive specific neurons wide-dynamic-range neurons	change of receptive fields and impulse pattern; sensitization and recruitment; change of inhibition
Abnormal neural regulation of **SYMPATHETIC EFFECTOR ORGANS** blood vessels, sweat glands	*Periphery:* neuroeffector apparatus sympathetic neurons afferent neurons	change of neuroeffector transmission; development of "adaptive supersensitivity" to nerve impulse, catecholamines, and local substances
	Spinal cord, supraspinal control: vasoconstrictor and sudomotor systems, etc.	change of reflex pattern; loss of functional specificity of sympathetic systems

Abnormal neural regulation of **SKELETAL MUSCLE** (active movement disorder; decrease of strength; tremor)	*Periphery:* Neuromuscular transmission?	unknown
	Spinal cord, supraspinal control: motoneurons, spinal/supraspinal circuits related to motoneurons, influence of nociceptive inputs	unknown
TROPHIC CHANGES (skin and appendage subcutis, bone, joint)	sympathetic postganglionic neurons afferent neurons	unknown; possibly "axon response (reflex)" (vasodilation, plasma extravasation); influence of sympathetic and afferent axons on non-neural cells (vascular, immune, others), activity dependent?
Beneficial effects of **SYMPATHETIC BLOCKS**	sympathetic postganglionic neurons afferent neurons central circuits	interruption of abnormal coupling between sympathetic and afferent axons; decrease of afferent activity, increase of threshold for afferent excitation; vasodilation

somatosensory system, in the sympathetic nervous system, in the somatomotor system, at the level of the autonomic effector organs, and also at the psychological level (Chapter 11, this volume) in patients with presumed CRPS; (5) the in vivo and in vitro animal models used to test the different hypotheses raised by the clinical observations are inadequate. To repeat, a valid global animal model for RSD does not exist.

Questions emerging from the clinical phenomenology of patients with CRPS I or II are as follows:

• What are the minimal criteria for early and late diagnosis of CRPS I and II? What are the criteria for showing that the sympathetic nervous system is actively involved in the generation of pain, changes in the reaction of the autonomic effector organs, somatomotor changes, and trophic changes (Chapters 2 and 3, this volume)?

• What is the essential difference of the neuronal mechanisms between CRPS I and CRPS II? The first may develop after trivial trauma without nerve lesion; the latter develops after major nerve lesion.

• How common is CRPS I and its subentities (CRPS type I with spontaneous pain, CRPS type I without spontaneous pain)?

• Is the staging of CRPS I valid, i.e., does a patient with RSD pass successively through different stages that are characterized by distinct clinical symptoms (Chapter 2, this volume)?

• CRPS I may be indistinguishable in its clinical phenomenology from posttraumatic reactions such as pain, swelling, and autonomic reactions. Are there transitions between CRPS I and general posttraumatic pain states? When does a posttraumatic pain state develop into CRPS I?

• Why does, in some cases, CRPS I develop after trivial trauma that affects peripheral parts of the extremity (Livingstone 1976)? Are more extensive traumas less likely to lead to CRPS? Why does CRPS II develop in only a small percentage (3–5%) of patients with typical "partial" nerve lesions at the extremities (Richards 1967; Sunderland 1991)?

• Why and how often do spontaneous remissions occur in CRPS I?

• Is the excitation of afferents from deep somatic structures (e.g., fascia, tendons, periost, joint capsule) important in the development of CRPS I? Is the activity in these afferents important for maintaining CRPS I? Is the activity in these afferents dependent on the sympathetic nervous system?

• Patients with CRPS I at the traumatized extremities commonly have a glove-like edema (swelling) that may disappear after sympathetic blocks. How is the sympathetic nervous system involved in the generation of the edema? Does the edema contribute to the excitation of nociceptive afferents from deep somatic structures and thus to the generation of pain and of the other associated phenomena?

• How are the somatomotor changes generated (reduction of active range of motion and muscular strength, increase of physiological tremor) that are observed in about 50% of the patients with RSD (Schwartzman and Kerrigan 1990; Deuschl et al. 1991) and that disappear after sympathetic blocks? What is the role of the sympathetic nervous system?
• Does genetic variability contribute to the development of CRPS?
• To what extent does the variability of symptoms reflect psychological and personality differences among patients?

SYNOPSIS FOR THIS VOLUME

Given the background just outlined, this volume concentrates on the following topics:

1. How can animal models contribute to understanding the involvement of the sympathetic nervous system in pain? What information, relevant for both a mechanistic hypothesis and the clinical diagnosis of CRPS, can be drawn from animal models? Which measurements made on the patients correspond to the animal models? What are the similarities and differences between the models and the clinical condition?

2. What clinical research questions are relevant to the subject "sympathetic nervous system in the generation of pain?" What should be measured? Clinical research should concentrate on the:
 • afferent/sensory system (not only related to pain but also to other sensory abnormalities)
 • sympathetic/autonomic effector
 • vascular/other peripheral structures (perhaps trophic changes), and
 • skeletomotor components

3. To what degree is the brain (psychological component) involved in the expression of CRPS?

4. Symptoms and signs of CRPS: What are the criteria for a precise clinical diagnosis of CRPS and its subdifferentiation? What is the differential diagnosis? What is the best way to differentiate pains that are dependent on the sympathetic nervous system from those that are not?

5. Which tests are critical to the accurate diagnosis of CRPS? Which can be recommended? Which tests have to be verified before they can be generally recommended and which tests need to be developed? How should we deal with the placebo problem?

ACKNOWLEDGMENTS

Supported by the Deutsche Forschungsgemeinschaft. The author thanks Dr. Howard Fields for his critique of this chapter.

REFERENCES

Ackerman, K.D., Bellinger, D.L., Felten, S.Y. and Felten D.L., Ontogeny and senescence of noradrenergic innervation of the rodent thymus and spleen. In: R. Ader, D.L. Felten and N. Cohen (Eds.), Psychoneuroimmunology, 2nd ed., Academic Press, San Diego, 1991, pp. 71–125.

Arnér, S., Intravenous phentolamine test: diagnostic and prognostic use in reflex sympathetic dystrophy, Pain, 46 (1991) 17–22.

Bandler, R. and Shipley, M.T., Columnar organization in the midbrain periaqueductal gray: modules for emotional expression? Trends Neurosci., 17 (1994) 379–388.

Bannister, R. and Mathias, C.J., Autonomic Failure, 3rd ed., Oxford University Press, Oxford, 1992.

Baumann, T.K., Simone, D.A., Shain, C.N. and LaMotte R.H., Neurogenic hyperalgesia: the search for the primary cutaneous afferent fibers that contribute to capsaicinized pain and hyperalgesia, J. Neurophysiol., 66 (1991) 212–227.

Bennett, G.J., Neuropathic pain, In: P.D. Wall and R. Melzack (Eds.), Textbook of Pain, 3rd ed., Churchill Livingstone, Edinburgh, 1994, pp. 201–224.

Blumberg, H., Zur Entstehung und Therapie des Schmerzsyndroms bei der sympathischen Reflexdystrophie, Der Schmerz, 2 (1988) 125–143.

Blumberg, H., Clinical and pathophysiological aspects of reflex sympathetic dystrophy and sympathetically maintained pain. In: W. Jänig and R.F. Schmidt (Eds.), Reflex Sympathetic Dystrophy: Pathophysiological Mechanisms and Clinical Implications, VCH Verlagsgesellschaft, Weinheim, 1992, pp. 29–49.

Blumberg, H., Hoffmann, U., Mohadjer, M. and Scheremet, R., Clinical phenomenology and mechanisms of reflex sympathetic dystrophy: emphasis on edema. In: G.F. Gebhart, D.L. Hammond and T.S. Jensen (Eds.), Proceedings of the 7th World Congress on Pain, Progress in Pain Research and Management, Vol. 2, IASP Press, Seattle, 1994, pp. 455–481.

Blumberg, H. and Jänig, W., Activation of fibers via experimentally produced stump neuromas of skin nerves: ephaptic transmission or retrograde sprouting? Exp. Neurol., 76 (1982) 468–482.

Blumberg, H. and Jänig, W., Changes of reflexes in vasoconstrictor neurons supplying the cat hindlimb following chronic nerve lesions: a model for studying mechanisms of reflex sympathetic dystrophy? J. Auton. Nerv. Syst., 7 (1983) 399–411.

Blumberg, H. and Jänig, W., Reflex patterns in postganglionic vasoconstrictor neurons following chronic nerve lesions, J. Auton. Nerv. Syst., 14 (1985) 157–180.

Blumberg, H. and Jänig, W., Clinical manifestations of reflex sympathetic dystrophy and sympathetically maintained pain. In: P.D. Wall and R. Melzack (Eds.), Textbook of Pain, 3rd ed., Churchill Livingstone, Edinburgh 1994, pp. 685–697.

Bond, M.R., J.E. Charlton and C.J. Woolf (Eds.), Proceedings of the VIth World Congress on Pain, Pain Research and Clinical Management, Vol. 4, Elsevier, Amsterdam, 1991.

Bonica, J.J., Causalgia and other reflex sympathetic dystrophies. In: J.J. Bonica, J.C. Liebeskind and D.G. Albe-Fessard (Eds.), Advances in Pain Research and Therapy, Vol. 3, Raven Press, New York, 1979, pp. 141–166.

Bonica, J.J., Causalgia and other reflex sympathetic dystrophies. In: J.J. Bonica (Ed.), The Management of Pain, 2nd ed., Lea & Febiger, Philadelphia, 1990, pp. 220–243.

Campbell, J.N., Meyer, R.A. and Raja, S.N., Is nociceptor activation by alpha-1 adrenoreceptors the culprit in sympathetically maintained pain? APS Journal, 1 (1992) 3–11.

Cannon, W.B., Organization for physiological homeostasis, Physiol. Rev., 9 (1929) 399–431.

Cannon, W.B., The Wisdom of the Body, Norton, New York, 1939.

Cervero, F., G.J. Bennett and P.M. Headley (Eds.), Processing of sensory information in the superficial dorsal horn of the spinal cord, Nato ASI Series, Series A: Life Sciences: 176, Plenum Press, New York, 1989.

Chabal, C., Jacobson, L., Russell, L.C. and Burchiel, K.J., Pain response to perineuromal injection of normal saline, epinephrine, and lidocaine in humans, Pain, 49 (1992) 9–12.

Chen, Y., Michaelis, M., Jänig, W. and Devor, M., Adrenoceptor subtype mediating sympathetic-sensory coupling in injected sensory neurons, J. Neurophysiol., in press.

Davis, K.D., Treede, R.D., Raja, S.N., Meyer, R.A. and Campbell, J.N., Topical application of clonidine relieves hyperalgesia in patients with sympathetically maintained pain, Pain, 47 (1991) 309–317.

Devor, M. and Jänig, W., Activation of myelinated afferents ending in a neuroma by stimulation of the sympathetic supply in the rat, Neurosci. Lett., 24 (1981) 43–47.

Devor, M., Jänig, W. and Michaelis, M., Modulation of activity in dorsal root ganglion (DRG) neurons by sympathetic activation in nerve injured rats, J. Neurophysiol., 71 (1994) 38–47.

Deuschl, G., Blumberg, H. and Lücking, C.H., Tremor in reflex sympathetic dystrophy, Arch. Neurol., 48 (1991) 1247–1252.

Drummond, P.D., Finch, P.M. and Smythe, G.A., Reflex sympathetic dystrophy: the significance of differing plasma catecholamine concentrations in affected and unaffected limbs, Brain, 114 (1991) 2025–2036.

Evans, J.A., Reflex sympathetic dystrophy. Surg. Clin. North Am., 26 (1946) 780–790.

Felten, S.Y. and Felten, D.L., Innervation of lymphoid tissue. In: R. Ader, D.L. Felten and N. Cohen (Eds.), Psychoneuroimmunology, 2nd ed., Academic Press, San Diego, 1991, pp. 27–69.

Gracely, R.H., Lynch, S.L. and Bennett, G.J., Painful neuropathy: altered central processing, maintained dynamically by peripheral input, Pain, 51 (1992) 175–194.

Häbler, H.-J., Jänig, W. and Koltzenburg, M., Activation of unmyelinated afferents in chronically lesioned nerves by adrenaline and excitation of sympathetic efferents in the cat, Neurosci. Lett., 82 (1987) 35–40.

Hannington-Kiff, J. G., Pain Relief, Philadelphia, Lippincott, 1974.

Hord, A.H., Rooks, M.D., Stephens, B.O., Rogers, H.G. and Fleming, L.L., Intravenous regional bretylium and lidocaine for treatment of reflex sympathetic dystrophy: a randomized, double-blind study, Anesth. Analg., 74 (1992) 818–821.

Jänig, W., Organization of the lumbar sympathetic outflow to skeletal muscle and skin of the cat hindlimb and tail, Rev. Physiol. Biochem. Pharmacol., 102 (1985a) 119–213.

Jänig, W., Causalgia and reflex sympathetic dystrophy: in which way is the sympathetic nervous system involved? Trends Neurosci., 8 (1985b) 471–477.

Jänig, W., Systemic and specific autonomic reactions in pain: efferent, afferent and endocrine components, Eur. J. Anaesthesthiol., 2 (1985c) 319–346.

Jänig, W., Pre- and postganglionic vasoconstrictor neurons: differention, types and discharge properties, Ann. Rev. Physiol., 50 (1988a) 525–539.

Jänig, W., Pathophysiology of nerve following mechanical injury. In: R. Dubner, G.F. Gebhart and M.R. Bond (Eds.), Proceedings of the Vth World Congress on Pain, Pain Research and Clinical Management, Vol. 3, Elsevier, Amsterdam, 1988b, pp. 89–109.

Jänig, W., The sympathetic nervous system in pain: physiology and pathophysiology. In: M. Stanton-Hicks (Ed.), Pain and the Sympathetic Nervous System, Kluwer Academic Publishers, Boston, 1990a, pp. 17–89.

Jänig, W., Activation of afferent fibers ending in an old neuroma by sympathetic stimulation in the rat, Neurosci. Lett., 111 (1990b) 309–314.

Jänig, W., Guest editorial: experimental approach to reflex sympathetic dystrophy and related disorders, Pain, 46 (1991) 241–245.

Jänig, W., Can reflex sympathetic dystrophy be reduced to an alpha-adrenoceptor disease? Am. Pain Soc. J., 1 (1992a) 16–22.

Jänig, W., Pain and the sympathetic nervous system: pathophysiological mechanisms. In: R. Bannister and C.J. Mathias (Eds.), Autonomic Failure, 3rd ed., Oxford University Press, Oxford, 1992b, pp. 231–251.

Jänig, W., Ganglionic transmission *in vivo*. In: G. Burnstock (Ed.), The Autonomic Nervous System, Vol. 6, Autonomic Ganglia (Ed. by E.M. McLachlan), Harwood Academic Publishers, Chur, Switzerland, 1995a, pp. 349–395.

Jänig, W., Spinal cord reflex organization: somatosympathetic responses, clinical pathology. In: R. Bandler and G. Holstege (Eds.), The emotional motor system, Prog. Brain Res., in press.

Jänig, W., Vegetatives Nervensystem, Chap. 19, In: R.F. Schmidt and G. Thews (Eds.), Physiologie des Menschen; 26th ed., Springer-Verlag, Heidelberg, Berlin, 1995b, pp. 340–369.

Jänig, W., The sympathetic nervous system in pain, Eur. J. Anaesthesiol., 12 (Suppl. 10) (1995c) 53–60.

Jänig, W. and Baron, R., General and specific reactions of the sympathetic nervous system in pain. In: B.B. Brown and C. Prys-Roberts (Eds.), General Anaesthesia, 6th ed., Butterworth-Heinemann Ltd., Oxford, in press.

Jänig, W. and Häbler, H.J., Visceral-autonomic integration. In: G.F. Gebhart (Ed.), Visceral Pain, Progress in Pain Research and Management, Vol. 5, IASP Press, Seattle, 1995, pp. 311–348.

Jänig, W. and Koltzenburg, M., What is the interaction between the sympathetic terminal and the primary afferent fiber? In: A.I. Basbaum and J.M. Besson (Eds.), Towards a New Pharmacotherapy of Pain, Dahlem Workshop Reports, John Wiley & Sons, Chichester, 1991a, pp. 331–352.

Jänig, W. and Koltzenburg, M., Sympathetic reflex activity and neuroeffector transmission change after chronic nerve lesions. In: M.R. Bond, J.E. Charlton and C.J. Woolf (Eds.), Proceedings of the VIth World Congress on Pain, Pain Research and Clinical Management, Vol. 4, Elsevier, Amsterdam, 1991b, pp. 365–371.

Jänig, W. and Koltzenburg, M., Plasticity of sympathetic reflex organization following cross-union of inappropriate nerves in the adult cat, J. Physiol., 436 (1991c) 309–323.

Jänig, W. and Koltzenburg, M., Possible ways of sympathetic afferent interactions. In: W. Jänig and R.F. Schmidt (Eds.), Reflex Sympathetic Dystrophy: Pathophysiological Mechanisms and Clinical Implications, VCH Verlagsgesellschaft, Weinheim, 1992, pp. 213–245.

Jänig, W. and McLachlan, E.M., Organization of lumbar spinal outflow to the distal colon and pelvic organs, Physiol. Rev., 67 (1987) 1332–1404.

Jänig, W. and McLachlan, E.M., Characteristics of function-specific pathways in the sympathetic nervous system. Trends Neurosci., 15 (1992a) 475–481.

Jänig, W. and McLachlan, E.M., Specialized functional pathways are the building blocks of the autonomic nervous system, J. Auton. Nerv. Syst., 41 (1992b) 3–14.

Jänig, W. and McLachlan, E.M., The role of modifications in noradrenergic peripheral pathways after nerve lesions in the generation of pain, In: H.L. Fields and J.C. Liebeskind (Eds.), Pharmacological Approaches to the Treatment of Chronic Pain: New Concepts and Critical Issues, Progress in Pain Research and Management, Vol. 1, IASP Press, Seattle, 1994, pp. 101–129.

Jänig, W. and F.R. Schmidt (Eds.), Reflex Sympathetic Dystrophy: Pathophysiological Mechanisms and Clinical Implications, VCH Verlagsgesellschaft, Weinheim, 1992.

Jänig, W., Blumberg, H., Boas, R.A. and Campbell, J.A., The reflex sympathetic dystrophy syndrome: consensus statement and general recommendations for diagnosis and clinical reseach. In: M.R. Bond, J.E. Charlton and C.J. Woolf (Eds.), Proceedings of the VIth World Congress on Pain, Pain Research and Clinical Management, Vol. 4, Elsevier, Amsterdam, 1991, pp. 372–375.

Jobling, P., McLachlan, E.M., Jänig, W. and Anderson, C.R., Electrophysiological responses in the rat tail artery during reinnervation following lesions of the sympathetic supply, J. Physiol., 454 (1992) 107–128.

Koltzenburg, M., Lundberg, L.E.R. and Torebjörk, H.E., Dynamic and static components of mechanical hyperalgesia in human hairy skin, Pain, 51 (1992) 207–219.

Koltzenburg, M., Häbler, H.-J. and Jänig, W., Functional reinnervation of the vasculature of the adult cat paw pad by axons originally innervating vessels in hairy skin, Neuroscience, 767, (1995) 245–252.

LaMotte, R.H., Lundberg, L.E.R. and Torebjörk, H.E., Pain, hyperalgesia and activity in nociceptive C units in humans after intradermal injection of capsaicin, J. Physiol., 448 (1992) 749–764.
Levine, J. and Taiwo, Y., Inflammatory pain. In: P.D. Wall and R. Melzack (Eds.) Textbook of Pain, 3rd ed., Churchill Livingstone, Edinburgh, 1994, pp. 45–56.
Levine, J.D., Fields, H.L. and Basbaum, A.I., Peptides and the primary afferent neuron, J. Neurosci., 13 (1993) 2273–2286.
Levine, J.D., Taiwao, Y.O., Collins, S.D. and Tam, J.K., Noradrenaline hyperalgesia is mediated through interaction with sympathetic postganglionic neurone terminals rather than activation of primary afferent nociceptors, Nature, 323 (1986) 158–160.
Livingston, W.K., Pain Mechanisms: A Physiological Interpretation of Causalgia and its Related States, Plenum Press, New York, 1976.
Low, P.A. (Ed.), Clinical Autonomic Disorders, Little, Brown & Company, Boston, 1993.
Lynch, M.E., Psychological aspects of reflex sympathetic dystrophy: a review of the adult and paediatric literature, Pain, 49 (1992) 337–347.
McLachlan, E.M., Jänig, W., Devor, M. and Michaelis, M., Peripheral nerve injury triggers noradrenergic sprouting within dorsal root ganglia, Nature, 363 (1993) 543–545.
Merskey, H. and N. Bogduk (Eds.), Classification of Chronic Pain: Descriptions of Chronic Pain Syndromes and Definition of Pain Terms, 2nd ed., IASP Press, Seattle, 1994.
Michaelis, M., Devor, M. and Jänig, W., Time course of sympathetic modulation of activity in dorsal root ganglion neurons with A and C fibers following peripheral nerve injury in rats, J. Neurophysiol., in press.
Miao, F.J.-P., Jänig, W. and Levine, J.D., Role of sympathetic postganglionic neurons in synovial extravasation induced by bradykinin, J. Neurophysiol., in press.
Ochoa, J.L., Reflex sympathetic dystrophy: a disease of medical understanding, Clin. J. Pain, 8 (1992) 363–366.
Ochoa, J.L. and Verdugo, R., Reflex sympathetic dystrophy: definitions and history of the ideas with a critical review of human studies. In: P.A. Low (Ed.), Clinical Autonomic Disorders, Little, Brown & Company, Boston, 1993, pp. 473–492.
Ochoa, J.L., Verdugo, R. and Campero, M., Pathophysiological spectrum of organic and psychogenic disorders in neuropathic pain patients fitting the description of causalgia or reflex sympathetic dystrophy. In: G.F. Gebhart, D.L. Hammond and T.S. Jensen (Eds.), Proceedings of the 7th World Congress on Pain, Progress in Pain Research and Management, Vol. 2, IASP Press, Seattle, 1994, pp. 483–494.
Perl, E.R., Alterations in the responsiveness of cutaneous nociceptors: sensitization by noxious stimuli and the induction of adrenergic responsiveness by nerve injury. In: W.D. Willis (Ed.), Hyperalgesia and Allodynia, Raven Press, New York, 1992, pp. 59–79.
Price, D.D., Bennett, G.J. and Raffii, A., Psychophysical observations on patients with neuropathic pain relieved by a sympathetic block, Pain, 36 (1989) 273–288.
Price, D.D., Long, S. and Huitt, C., Sensory testing of pathophysiological mechanisms of pain in patients with reflex sympathetic dystrophy, Pain, 49 (1992) 163–173.
Raja, S.N., Treede, R.D., Davis, K.D. and Campbell, J.N., Systemic alpha-adrenergic blockade with phentolamine: a diagnostic test for sympathetically maintained pain, Anesthesiology, 74 (1991) 691–698.
Richards, R.L., Causalgia: a centennial review, Arch. Neurol., 16 (1967) 339–350.
Roberts, W.J., A hypothesis on the physiological basis for causalgia and related pains, Pain, 24 (1986) 297–311.
Sato, J. and Perl, E.R., Adrenergic excitation of cutaneous pain receptors induced by peripheral nerve injury, Science, 251 (1991) 1608–1610.
Schaible, H.G. and Grubb, B.D., Afferent and spinal mechanisms of joint pain, Pain, 55 (1993) 5–54.
Schwatzman, R.J. and Kerrigan, J., The movement disorder of reflex sympathetic dystrophy, Neurology, 40 (1990) 57–61.
Shortland, P. and Woolf, C.J., Chronic peripheral nerve section results in a rearrangement of the central axonal arborizations of axotomized A beta primary afferent neurons in the rat spinal cord, J. Comp. Neurol., 330 (1993) 65–82.

Stanton-Hicks, M., Pain and the Sympathetic Nervous System, Kluwer Academic Publishers, Boston, 1990.
Stanton-Hicks, M., Jänig, W., Hassenbusch, S., Haddox, J.D., Boas, R. and Wilson, P., Reflex sympathetic dystrophy: changing concepts and taxonomy, Pain, 63 (1995) 127–133.
Sunderland, S., Nerve Injuries and Their Repair, Churchill Livingstone, Edinburgh, 1991.
Torebjörk, E., Clinical and neurophysiological observations relating to psychophysiological mechanisms in reflex sympathetic dystrophy. In: M. Stanton-Hicks, W. Jänig and R.A. Boas (Eds.), Reflex Sympathetic Dystrophy, Kluwer Academic Publishers, Boston, 1990, pp. 71–80.
Torebjörk, E., Lundberg, L.E. and LaMotte, R.H., Central changes in processing of mechanoreceptive input in capsaicin-induced secondary hyperalgesia in humans, J. Physiol. (Lond), 448 (1992) 765–780.
Torebjörk, E., Wahren, L.K., Wallin, G., Hallin, R. and Koltzenburg, M., Noradrenalin-evoked pain in neuralgia, Pain, 63 (1995) 11–20.
Verdugo R.J. and Ochoa, J.L., "Sympathetically maintained pain." I. Phentolamine block questions the concept, Neurology, 44 (1994) 1003–1010.
Verdugo, R.J., Campero, M. and Ochoa, J.L., Phentolamine sympathetic block in painful polyneuropathies. II. Further questioning of the concept of "sympathetically maintained pain," Neurology, 44 (1994) 1010–1014.
Wahren, L.K., Gordh, T. and Torebjörk, E., Effects of regional intravenous guanethidine in patients with chronic neuralgia in the hand: a follow-up study over a decade, Pain, 62 (1995) 379–385.
Walker, A.E. and Nulsen, F., Electrical stimulation of the upper thoracic portion of the sympathetic chain in man, Arch. Neurol. Psychiat., 59 (1948) 559–560.
Wall, P.D. and R. Melzack (Eds.), Textbook of Pain, 3rd ed, Churchill Livingstone, Edinburgh, 1994.
Wallin, G., Torebjörk, H.E. and Hallin, R.G., Preliminary observations on the pathophysiology of hyperalgesia in the causalgic pain syndrome. In: Y. Zottermann (Ed.), Sensory Functions of the Skin in Primates, Pergamon, Oxford, 1976, pp. 489–499.
White, J.C. and Sweet, W.H., Pain and the Neurosurgeon, Charles C. Thomas, Springfield, 1969.
Willis, W.D., Hyperalgesia and Allodynia, Raven Press, New York, 1992.
Willis, W.D. and Coggeshall, R.E., Sensory Mechanisms of the Spinal Cord, Plenum Press, New York, 1991.
Willner, C.L., Pain and the sympathetic nervous system: clinical considerations. In: P.A. Low (Ed.), Clinical Autonomic Disorders, Little, Brown & Company, Boston, 1993, pp. 493–503.
Woolf, C.J., Shortland, P. and Coggeshall, R.E., Peripheral nerve injury triggers central sprouting of myelinated afferents, Nature, 355 (1992) 75–78.

Correspondence to: Wilfrid Jänig, Dr med, PD, Physiologisches Institut, Christian-Albrechts-Universität zu Kiel, Olshausenstr. 40, 24098 Kiel, Germany. Tel: 49-431-880-2036; Fax: 49-431-880-4580; E-mail: w.janig@physiologie.uni-kiel.de.

2

Clinical Characteristics of Patients with Complex Regional Pain Syndrome in Germany with Special Emphasis on Vasomotor Function

Ralf Baron,[a] Helmut Blumberg,[b] and Wilfrid Jänig[c]

[a]Klinik für Neurologie, Christian-Albrechts-Universität zu Kiel, Kiel, Germany, [b]Neurochirurgische Universitätsklinik, Klinikum der Albert-Ludwigs-Universität, Freiburg, Germany, [c]Physiologisches Institut, Christian-Albrechts-Universtät zu Kiel, Kiel, Germany

Sometimes complex painful disorders may develop as a disproportionate consequence of trauma affecting the limbs with or without obvious nerve lesion. Clinical signs and symptoms are extremely variable (Schwartzman and McLellan 1987; Gibbons and Wilson 1992; Blumberg and Jänig 1994). Three major components can be distinguished: (1) sensory abnormalities including spontaneous burning pain, hyperalgesia, and allodynia (Blumberg 1988; Price et al. 1989, 1992; Jänig et al. 1991; Wahren et al. 1991; Wahren and Torebjörk 1992); (2) vascular and sweating abnormalities, edema and trophic changes in skin, subcutaneous tissues, joints, and bone (Sudeck 1902; Campbell et al. 1988; Low et al. 1994); and (3) motor abnormalities including impairment of active and passive function, tremor, or dystonia (Marsden et al. 1984; Deuschl et al. 1991; Bhatia et al. 1993). According to the *Classification of Chronic Pain* (Merskey and Bogduk 1994) these disorders are called complex regional pain syndromes (CRPS).

The pathophysiological mechanisms of the symptoms and the role of the sympathetic nervous system in the cause of the disease and in the generation and maintenance of pain are not clear (Sunderland 1976; Roberts 1986; Schott 1986, 1989). Some investigators pointed out that the patients are characterized by sympathetic overactivity in the affected limb (Bonica 1990). This conclusion is erroneously based upon the observation that skin blood flow and temperature are reduced in many patients and that blocking the sympathetic supply to the affected part may relieve the symptoms (for reviews, see Bonica 1990; Nathan 1983; Schott 1986, 1989; Jänig and Schmidt 1992; Wallin et al. 1976; Loh and Nathan 1978; Loh et al. 1980; cf. Davis et al. 1991). Others hypothesized more complex changes in reflex patterns of different sympathetic systems (Blumberg 1988, 1992; Jänig 1990). Peripheral interactions between efferent sympathetic and afferent nociceptive pathways were suggested to maintain a central "vicious circle" accounting for vascular, sensory, and motor disturbances (Jänig 1990; Treede et al. 1992).

In recent studies patients presenting with similar clinical signs and symptoms, without or with obvious nerve damage, could be distinguished by the effect of sympathetic blockade, regional guanethidine blocks, or intravenous phentolamine injections (Campbell et al. 1988; Arnér 1991; Raja et al. 1991, 1992; Treede et al. 1992). Pain relieved by specific sympatholytic procedures is therefore now considered "sympathetically maintained pain" (SMP). Thus, SMP is defined to be a symptom of CRPS and not a clinical entity.

Other authors, however, do not support the idea that the sympathetic nervous system is actively involved in the generation of pain, but claim that its role has to be reconsidered or even discarded (Schott 1994; Verdugo and Ochoa 1994; Verdugo et al. 1994). They argue that the effects resembling sympathetic dysfunction at the affected limb relate neither to the pain itself nor to pain relief following sympathetic blockade. Moreover, the techniques and results of sympathetic blockade have rarely been adequately evaluated and are in most cases not placebo-controlled (Chapters 10 and 11, this volume). Schott (1994) believes that the idea of the involvement of the sympathetic nervous system in pain in CRPS is a misconception and that the pain as well as the associated changes are related to activity in a special set of peptidergic afferents that innervate blood vessels and project with the sympathetic supply to the spinal cord. This idea lacks any experimental basis.

In the past the general problem was a lack of consensus about the criteria leading to a reliable diagnosis of CRPS. This was related, first, to the lack of systematic clinical investigations of patients and, second, to the lack of quantitative studies of pain, changes of blood flow and sweating, trophic changes, edema, and motor disturbances in these patients.

Our description is based upon patients with CRPS who were diagnosed and treated in the Neurological Clinic of the university in Freiburg (203 patients, see Blumberg and Jänig 1994) and in the Neurological Clinic and Anesthesiological Clinic of the university in Kiel (35 patients) during the last five years. Low and colleagues performed a companion study in Rochester (Minnesota) and report their results on patients with presumed CRPS in Chapter 3 (this volume).

CRPS TYPE I (REFLEX SYMPATHETIC DYSTROPHY)

EPIDEMIOLOGY

The frequency of CRPS I with respect to age shows a normal distribution with a peak at 50 years, which agrees with previous reports. Both children (Chapter 4, this volume) and very old persons may suffer from CRPS I. Female patients somewhat outnumber male patients.

The onset of CRPS I is in almost all cases preceded by noxious events at the distal affected extremity. These include minor trauma (e.g., distortion, bruising, or skin lesions), bone fracture, operations (e.g., of carpal tunnel, Dupuytren's contracture), and other lesions (e.g., shoulder trauma, myocardial infarction, or even a contralateral cerebrovascular lesion). An important feature is that often the symptoms of CRPS I are apparently disproportionate to the inciting event with a tendency to generalize at the distal limb. Thus, all symptoms of CRPS I may occur irrespective of the type of the preceding lesion. Furthermore, the site of the lesion at the limb does not determine the location of symptoms (Blumberg 1988; Blumberg and Jänig 1994). The upper extremity is affected more often than the lower extremity in a ratio of about 2:1.

CLINICAL PHENOMENOLOGY

The clinical picture of CRPS I is characterized by a triad of autonomic (sympathetic), motor, and sensory symptoms (Table I, Blumberg 1988; Blumberg and Jänig 1994; Veldman et al. 1993). These symptoms develop in the distal region of the affected extremity following a noxious event, irrespective of its type and location. They are not confined to the innervation zone of an individual nerve and show a distally generalized distribution. Symptoms are present in tissues that are not directly affected by the preceding lesion. In 5% of the patients, the symptoms of CRPS I are localized, e.g., the triad of symptoms is only present in one finger (Blumberg et al. 1993). Rarely, CRPS I may also be present in more proximal regions such as the knee, hip or shoulder, and in extreme cases of CRPS I the entire extremity may become symptomatic.

Somatosensory functions and pain

Spontaneous pain is a prominent feature in most patients. The quality of the spontaneous pain varies and may be burning, throbbing, pressing, shooting, or aching. In nearly all cases, the pain is felt deeply inside the distal part of the affected extremity. It always shows a diffuse distribution and is unrelated

Table I
Criteria for differential diagnosis of complex regional
pain syndromes (CRPS) type I and II

	CRPS I	CRPS II
Etiology	Any kind of lesion	Partial nerve lesion
Localization	Distal part of extremity	Any peripheral site of body
	Independent from site of lesion	Mostly confined to the territory of affected nerve
Spreading of symptoms	Obligatory	Rare
Spontaneous pain	Common	Obligatory
	Mostly deep and superficial	Predominately superficial
	Orthostatic component	No orthostatic component
Mechanical allodynia	Most of patients with spreading tendency	Obligatory in nerve territory
Autonomic symptoms	Distally generalized with spreading tendency	Related to nerve lesion
Motor symptoms	Distally generalized	Related to nerve lesion
Sensory symptoms	Distally generalized with spreading tendency	Related to nerve lesion

to the territories of individual nerves. It is apparently disproportionate to the inciting event. The pain usually decreases when the extremity is elevated and increases when it is lowered (orthostatic component). One of us (H.B.) maintains that spontaneous pain is absent or not prominent in a small fraction of patients with CRPS I (but these patients may have evoked abnormal pain and the other changes that are typical of CRPS I). Future investigations will show whether these patients are a subgroup of patients with CRPS I (Merskey and Bogduk 1994; Stanton-Hicks et al. 1995).

Various kinds of evoked abnormal sensations are found. In the skin, these are mechanical allodynia, hyperpathia (pain elicited by painful stimuli that appears with a delay, outlasts the stimulus, and spreads beyond the site of the stimulus), hyperalgesia and hypoalgesia, and hyeresthesia and hypoesthesia, all showing a diffuse distribution with no spatial relationship to individual nerve territories and to the site of the preceding lesion (in contrast to allodynia in CRPS II, see page 33). Usually, these sensations are more pronounced on the distal palmar/plantar side than on the dorsal side of the hand or foot; in particular, allodynia is sometimes most prominent at the fingertips. However, the latter observation is somewhat controversial, because allodynia was not a prominent symptom in the patients with CRPS I in Freiburg (Blumberg and Jänig 1994). In about 90% of the cases pain is elicited by movements and pressure at one or more finger/hand or toe/foot joints, even when these are not affected by the preceding lesion.

Autonomic (sympathetic) functions

The *skin blood flow* is abnormal in most cases of CRPS I: the skin is often marbled/reddish or bluish/pale. At normal room temperature the skin temperature on the palmar or plantar side of the ipsi- and contralateral finger or toe tips, respectively, shows a systematic side difference in about 80% of the patients, i.e., all fingers or toes of the affected extremity being either warmer or colder when compared with the corresponding contralateral fingers or toes. The mean side difference of skin temperature in these patients is about 2.5°C. Only 20% of controls show a systematic side difference of 1.6°C under room temperature conditions. Temperature differences in CRPS patients are not static values. They largely depend on various environmental conditions (see pages 12–16). Therefore, this symptom has only limited diagnostic value. For comparison, the conditions under which skin temperature measurements were performed should always be mentioned.

The *sweating* is also disturbed in many patients with CRPS I. The palmar or plantar side of the hands or feet is either hypo- or hyperhidrotic.

The *edema* (swelling) is a major symptom of CRPS I. Almost all patients describe a swelling of the distal part of the affected limb at least at some time during the course of the disease. In some cases the swelling depends critically on aggravating stimuli. It sometimes diminishes after sympathetic blocks and is considered to be a sign of a disturbed sympathetic function in some patients (Blumberg et al. 1994). In cases with severe swelling it is often combined with shiny skin. Slight swelling is indicated by a loss of skin folds.

Skeletomotor functions

In 90% of CRPS I cases, active muscular strength is decreased and often involves all muscles of the affected distal extremity, especially those exerting the strength of the hand grip. In most cases this disability is not explained by passive impairment of motion due to pain, edema, or contractures. No tendon reflex abnormalities can be documented. Complex movements of the affected distal extremity are considerably reduced, in particular the ability to close the fist and to oppose the tips of thumb and fifth finger. Furthermore, tremor (postural or action) is present in about half of the patients with an affected upper extremity. The postural tremor is an increased physiological tremor (Deuschl et al. 1991). These motor disturbances, in particular the tremor, are more obvious and severe at the upper extremity than at the lower extremity. Rare cases with long-standing CRPS I may develop dystonia at the affected extremity (Bhatia et al. 1993).

Trophic changes and changes in bone

In 30% of the CRPS I patients, *trophic skin changes* (e.g., disturbed nail growth, increased hair growth, palmar/plantar fibrosis, thin glossy skin, and hyperkeratosis) are present. None of these changes were observed during the first 10 days after the onset of CRPS I. Thus, trophic changes cannot be used for early diagnosis of CRPS I. Whether the passive movement restrictions (stiff joints) are related to the trophic changes of joints and tendons, which are seen in cases with long-standing CRPS I, or to functional motor disturbances (e.g., flexor-extensor co-contractions), or to both remains to be clarified.

The work of Sudeck (1902) first showed that patchy bone demineralization (osteoporosis) may occur in CRPS I. Plain radiographs show a diffuse and spotty distal distribution of demineralization of small bones with a periarticular dominance at the longer bones. These changes are not seen in early CRPS I but are likely to occur months after its beginning.

In contrast, three-phase bone scan demonstrated early changes in bone metabolism with high specificity and sensitivity. The uptake of an intravenously injected radionuclide tracer into the bone is measured at various times (seconds/minutes/hours) after injection of the tracer. The three phases are arterial, soft-tissue, and mineral. For all three phases, characteristic scintigraphic findings seem to occur in CRPS I; i.e., a diffuse increase in uptake of tracer is found periarticular around distal joints on the ipsilateral side (Kozin et al. 1981; Demangeat et al. 1988).

Sudeck (1902) first discussed an inflammatory pathogenesis of CRPS I, in particular of the trophic changes in deep somatic tissues. This idea of an inflammatory pathogenesis is based on the observation that in the acute phase all classical signs and symptoms of inflammation—rubor, calor, dolor, tumor, and functio laesa—are present. Moreover, the therapeutic effect of corticosteroids in some patients supports this idea (Christensen et al. 1982). Recently, scintigraphic investigations with marked immunoglobulins showed an intra-ossary plasma extravasation in patients with CRPS I, which supports an inflammatory component of the disorder (Oyen et al. 1993).

Combination and variability of symptoms

The clinical picture of CRPS I is characterized by a combination of autonomic, motor and sensory symptoms. Such a triad is present in about 90% of our sample of CRPS I patients. In the other cases, symptoms of only two parts of the triad are present. In each part of the triad the combination of symptoms varies from patient to patient. For example, swelling might be combined with normal skin temperature and normal sweating, normal movement ability with tremor and paresis.

The expression of CRPS I symptoms may vary considerably from mild to severe. In most cases, superficial and deep symptoms of CRPS I are about equally represented, but in some cases severe superficial symptoms (e.g., strong swelling, large differences of skin temperature, strong numbness) may be combined with less prominent deep symptoms (e.g., no osteoporosis, little paresis) or vice versa. The expression of symptoms, in particular those presumably associated with the sympathetic nervous system, may also spontaneously vary in the same patient (see pages 36–39).

Aggravation of symptoms in CRPS I by external stimuli

Several events may aggravate the symptoms in CRPS I, including physical load, painful stimuli or movements (e.g., during physiotherapy sessions), environmental temperature changes, local temperature changes (e.g., by application of cold or warm water), and increase in hydrostatic pressure (e.g., in orthostasis). The symptom swelling depends critically on aggravating stimuli. Noxious movements of the fingers may considerably increase the edema and the spontaneous pain. Other stimuli, such as environmental and local temperature changes, mostly affect blood flow through skin (which is reflected in the skin temperature) and may aggravate the spontaneous pain.

TIME COURSE OF THE DISORDER

For therapeutic reasons, every effort should be made to diagnose CRPS I as early as possible. In this context it is important to know whether CRPS I has an acute or slow onset. CRPS I mostly starts acutely, i.e., the cardinal symptoms may appear within hours or days. At the onset, the main symptoms of CRPS I are spontaneous pain, generalized swelling, and the systematic side difference of skin temperature. These early symptoms develop in areas and tissues that are *not* affected by the preceding lesion.

Swelling and pain provide valuable information for an early diagnosis of CRPS I; before the onset of CRPS I, pain is felt inside the area of the preceding lesion. With the onset of CRPS I, the pain is diffuse and deep inside the distal extremity and the swelling generalized, yet the initial pain may already have disappeared. In some cases, spontaneous diffuse pain may not be present at the onset of CRPS I but develops later.

To some extent the generalizing tendency of symptoms may be a physiological phenomenon in posttraumatic pain states and will disappear without any treatment. An exact differentiation of these physiological diffuse posttraumatic reactions and the development of "real" CRPS I is not possible. Therefore, results of treatment studies that started in very early stages are hardly valuable. However, general agreement exists that if CRPS I develops, specific treatment should start as early as possible. There still is no way to resolve this dilemma.

If the CRPS I syndrome is untreated, its symptoms, in many cases, will be more or less continuous over months or years. In this "permanent" form of CRPS I trophic changes and diffuse allodynia and hyperalgesia may occur. If the syndrome finally subsides, the swelling decreases but severe restrictions of passive movements together with muscular atrophy are likely to remain. In this condition, spontaneous pain may still be present or may subside.

About 30% of patients exhibit an intermittent form of CRPS I: the symptoms appear and disappear spontaneously or, more commonly, in relation to various kinds of strain, as noted above. Finally, patients can experience spontaneous remissions in which the symptoms disappear days or weeks after onset of CRPS I. The frequency of these spontaneous remissions is unknown; however, it does not seem to be negligible.

STAGING OF CRPS I

According to literature reports, untreated CRPS I may pass through three stages (Bonica 1990). The first (acute) stage is presumed to be characterized by the key symptoms of pain, edema, and warm skin, the second (dystrophic) stage by cold skin and trophic changes, and the third (atrophic) stage by atrophy of skeletal muscles and bone and contractures of joints. The duration of the first two stages is reported to be variable, lasting from weeks to months. It is impossible to predict whether CRPS I patients, if untreated, will reach the second or third stage or whether spontaneous remissions will occur. Furthermore, recovery from the third stage is unlikely. Symptoms that are specific for the first and the second stages do not exist. It is unclear whether individual patients consecutively pass through all three stages. Therefore, it is generally questionable whether staging of CRPS I is appropriate. What is probably more important, is that patients with CRPS I should be graded, according to the intensity of the sensory, autonomic, motor, and trophic changes, as being mild, moderate, or severe (Bonica 1990).

CRPS TYPE II*

EPIDEMIOLOGY

CRPS II is always preceded by a partial injury of a peripheral nerve or its major branches. The onset usually occurs immediately after the nerve injury. If untreated, the syndrome may last for years without any change of symptoms.

CLINICAL PHENOMENOLOGY

Patients with CRPS II usually exhibit a less complex clinical picture than do patients with CRPS I (Table I). The cardinal symptoms of CRPS II are spontaneous burning pain, hyperalgesia, and mechanical and cold allodynia (Chapter 9, this volume). These sensory symptoms are most intense in the territory of the affected peripheral nerve, and the tendency to spread is less obvious than in CRPS II, although allodynia may extend to a certain degree beyond the border of nerve territories. Pain may be exacerbated by temperature change or movement of the involved limb, stress, and emotional stimuli. Spontaneous and evoked pain are felt superficially, not deep inside the extremity, and the intensity of both is not dependent on the position of the extremity (absence of the orthostatic component). Pain elicited by movement and pressure of joints is absent.

The triad of sensory, autonomic, and motor symptoms that extends, at the affected extremity, into territories outside of the lesioned site and that is typical for most cases with CRPS I, is less frequent or even absent in CRPS II. Abnormalities in skin blood flow, most often vasodilatation in early stages and considerable vasoconstriction in late stages, changes in skin temperature and skin color, and sweating abnormalities may develop and are most intense in the zone of the lesioned nerve. Vasodilatation and vasoconstriction within the area of the lesioned nerve are thought to be at least in part due to impairment of sympathetic function following interruption and regeneration of vasoconstrictor fibers and due to consecutive hyperreactivity of cutaneous blood vessels to circulating catecholamines and environmental (e.g., thermal) stimuli (see pages 36–39).

Impairment of motor function is sometimes seen and may in part be explained by lesions of motor axons. Swelling and trophic changes are discrete. Usually, there are no changes in bone metabolism as demonstrated with plain radiographs or three-phase bone scan.

---

*CRPS II was formerly called SMP by one of us (cf. Blumberg and Jänig 1994).

COMBINATION OF BOTH TYPES OF CRPS

Sometimes CRPS I and CRPS II are simultaneously present in the same patient. The pain syndrome may start with CRPS II and then develop into CRPS I. For example, an accidental trauma or a carpal tunnel syndrome (or its surgical treatment) with peripheral nerve injury may lead to spontaneous pain and allodynia inside the area of the lesioned nerve. Later, the whole hand distally may exhibit the generalized triad of sensory, autonomic, and motor changes that is typical for CRPS I. In these patients, the pain consists of superficial spontaneous pain and evoked pain (allodynia), which are related to the lesioned nerve zone (CRPS II type of pain), and of deep diffuse spontaneous and movement-related pain, which are typical for CRPS I and which may be aggravated by various maneuvers (orthostasis, physical exercise, thermal load).

CRPS II also may occur following CRPS I. For example, if CRPS I with its typical triad has developed following a radial fracture, which is treated by a plaster cast, secondarily a partial superficial radial nerve lesion may occur. This can result in additional (superficial) spontaneous pain and allodynia, restricted to the territory of the lesioned nerve (CRPS II symptoms).

Finally, one caveat should be kept in mind concerning this classification and the clinical characteristics presented here: CRPS II patients may also develop CRPS I (or vice versa) and CRPS I may be locally restricted in some cases. Therefore, we may discover transitory states between CRPS I and CRPS II (Table I).

DIAGNOSTIC TESTS

The clinical symptomatology of CRPS alone does not allow us to conclude whether the sympathetic nervous system is involved in the generation of pain and other symptoms. Moreover, it is particularly important to decide whether and which components of pain may be related to sympathetic activity. Therefore, special diagnostic tests should be applied before treatment is started. At our clinics we propose four tests, two well established and two still being independently verified before they can be generally recommended or refuted. The relief of spontaneous pain and evoked pain should be measured quantitatively by the visual analogue scale or other scales. Placebo effects should be checked by injection of sodium chloride solution, for example, when sympathetic ganglia are blocked by a local anesthetic or in the phentolamine test (Arnér 1991; Raja et al. 1991; Price et al. 1992; Chapter 10, this volume).

Sympathetic blocks with local anesthetics

To block impulse activity in sympathetic neurons to the upper or lower extremity, a local anesthetic is applied ipsilaterally to the stellate ganglion or the lumbar paravertebral sympathetic ganglia, respectively (Bonica 1990). A complete block is assumed when the skin temperature of ipsilateral finger or toe tips increases to ≥ 35°C. An ipsilateral Horner's sign does not prove that the sympathetic impulse transmission through the stellate ganglion to the upper extremity is blocked. Temporary relief of pain indicates that the (efferent) sympathetic system may be involved in the generation of pain (by whatever mechanism) (Chapter 12, this volume). False positives, which may be generated by blockade of impulse activity in nociceptive afferents of adjacent nerve trunks (plexus brachialis, plexus lumbalis), can be excluded by careful clinical testing of sensory functions. Afferents projecting through the paravertebral ganglia to upper and lower extremities most likely do not exist and can not be responsible for the pain-relieving effects of the sympathetic blocks by local anesthetics (Jänig 1990).

Guanethidine test

One treatment is intravenous injection of guanethidine into an extremity with CRPS distal to a suprasystolic cuff (Hannington-Kiff 1977; Loh et al. 1980; Blumberg and Hoffmann 1994; Hoffmann and Blumberg 1994). This procedure can also be applied to test whether the sympathetic nervous system is involved in the generation of pain. The guanethidine test is positive, first, if the injection is followed by a short-lasting (burning) pain or by a sensation of pressure or heat, which have the same distribution as the spontaneous pain experienced by the patient and, second, if the spontaneous pain is relieved after opening the cuff (about 15 minutes after injection of the guanethidine). Both effects of the guanethidine are assumed to be related to the pharmacological actions of the drug. First, it is taken up by the noradrenergic varicosities of postganglionic axons and depletes noradrenaline from its stores, which leads to excitation of nociceptors. Second, it prevents further release of noradrenaline from the depleted postganglionic axons for up to one to two days.

Phentolamine test

Recently, Arnér (1991) and Raja et al. (1991) independently introduced the phentolamine test as a tool for diagnosis of CRPS (see also Campbell et al. 1992). Phentolamine is an α-adrenoceptor antagonist ($\alpha 1$, $\alpha 2$). The rationale of this test is that excitation of nociceptive afferent neurons by noradrenaline, which is released from postganglionic axons, is prevented by blockade of α-adrenoceptors. During intravenous infusion of phentolamine, pain is measured continuously by a visual analogue scale. If pain is reduced, the sympathetic nervous system is likely to be involved in the generation of pain. Arnér (1991) has shown that patients who obtained transient pain relief during intravenous infusion of phentolamine were likely to respond favorably to treatment with intravenous regional guanethidine. However, this test needs confirmation by further independent investigations before it can be universally recommended as diagnostic test (Verdugo and Ochoa 1994).

Ischemia test

Interruption of the circulation in the distal part of the affected extremity by a suprasystolic cuff (after an Esmarch bandage or equivalent is wrapped around the hand or foot from distal to proximal up to the cuff to reduce the volume of the distal extremity) suppresses or reduces the deep diffuse pain after one to two minutes. This pain-suppressing effect has occasionally been reported in the literature (Loh et al. 1980; Gracely et al. 1990) and is used as a supplementary test for diagnosis (Blumberg and Hoffmann 1994; Hoffmann and Blumberg 1994).

The pain suppression is not due to blockade of A or C fibers. A positive test has a high prognostic value for pain relief generated by sympatholytic interventions. However, these observations need independent confirmation by studies in which the clinical diagnosis (including the response to a sympathetic block) and the ischemia test are conducted independently on the same group of patients. Preliminary results show that the test is negative in CRPS II and in patients who have pain in the extremities that is not dependent on activity in the sympathetic nervous system (e.g., in patients with diabetic sensory neuropathy). The mechanism of the pain-relieving effect of this test is unclear, but it may be related to microvascular conditions in the deep somatic tissues of the extremities. It is unlikely that the ischemia itself elicits the pain-relieving effect; more likely it is related to a decrease in activity in small-diameter deep somatic afferents as a consequence of decrease in vascular filling.

SKIN TEMPERATURE, SKIN BLOOD FLOW, AND SYMPATHETIC INNERVATION OF CUTANEOUS BLOOD VESSELS IN CRPS

CRPS II

A partial nerve lesion is the important preceding event in CRPS II. Therefore, it is generally assumed that abnormalities in skin blood flow within the territory of the lesioned nerve, most often vasodilatation in early stages and considerable vasoconstriction in late stages, are due to *peripheral* impairment of sympathetic function and sympathetic denervation. During the first weeks after transection of vasoconstrictor fibers, vasodilatation is present within the affected area. Later the vasculature may develop an increased sensitivity that amplifies the response to local cold temperature stimuli and to catecholamines, presumably due to up-regulation of adrenoceptors (Fleming and Trendelenburg 1961; Jobling et al. 1992; Jänig and Koltzenburg 1991; Koltzenburg et al. 1995).

Similar observations were recently described in the chronic nerve constriction model in rats (Wakisaka et al. 1991). The skin on the lesioned side was abnormally warm for about the first postoperative week and then evolved to a chronically cold status. The late-stage cold skin was present despite a complete absence of fluorescence for noradrenaline. Thus, in this animal model, the cold skin is definitely not due to excessive noradrenergic sympathetic vasoconstrictor activity. Denervation supersensitivity is thought to be the likely explanation.

Evidence has been presented that similar mechanisms are responsible for the cold skin in patients with poly- and mononeuropathy (Ochoa and Yarnitsky 1994). These so-called triple-cold patients showed a considerable impairment of sympathetic reflexes, indicating small-fiber injury, sympathetic denervation, and consecutive denervation supersensitivity. Furthermore, reinnervated blood vessels may maintain the hyperreactivity to circulating catecholamines and to nerve impulses (Koltzenburg et al. 1995).

CRPS I

In contrast to CRPS II, most of the CRPS I patients have had only minor trauma without overt nerve injury. Changes in skin temperature, skin blood flow, and sweating also occur in regions not innervated by the peripheral nerve whose branches might be affected by the minor trauma. These symptoms show a generalized distribution and are not restricted to peripheral nerve territories.

It is generally assumed that sympathetic functions are disturbed in CRPS I. The abnormalities should be due to either hyper- or hypoactivity in sympathetic vasoconstrictor and sudomotor neurons on the affected side. However, we have lacked direct evidence for such behavior of sympathetic neurons. Bilateral microneurographic recordings from sympathetic postganglionic fibers of CRPS I patients could not demonstrate any side difference in overall activity or in discharge patterns to arousal stimuli and mental stress (Wallin et al. 1976; Torebjörk 1989; Casale and Elam 1992). Thus, any of the changes in sympathetic function observed in patients can only be taken as indirect evidence for disturbed sympathetic neuronal activity in CRPS I.

To test these phenomena in more detail and to answer the question whether and in which way the sympathetic nervous system may contribute to changes of its effector responses, we studied resting and reflex behavior of sympathetic effector organ function, i.e., skin temperature and skin blood flow (cf. Blumberg 1988, 1992; Baron et al. 1993; Baron and Engler, in press). In general we documented the following clinical characteristics:

• The skin temperature at distal parts of the extremities, that is dependent on the overall blood flow through the skin, characteristically shows a difference between sides with the affected extremity being either warmer or colder. The patients usually report a distorted reaction of the skin temperature to a change in environmental temperature and emotional stress, e.g., the affected hand cools down too slowly or too fast if the limb is exposed to a cold environment or if the patient is freezing or under stress.

• When systematic measurements of skin temperature are applied, it is obvious that temperature side differences are not static descriptors but comprise dynamic changes critically dependent on environmental temperature, local temperature, and emotional stress. In contrast to controls, the affected limb has unstable temperatures typically fluctuating by more than 2°C.

Data presented in the following sections were obtained in a limited number of patients. We are aware of the tentativeness of the hypotheses derived from these experiments. Nevertheless, we think it is worthwhile to discuss possible pathophysiological mechanisms, although not all patients reacted exactly in the same manner. We are now conducting studies with more patients.

Skin temperature under resting conditions

To characterize different groups of patients according to their skin temperature dynamics and underlying pathophysiological mechanisms, it was necessary to define criteria of skin temperature measurements. First, we determined skin temperature in a standardized manner with an infrared thermometer at the tips of all fingers or toes and at two additional sites of the palmar or plantar skin. Second, we defined patients who described their affected limb as being warm at room temperature (about 20°C environment) and under neutral emotional conditions (resting conditions) as "warm patients" and those who described their affected limb as being cold under these conditions as "cold patients." In most patients this subjective estimation of skin temperature could also be objectified by infrared skin temperature measurements.

Using this definition of resting skin temperature, we classified 60% of the entire group of patients as "warm" and 20% as "cold;" in 20% no difference could be demonstrated (Blumberg and Jänig 1994). The warm status seems to be a typical feature of acute phases of CRPS I. Most patients with cold limbs in late stages reported a warm or hot affected limb during the first weeks of the disorder. It is a general observation that most patients with cold limbs are difficult to treat.

Skin temperature under thermal load

To explore skin temperature and skin blood flow dynamics of the two different types of patients (warm and cold) in more detail, we analyzed these parameters in relation to changes of environmental temperature. Whole-body cooling and warming were achieved with a thermal suit that changed environmental temperature in a standardized way and reflexly altered skin sympathetic vasoconstrictor activity. The subject lay in a suit supplied by tubes, in which running water with an inflow temperature of 12°C and 50°C (inflow temperature), was used to cool or warm the whole body. During the experiment, the skin temperature and skin blood flow of both hands were monitored at regular intervals. At the beginning, measurements were obtained under resting conditions (20°C environmental temperature).

Most of the patients showed characteristic dynamic changes in vascular responses on the affected side compared to the healthy side. However, as mentioned above, not all patients react in such a standardized way. Therefore, we only report the typical thermoregulatory patterns of most patients with CRPS I. The differential reaction patterns are a subject of further investigation.

Warm patients. Under resting conditions, at 20°C environmental temperature, the affected side was on average 2–3°C warmer than the healthy side. Under cooling conditions the skin temperature decreased more slowly on the affected side. The temperature difference slowly increased and reached a maximum of 4–5°C with the affected limb being warmer. During warming, the skin temperature also increased more slowly on the affected side. Finally, the same level of temperature was measured on both sides (Fig. 1A).

Cold patients. Under resting conditions in a 20°C environment the affected limb was about 2–3°C colder compared with the unaffected side. After whole-body cooling the skin temperature on the affected limb decreased more quickly to lower values than it did on the healthy side. The maximum temperature difference under these conditions was about 4–5°C. After whole-body warming side differences were no longer present (Fig. 1B).

Skin blood flow and sympathetic vasoconstrictor function under thermal load

Warm patients. Skin blood flow at two corresponding fingertips on the affected and healthy side was recorded using pulse plethysmography. Sympathetic vasoconstrictor reflexes were induced by asphyxia and stimulation of skin by using noxious heat. Data are only available after whole-body warming. Under these conditions no differences in baseline blood flow and reflexes could be recorded.

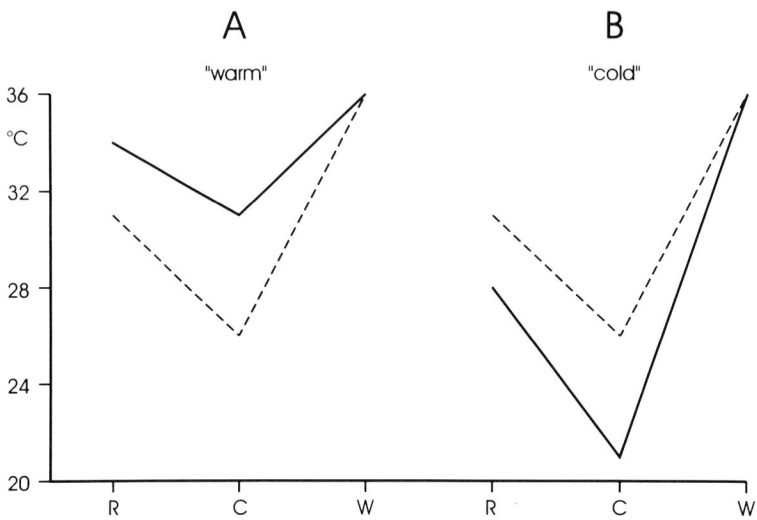

Fig. 1. Characteristics of skin temperature of hands in patients with CRPS I in resting conditions (R), during whole-body cooling (C), and during whole-body warming (W). The skin temperature of the healthy side (– – –) and the affected side (——) was measured. Resting conditions (R) are defined by room temperature of about 20°C and neutral emotional condition (the patient has adapted to the laboratory). Whole-body cooling and warming were applied by means of a thermal suit to change environmental temperature in a standardized way and reflexly alter skin sympathetic vasoconstrictor activity. The subject was lying in a suit supplied by tubes, in which running water of 12°C or 50°C (inflow temperature) was used to cool or warm the whole body. During the experiment, the skin temperature of both hands was monitored at regular intervals. **A:** "warm" patient: temperature of affected limb warmer than contralateral control under resting conditions. **B:** "cold" patient: temperature of affected limb colder under resting conditions than contralateral healthy one. Scheme

Cold patients. Skin blood flow was measured at two corresponding fingertips on the affected and contralateral limbs using laser Doppler flowmetry. Sympathetic vasoconstrictor reflexes were induced by deep inspiration. Under resting conditions (20°C environmental temperature), after whole-body cooling, and in combination with mental activity, baseline blood flow and skin temperature were considerably lower on the affected side. Under these conditions, vasoconstriction was almost complete and no additional vasoconstrictor reflexes could be elicited (Fig. 2A). After patients went through whole-body warming and emotional acclimatization, their baseline blood flow demonstrated no significant side differences. Under these conditions sympathetic vasoconstrictor responses were quantitatively the same on both sides (Fig. 2B).

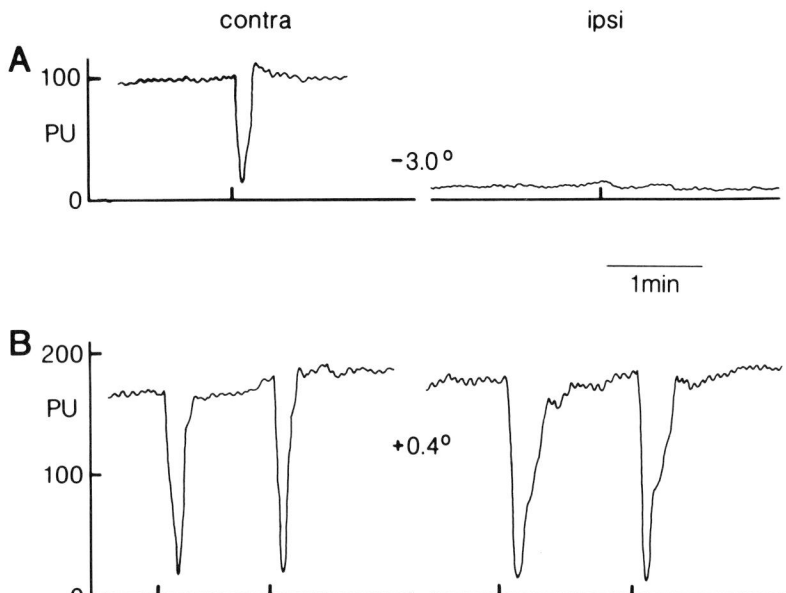

Fig. 2. Blood flow characteristics in a cold patient with CRPS I. Vasomotor reflexes were induced by deep inspiration (vertical marks on x-axis). **A:** Baseline blood flow in cold environment on the unaffected (contra) and affected (ipsi) side. Note the considerable vasoconstriction on the affected side that was 3°C colder than the contralateral side. No additional vaso-constrictor reflexes could be elicited. **B:** Baseline blood flow and sympathetic vaso-constrictor reflexes after whole-body warming. Baseline blood flow and sympathetic reflexes were the same on both sides. There was almost no temperature difference. The affected side (ipsi) was 0.4°C warmer than the contralateral side (contra). (PU = perfusion units)

Pathophysiological mechanisms of vascular abnormalities: a hypothesis indicating central nervous system pathology

Concerning a possible sympathetic contribution to the autonomic symptoms in CRPS, there seems to be a complex deterioration rather than any evidence for a general increase or decrease of activity in sympathetic neurons, as it is still widely assumed. We can distinguish warm and cold patients. However, this typical temperature side difference is not a static descriptor but comprises a dynamic descriptor that is critically dependent on environmental temperature, local temperature, and emotional setting. It is only present at room temperature (20°C) or in a cold environment and possibly under emotional stress. After whole-body warming and emotional relaxation, patients in both groups showed no systematic side differences in skin temperature. The skin temperature dynamics were paralleled by skin blood flow reactions. How can these phenomena be explained?

Cutaneous vasoconstrictor neurons supplying the hands and feet are mainly involved in thermoregulation. They do not exhibit spontaneous activity after whole-body warming and are active during body cooling and in a cold environment. Therefore, no side difference is present after whole-body warming, in cold as well as in warm patients. Furthermore, nonthermoregulatory sympathetic reflexes elicited, for example, by deep inspiration, are identical on both sides. In cold patients whole-body cooling and perhaps also emotional stimuli may lead to a more vigorous reaction of sympathetic vasoconstrictor neurons on the affected side. In warm patients whole-body cooling and emotional stimuli may lead to decreased reaction of sympathetic vasoconstrictor neurons.

These findings support the idea that CRPS I may be associated with an disturbed unilateral thermoregulation of the extremities. An abnormal unilateral reflex pattern of sympathetic vasoconstrictor neurons due to thermoregulatory and emotional stimuli may be present. The pathophysiological mechanisms underlying such disturbed sympathetic reflex activity must be located in the central nervous system, probably in the spinal cord. This interpretation is consistent with experimental findings obtained in animals, which show that the reflex pattern in cutaneous vasoconstrictor neurons may change after peripheral nerve lesion (Blumberg and Jänig 1985; Jänig and Koltzenburg 1991).

Other symptoms in CRPS I indicating pathophysiological mechanisms within the central nervous system

• Symptoms of CRPS I develop in the distal region of the affected extremity most often following a noxious event, irrespective of its type and location. They are not confined to the innervation zone of an individual nerve and show a distally generalized distribution. They are present in tissues that are not directly affected by the preceding lesion. This spreading tendency of symptoms argues for a central origin of the disorder.

• Hyperhidrosis, a typical feature of many CRPS I patients, cannot be explained by a peripheral mechanism because, in contrast to blood vessels, sweat glands do not develop a denervation supersensitivity (Fleming and Westphal 1988). Therefore, increase of sweating in patients with CRPS I is generated by an increase of activity in sympathetic sudomotor neurons of central origin.

• Impairment of muscle strength involving all muscles of the affected distal extremity, which cannot be explained by pain, edema or severance of peripheral nerves, also seems to be the result of a centrally mediated impulse abnormality in the motoneuron pool projecting to the distal extremity. Moreover, an increased physiological tremor, present in about 50% of the patients with CRPS I, must be due to central changes.

• Results of animal experiments suggest that positive sensory phenomena such as dynamic mechanical allodynia can be explained by a reorganization of synaptic structures in the central nervous system. These touch-evoked pain sensations are thought to involve changes in the CNS processing that strengthen the synaptic ties between central pain-signaling pathways and input from low-threshold mechanoreceptors with Aß fibers (cf. Baron and Saguer 1993; Koltzenburg et al. 1994; for review see Bennett 1994; Baron and Maier 1995a,b; Chapter 10, this volume). However, this explanation can only be half the truth, because it could barely explain how dynamic, mechanical (Aß-fiber-mediated) allodynia can be alleviated in some patients within minutes after sympathetic blocks (Wahren et al. 1991; Price et al., this volume). The latter observation supports the idea that the activation of the central nervous nociceptive system by Aß fibers is a dynamic process and critically dependent on an additional synaptic input (e.g., in nociceptive C afferents) that is maintained by sympathetic activity. This hypothesis is fully consistent with experimental results on humans showing that capsaicin application to skin can elicit Aß-mediated allodynia that develops and disappears within one to two hours (LaMotte et al. 1992; Torebjörk et al. 1992).

SUMMARY

CRPS I

1. CRPS I develops after several types of initiating noxious events. It is defined by a triad of sensory, autonomic, and motor symptoms, which occur distally at the affected extremity in a generalized distribution independent of type and location of the preceding trauma. The symptoms are not limited to the distribution of a single peripheral nerve and are apparently disproportionate to the inciting event.

2. CRPS I is mostly acute in its onset and can be diagnosed early. Its clinical picture is characterized as follows:

• Spontaneous, deep, diffuse pain is present in most patients. Cutaneous and deep hyperalgesia and changes of other sensations are almost regularly found. Allodynia seems to be present in most of the patients depending on the time of the initiating event.

• The autonomic changes consist of swelling (edema), disturbances of blood flow through skin (side differences of skin temperature), and disturbances of sweating (hyper- and hypohidrosis).

• The motor changes are represented by a reduction of the range of active movement and of muscular strength and by an increase in physiological tremor of the distal extremity.

• Most trophic disturbances (changes of skin and its appendages, atrophy of muscles, and contractures of joints) and changes in bones (osteoporosis) are late consequences of CRPS I. In contrast, changes in bone metabolism can be demonstrated early by three-phase bone scanning with high specificity and sensitivity.

3. If untreated, CRPS I may continuously be present for months to years or may change into an intermittent form. Spontaneous remissions of CRPS I also occur.

CRPS II

CRPS II is a pain syndrome that develops after a peripheral nerve lesion. Its cardinal symptoms are spontaneous pain and mechanical and cold allodynia. These sensory symptoms are preferentially restricted to the territory of the affected nerve but may also show a spreading tendency. Abnormalities in skin blood flow and sweating may develop and are usually restricted to the zone of the lesioned nerve. Impairment of motor function is sometimes seen and may in part be explained by lesions of motor axons. Swelling and trophic changes are discrete. A combination of symptoms of CRPS II and CRPS I may be present in the same patient.

PATHOPHYSIOLOGICAL MECHANISMS

Several lines of evidence indicate that in CRPS I *central nervous system* factors are mainly involved in the generation of autonomic, motor, and sensory abnormalities. Vascular abnormalities, for example, may be associated with a disturbed unilateral thermoregulation of the extremities. An abnormal reflex pattern of sympathetic vasoconstrictor neurons due to body temperature stimuli may be present on the affected side. Vascular abnormalities in CRPS II within the territory of the lesioned nerve may be due to *peripheral* impairment of sympathetic function and sympathetic denervation.

ACKNOWLEDGMENTS

This work was supported by the Wilhelm Sander-Stiftung (R.B.), the Bundesministerium für Forschung und Technologie (H.B.), and the Deutsche Forschungsgemeinschaft (W.J.). We are grateful for the good cooperation of Priv. Doz. Dr. C. Maier, Clinic for Anesthesiology, Kiel, Germany.

REFERENCES

Arnér, S., Intravenous phentolamine test: diagnostic and prognostic use in reflex sympathetic dystrophy, Pain, 46 (1991) 17–22.
Baron, R. and Engler, F., Postganglionic dysautonomia with incomplete recovery: a clinical, neurophysiological and immunological case study, J. Neurol., in press.
Baron, R. and Maier, C., Phantom limb pain: are cutaneous nociceptors and spinothalamic neurons involved in the signaling and maintenance of spontaneous and touch-evoked pain? A case report, Pain, 60 (1995a) 223–228.
Baron, R. and Maier, C., Painful neuropathy: C-nociceptor activity may not be necessary to maintain central mechanisms accounting for dynamic mechanical allodynia, Clin. J. Pain, 11 (1995b) 63–69.
Baron, R. and Saguer, M., Postherpetic neuralgia: are C-nociceptors involved in signalling and maintenance of tactile allodynia? Brain, 116 (1993) 1477–1496.
Baron, R., Feldmann, R. and Lindner, V., Small fiber function in autonomic failure, J. Neurol., 241 (1993) 87–91.
Bennett, G.J., Neuropathic pain. In: P.D. Wall and R. Melzack, (Eds.), Textbook of Pain, 3rd ed., Churchill Livingstone, Edinburgh, 1994, pp. 210–224.
Bhatia, K.P., Bhatt, M.H. and Marsden, C.D., The causalgia-dystonia syndrome, Brain, 116 (1993) 843–851.
Blumberg, H., Zur Entstehung und Therapie des Schmerzsyndroms bei der sympathischen Reflexdystrophie, Der Schmerz, 2 (1988) 125–143.
Blumberg, H., Clinical and pathophysiological aspects of reflex sympathetic dystrophy and sympathetically maintained pain. In: W. Jänig and R.F. Schmidt (Eds.), Reflex Sympathetic Dystrophy. Pathophysiological Mechanisms and Clinical Implications, VCH Verlagsgesellschaft, Weinheim, New York, 1992, pp. 29–50.
Blumberg, H. and Hoffmann, U., Der "Ischämie-Test:" ein neues Verfahren in der klinischen Diagnostik der sympathischen Reflexdystrophie (Kausalgie, M. Sudeck), Der Schmerz, 6 (1992) 196–198.
Blumberg, H. and Jänig, W., Reflex patterns in postganglionic vasoconstrictor neurons following chronic nerve lesions, J. Auton. Nerv. Syst., 14 (1985) 157–180.
Blumberg, H. and Jänig, W., Clinical manifestations of reflex sympathetic dystrophy and sympathetically maintained pain. In: P.D. Wall and R. Melzack (Eds.), Textbook of Pain, Churchill, Livingstone, 1994, pp. 685–697.
Blumberg, H. and Hoffmann, U., Zur Diagnostik der sympathischen Reflexdystrophie, Nervenarzt, 65 (1994) 370–374.
Blumberg, H., Wakhloo, A.K., Hoffmann, U. and Wokalek, H., Die lokalisierte Form der sympathischen Reflexdystrophie, Der Schmerz, 7 (1993) 178–181.
Blumberg, H., Hoffmann, U., Mohadjer, M. and Scheremet, R., Clinical phenomenology and mechanisms of reflex sympathetic dystrophy: emphasis on edema. In: G.F. Gebhart, D.L. Hammond and T.S. Jensen (Eds.), Proceedings of the 7th World Congress on Pain, Progress in Pain Research and Management, Vol. 2, IASP Press, Seattle, 1994, pp. 455–481.
Bonica, J.J., Causalgia and other reflex sympathetic dystrophies. In: J.J. Bonica (Ed.), The Management of Pain, Vol. 2, Lea & Febiger, Philadelphia, 1990, pp. 220–243.
Campbell, J.N., Raja, S.N. and Meyer, R.A., Painful sequelae of nerve injury. In: R. Dubner, G.F. Gebhart, R.F. Bond (Eds.), Proceedings of the Vth World Congress on Pain, Pain Research and Clinical Management, Vol. 3, Elsevier, Amsterdam, 1988, pp. 135–143.
Campbell, J.N., Meyer, R.A. and Raja, S.N., Is nociceptor activation by alpha-1 adrenoreceptors the culprit in sympathetically maintained pain? APS Journal, 1 (1992) 3–11.
Casale, R. and Elam, M., Normal sympathetic nerve activity in a reflex sympathetic dystrophy with marked skin vasoconstriction, J. Autonom. Nerv. Syst., 41 (1992) 215–220.
Christensen, K., Jensen, E.M. and Noer, I., The reflex sympathetic dystrophy syndrome: response

to treatment with corticosteroids, Acta Chir. Scand., 148 (1982) 653–655.
Davis, K.D., Treede, R.D., Raja, S.N., Meyer, R.A. and Campbell, J.N., Topical application of clonidine relieves hyperalgesia in patients with sympathetically maintained pain, Pain, 47 (1991) 309–317.
Demangeat, J.L., Constantinesco, A., Brunot, B., Foucher, G. and Farcot, J.M., Three-phase bone scanning in reflex sympathetic dystrophy of the hand, J. Nucl. Med., 29 (1988) 26–32.
Deuschl, G., Blumberg, H. and Lücking, C.H., Tremor in reflex sympathetic dystrophy, Arch. Neurol., 48 (1991) 1247–1258.
Fleming, W.W. and Trendelenburg, U., The development of supersensitivity to norepinephrine after pretreatment with reserpine, J. Pharmacol. Exp. Ther., 133 (1961) 41–51.
Fleming, W.W. and Westfall, D.P., Adaptive supersensitivity. In: U. Trendelenburg and N. Weiner (Eds.), Handbook of Experimental Pharmacology, Vol. 90/I catecholamines, Springer-Verlag, New York, 1988, pp. 509–559.
Gibbons, J.J. and Wilson, P.R., RSD score: criteria for the diagnosis of reflex sympathetic dystrophy and causalgia, Clin. J. Pain, 8 (1992) 260–263.
Gracely, R.H., Lynch, S. and Bennett, G.J., Ischemic blocks of large fiber function in reflex sympathetic dystrophy: a paradox, Soc. Neurosci. Abstr., 16 (1990) 1280.
Hannington-Kiff, J.G., Relief of Sudeck's atrophy by regional intravenous guanethidine, Lancet I, (1977) 1132–1133.
Hoffmann, U. and Blumberg, H., Modifikation der Guanethidin-Blockade zur Diagnostik der sympathischen Reflexdystrophie (Morbus Sudeck), Der Schmerz, 8 (1994) 95–99.
Jänig, W., The sympathetic nervous system in pain: physiology and pathophysiology. In: M. Stanton-Hicks (Ed.), Pain and the Sympathetic Nervous System, Kluwer Academic Publishers, Boston, 1990, pp. 17–89.
Jänig, W. and Koltzenburg, M., Sympathetic reflex activity and neuroeffector transmission change after chronic nerve lesions. In: M.R. Bond, J.E. Charlton and C.J. Woolf (Eds.), Proceedings of the VIth World Congress on Pain, Pain Research and Clinical Management, Vol. 4, Elsevier, Amsterdam, 1991, pp. 365–371.
Jänig, W. and Schmidt, R.F., Reflex sympathetic dystrophy: pathophysiological mechanisms and clinical implications, VCH Verlagsgesellschaft, Weinheim, New York, 1992.
Jänig, W., Blumberg, H., Boas, R.A. and Campbell, J.A., The reflex sympathetic dystrophy syndrome: Consensus Statement and general recommendations for diagnosis and clinical research. In: M.R. Bond, J.E. Charlton and C.J. Woolf (Eds.), Pain Research and Clinical Management: Proceedings of the VIth World Congress on Pain, Pain Research and Clinical Management, Vol. 4, Elsevier Science Publishers, Amsterdam, 1991, pp. 372–375.
Jobling, P., McLachlan, E.M., Jänig, W. and Anderson, C.R., Electrophysiological responses in the rat tail artery during reinnervation following lesions of the sympathetic supply, J. Physiol. (Lond.), 454 (1992) 107–128.
Koltzenburg, M., Torebjörk, H.E. and Wahren, L.K., Nociceptor-modulated central sensitization causes mechanical hyperalgesia in acute chemogenic and chronic neuropathic pain, Brain, 117 (1994) 579–591.
Koltzenburg, M., Häbler, H.-J. and Jänig, W., Functional reinnervation of the vasculature of the adult cat paw pad by axons originally innervating vessels in hairy skin, Neuroscience, 67 (1995) 245–252.
Kozin, F., Soin, J.S., Ryan, L.M., Carrera, G.F. and Wortmann, R.L., Bone scintigraphy in the reflex sympathetic dystrophy syndrome, Radiology, 138 (1981) 437–443.
LaMotte, R.H., Lundberg, L.E.R. and Torebjörk, H.E., Pain, hyperalgesia and activity in nociceptive C units in humans after intradermal injection of capsaicin, J. Physiol., 448 (1992) 749–764.
Loh, L. and Nathan, P.W., Painful peripheral states and sympathetic blocks, J. Neurol. Neurosurg. Psychiatry, 41 (1978) 664–671.
Loh, L., Nathan, P.W., Schott, G.D. and Wilson, P.G., Effects of regional guanethidine infusion in certain painful states, J. Neurol. Neurosurg. Psychiatry, 43 (1980) 446–451.
Loh, L., Nathan, P.W. and Schott, G.D., Pain due to lesions of central nervous system removed by

sympathetic block, Brit. Med. J., 282 (1981) 1026–1028.

Low, P.A., Amadio, P.C., Wilson, P.R., McManis, P.G. and Willner, C.L., Laboratory findings in reflex sympathetic dystrophy: a preliminary report, Clin. J. Pain, 10 (1994) 235–239.

Marsden, C.D., Obeso, J.A., Traub, M.M., Rothwell, J.C., Kranz, H. and La Cruz, F., Muscle spasms associated with Sudeck's atrophy after injury, Br. Med. J. Clin. Res., 288 (1984) 173–176.

Merskey, H. and Bogduk, N. (Eds.), Classification of Chronic Pain: Descriptions of Chronic Pain Syndromes and Definition of Terms, 2nd ed., IASP Press, Seattle, 1994.

Nathan, P.W., Pain and the sympathetic system, J. Auton. Nerv. Syst., 7 (1983) 363–370.

Ochoa, J.L. and Yarnitsky, D., The triple cold syndrome: cold hyperalgesia, cold hypoaesthesia and cold skin in peripheral nerve disease, Brain, 117 (1994) 185–197.

Oyen, W.J.G., Arntz, I.E., Claessens, R.A.M.J., Van der Meer, J.W.M., Corstens, F.H.M. and Goris, R.J.A., Reflex sympathetic dystrophy of the hand: an excessive inflammatory response? Pain, 55 (1993) 151–157.

Price, D.D., Bennett, G.J. and Rafii, A., Psychophysical observations on patients with neuropathic pain relieved by a sympathetic block, Pain, 36 (1989) 273–288.

Price, D.D., Long, S. and Huitt, C., Sensory testing of pathophysiological mechanisms of pain in patients with reflex sympathetic dystrophy, Pain, 49 (1992) 163–173.

Raja, S.N., Treede, R.D., Davis, K.D. and Campbell, J.N., Systemic alpha-adrenergic blockade with phentolamine: a diagnostic test for sympathetically maintained pain, Anesthesiology, 74 (1991) 691–698.

Raja, S.N., Davis, K.D. and Campbell, J.N., The adrenergic pharmacology of sympathetically-maintained pain, Microsurgery, 8 (1992) 63–69.

Roberts, W.J., A hypothesis on the physiological basis for causalgia and related pains, Pain, 24 (1986) 297–311.

Schott, G.D., Mechanisms of causalgia and related clinical conditions. The role of the central and of the sympathetic nervous systems, Brain, 109 (1986) 717–738.

Schott, G., Clinical features of algodystrophy: is the sympathetic nervous system involved? Funct. Neurol., 4 (1989) 131–134.

Schott, G.D., Visceral afferents: their contribution to "sympathetic dependent" pain, Brain, 117 (1994) 397–413.

Schwartzman, R.J. and McLellan, T.L., Reflex sympathetic dystrophy: a review, Arch. Neurol., 44 (1987) 555–561.

Stanton-Hicks, M., Jänig, W., Hassenbusch, S., Haddox, J.D., Boas, R. and Wilson, P., Reflex sympathetic dystrophy: changing concepts and taxonomy, Pain, 63 (1995) 127–133.

Sudeck, P., Über die akute (trophoneurotische) Knochenatrophie nach Entzündungen und Traumen der Extremitäten, Deut. Med. Wschr., 28 (1902) 336–342.

Sunderland, S., Pain mechanisms in causalgia, J. Neurol. Neurosurg. Psychiatry, 39 (1976) 471–480.

Torebjörk, E., Clinical and neurophysiological observations relating to pathophysiological mechanisms of reflex sympathetic dystrophy. In: M. Stanton-Hicks, W. Jänig and R.A. Boas (Eds.) Reflex Sympathetic Dystrophy, Kluwer, Boston, Dordrecht, London, 1989, pp. 71–80.

Torebjörk, H.E., Lundberg, L.E. and LaMotte, R.H., Central changes in processing of mechanoreceptive input in capsaicin-induced secondary hyperalgesia in humans, J. Physiol., 448 (1992) 765–780.

Treede, R.D., Davis, K.D., Campbell, J.N. and Raja, S.N., The plasticity of cutaneous hyperalgesia during sympathetic ganglion blockade in patients with neuropathic pain, Brain, 115 (1992) 607–621.

Veldman, P.H.J.M., Reynen, H.M., Arntz, I.E. and Goris, R.I.A., Signs and symptoms of reflex sympathetic dystrophy: prospective study of 829 patients, Lancet, 342 (1993) 1012–1016.

Verdugo, R.J. and Ochoa, J.L., "Sympathetically maintained pain." I. Phentolamine block questions the concept, Neurology, 44 (1994) 1003–1010.

Verdugo, R.J., Campero, M. and Ochoa, J.L., Phentolamine sympathetic block in painful polyneuropathies. II. Further questioning of the concept of "sympathetically maintained pain," Neurology, 44 (1994) 1010–1014.

Wahren, L.K. and Torebjörk, E., Quantitative sensory tests in patients with neuralgia 11 to 25 years after injury, Pain, 48 (1992) 237–244.

Wahren, L.K., Torebjörk, E. and Nyström, B., Quantitative sensory testing before and after regional guanethidine block in patients with neuralgia in the hand, Pain, 46 (1991) 23–30.

Wakisaka, S., Kajander, K.C. and Bennett, G.J., Abnormal skin temperature and abnormal sympathetic vasomotor innervation in an experimental painful peripheral neuropathy, Pain, 46 (1991) 299–313.

Wallin, G., Torebjörk, E. and Hallin, R., Preliminary observations on the pathophysiology of hyperalgesia in the causalgic pain syndrome. In: Y. Zotterman (Ed.), Sensory Functions of the Skin in Primates, Pergamon, New York, 1976, pp. 489–502.

Correspondence to: Ralf Baron, Dr med, PD, Klinik für Neurologie, Christian-Albrechts-Universität zu Kiel, Niemannsweg 147, 24105 Kiel, Germany. Tel: 49-431-597-2633; Fax: 49-431-597-2712.

3

Clinical Characteristics of Patients with Reflex Sympathetic Dystrophy (Sympathetically Maintained Pain) in the USA

Phillip A. Low,[a] Peter R. Wilson,[b] Paola Sandroni,[a] Catherine L. Willner,[a] and Thomas C. Chelimsky[c]

[a]Autonomic Disorders Research Center, Department of Neurology, and [b]Pain Clinic, Mayo Clinic, Rochester, Minnesota, and [c]Department of Neurology, Case Western Reserve University, Cleveland, Ohio, USA

Reflex sympathetic dystrophy/sympathetically maintained pain (RSD/SMP*) is characterized by diffuse limb pain, maximal distally, developing following injury, with allodynia (pain perception in response to a nonpainful stimulus) and hyperalgesia, and is commonly associated with vasomotor, sudomotor, swelling, and trophic changes (Bonica 1973; Willner 1993). The common association with manifestations of sympathetic dysfunction combined with the special characteristics of the pain (distribution and quality) permit the diagnosis of RSD/SMP (Low et al. 1994). Although the pathogenesis is uncertain and the pathophysiologic role of the sympathetic nervous system in this condition continues to be controversial (Verdugo and Ochoa 1994; Verdugo et al. 1994), most pain clinicians are impressed with the at least transient response to sympathetic block (Raja et al. 1991).

This chapter summarizes the Mayo Autonomic Laboratory experience over three study phases. We will review our initial experience with laboratory evaluation of 12 patients with presumed RSD/SMP, followed by an extensive review of 407 patients, and finally, a prospective evaluation of 102 patients who were referred for autonomic testing and considered to have possible RSD/SMP.

---

*The term CRPS (complex regional pain syndrome) is the preferred term, but because of the large amount of retrospective data, we have used the term RSD/SMP in this chapter.

PERIOD I: INITIAL EXPERIENCES, 1982-1984

The Mayo Autonomic Reflex Laboratory commenced in 1982. The initial experience spanned a period of two years ending in 1984. In our initial evaluation, we examined the agreement between the clinical features of RSD/SMP, based on the presence of diffuse chronic limb pain associated with allodynia, and laboratory indices of asymmetry in side-by-side comparison of vasomotor and sudomotor indices. We postulated that we should be able to use this laboratory sensitivity and specificity of measurements to enhance our clinical diagnosis. The hypothesis is that if good agreement is obtained, then we can use the improved sensitivity of laboratory quantitation to diagnose lesser degrees of sympathetic dysfunction. The specific aims of the evaluation have remained unchanged through the three phases of our research, although refinements of testing have occurred.

We thus did a side-by-side comparison of sudomotor and vasomotor indices in 12 patients who clinically had reflex sympathetic dystrophy (RSD/SMP; Tables I and II). The specific aims of the evaluation have remained unchanged to the present time, although refinements of testing have occurred. We compared sudomotor and vasomotor tone simultaneously from the affected and non-affected extremity. Sudomotor evaluation consisted of a recording of unstimulated resting sweat output (RSO) and the quantitative sudomotor axon reflex test (QSART). One component is a somatosympathetic (somatosudomotor) response, where a somatic stimulus (electrical current) evokes a sympathetic response. The somatic afferent limb is carried by type II to IV afferents. It can be activated by maneuvers such as an inspiratory gasp, an electrical stimulus, or a loud noise (Shahani et al. 1984). It has spinal, bulbar, and suprabulbar components. The final common pathway of the efferent limb

Table I
Characteristic of patients with RSD/SMP (Period 1)

Number of patients	12
Age (mean ± SD)	36.8 ± 16.5
Gender	M = 4; F = 8
Affected limb	Lower extremity = 11 (L = 7; R = 4) Upper extremity = 1 (right)
Duration of symptoms	<12 months, n = 8 >12 months, n = 4
Initiating injury	Trauma, n=10 Surgery, n=1 None, n=1

Table II
Clinical details in 12 patients with RSD/SMP

Case	Age (years)	Duration of Pain (months)	Pain	Swelling	VM	X-Ray Demin.	Bone Scan	Severity	Response to Treatment
1	51	17	+	+	+	+	?	mild	?
2	26	4	+	++	+	-	ND	mild	Y (PM&R)
3	37	4	+	+	+	-			
4	38	4	++	?	?	-	-	moderate	Y (Sym bl)
5	73	6	++	+	+	-	-	moderate	
6	50	10	++	+	++	-	ND	severe	Y (Sym bl)
7	26	9	+	+	+	-			
8	19	10	++	+	+	+	ND	severe	Y (Sym bl)
9	39	18	+	+	++	+	ND	moderate	
10	44	36	++	++	?	-	ND	severe	Y (Sym bl)
11	24	2	++	++	++	-		severe	Y (Sym bl)
12	14	12	+	+	?	-	-	mild	Y (TENS)

Note: VM, vasomotor; +, present on history; ++, marked or confirmed on examination; ?, equivocal; ND, not done; Y, yes; PM&R, physical medicine and rehabilitation; Sym bl, sympathetic block; TENS, transcutaneous electrical nerve stimulation

comprises sympathetic preganglionic and postganglionic efferent fibers (Sato and Schmidt 1973). The second is an "axon-reflex" sweat response, mediated by the postganglionic sudomotor axon. Acetylcholine activates postganglionic sympathetic sudomotor fibers, initially antidromically; the impulse, on reaching a branch-point, is thought to then travel orthodromically, to release acetylcholine, which then binds to M_3 receptors (Low et al. 1993). All recordings were done simultaneously, bilaterally, so as to compare the amplitude, volume, and dynamic properties of the sudomotor responses of the two sides. In all descriptions of QSART, sweat volumes will refer to combined volumes.

METHODS

Patient selection and preparation

We studied 12 patients who were considered to have reflex sympathetic dystrophy (RSD/SMP). These patients had pain that was diffuse, maximal distally, and aggravated by touch or pressure (Tables I and II). All evaluations in this and subsequent studies were done in a controlled-temperature environment of 23°C.

Measurement of resting sweat output

RSO for upper extremity studies was recorded over nonstimulated skin by using large capsules (5.31 cm^2) attached bilaterally to the medial distal forearm and hypothenar eminence. For lower extremity studies, bilateral recordings were made over the extensor digitorum brevis muscle and the medial distal leg (Low 1993). All recordings were done simultaneously. The unstimulated, resting sweat content (RSO) was measured by a console of four sudorometers (Low and Zimmerman 1993). RSO was recorded over five minutes in the four sites simultaneously, and RSO values over the last of the five minutes were read by the computer. We selected the fifth minute because steady-state conditions were attained by that time.

QSART recordings

In contrast to RSO, QSART measures evoked sweat response. The stimulus was the iontophoresis of 10% acetylcholine applied through one compartment and the response recorded with a sudorometer connected to a different compartment (Low 1993; Low et al. 1983). The stimulus evokes a somatosympathetic response, mediated by somatic afferents and sympathetic sudomotor efferents. The somatosympathetic response is not recordable in normal subjects. In some patients with RSD/SMP, the response is recordable. This larger sudomotor output is presumed to be in response to a sympathetic volley that is larger or better synchronized. The somatosympathetic response, with a latency of 0.1–0.2 minutes, is clearly separable from the QSART response, mediated by the postganglionic axon alone. The latter has a latency greater than 0.5 minutes (Low et al. 1983; Low 1993). The ultra-short latency is too short to be mediated by the axon-reflex response (Low et al. 1993). Finally, the sweat volume of the somatosympathetic response is very small (< 0.04 µl/cm^2). QSART is recorded over the medial distal forearm bilaterally for upper extremity studies. For lower extremity studies, recordings were made bilaterally over the extensor digitorum brevis muscle and the medial distal leg. All recordings were done simultaneously. The normal response has a latency of 1–2 minutes and is symmetric (Low 1993; Low et al. 1994). In some patients with RSD/SMP an augmented somatosympathetic response will manifest as a recordable sudomotor response within the first 10 seconds, often with persistent sweat activity (Fig. 1).

Measurement of skin vasomotor function

Skin vasomotor tone was determined in two ways. First, we measured skin blood flow using laser doppler flowmeters. Four skin sites were done

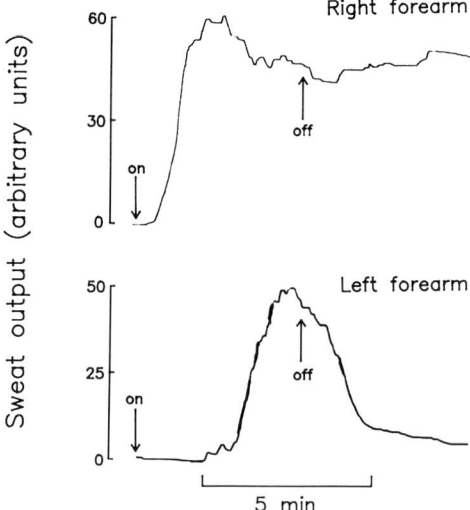

Fig. 1. QSART recordings from the painful (upper) and normal (lower) forearm of a patient with RSD/SMP. The top recording shows an ultrashort latency and persistent sweat activity. (Low 1993b)

over both the forearm and the lower extremity. The second method comprised the recording of skin temperature distribution using infrared thermometry. For the upper extremity, the ventral aspect of the forearm was divided horizontally into medial and lateral halves and vertically into upper, middle, and lower thirds, resulting in six areas. The thenar, midpalm, and hypothenar areas of the palm were studied as were the distal pads of each of the fingers.

For the lower extremity, the thigh and anterior leg were each divided into six areas. The skin over the extensor digitorum brevis was studied as were the pads on each toe. Each area of skin temperature was compared with the identical contralateral areas and charted. For each area, a computer program accepted the temperature once it remained stable over five sets of recordings over five seconds.

Controls and criteria for abnormality

RSO was recorded from the hypothenar eminence, distal forearm, distal leg, and foot in 124 subjects. There were no significant sex or age differences so data were pooled. Median values with 5–95% in brackets were 0.54 (0.20–1.02), 0.09 (0.04–0.15), 0.11 (0.06–0.56), and 0.14 (0.03–0.56) $\mu l/cm^2$ for hypothenar, forearm, distal leg, and foot, respectively. Responses were considered asymmetric when a difference of 40% occurred.

Control values for QSART were derived from studies on 223 normal subjects aged 10–83 years (Low et al. 1990; Low 1993; see earlier discussion). Latency, volume, and morphologic differences of QSART responses were compared between sides. The presence of an ultrashort latency (≤ 0.2 min) was considered abnormal, and likely comprises an augmented somato-sympathetic response (Low 1993). A difference in sweat volume of ≥ 50% or a response showing persistent sweat activity were also considered abnormal, as was a value that fell outside of the control range, corrected for age and gender.

Control data for skin temperature were based on age- and sex-matched controls (N = 25). In controls, differences between sides did not exceed 0.8°C. A difference ≥ 1°C between homologous sites was considered abnormal if it was seen in several different sites, indicating a diffuse distribution of vasomotor changes. The changes seen were usually distal, but if asymmetry was seen only in the pads, a difference of 2°C was required.

RESULTS

Demographic data and autonomic and pain symptoms are shown in Tables I and II. All patients had diffuse pain with hyperalgesia and allodynia. All patients had a history of swelling, although only three of 12 had objective evidence of swelling. Ten of 12 patients had some evidence of vasomotor abnormalities. Three of the 12 patients had evidence of demineralization on X-ray. Seven of the 12 patients had some response to treatment (Table II).

The pattern of abnormality was characteristic. Patients typically had vasomotor abnormalities that were diffuse, extending beyond peripheral nerve dermatomes, and maximal distally. The affected limb was either cooler or warmer, and typically demonstrated marked fluctuations in skin temperatures, often greater than 2°C in two series of thermograms taken 20 minutes apart, in contrast to stable recordings in controls. The sudomotor changes usually, but not invariably, paralleled the vasomotor changes.

Fig. 2 shows the frequency of abnormal autonomic indices. Abnormalities of skin blood flow were seen in only 44% of patients and may relate to the limited sampling of sites, whereas approximately two of every three patients had abnormalities in skin temperature distribution. Resting sweat asymmetry was seen in two of every three patients, QSART abnormalities in three of four patients; when QSART and RSO were combined more than 90% of patients were abnormal. When skin temperature was combined with sudomotor abnormalities, all patients demonstrated abnormalities.

Skin temperature was reduced in four patients, increased in four, unchanged in two, and technically unsatisfactory in two. RSO showed differences in excess of 40% in six of nine patients studied; it was increased in the affected side in four patients, and reduced in two. QSART responses were asymmetric or abnormal in nine of 12 patients studied. The volume was increased in six, reduced in two and showed an ultrashort latency alone in one. Five of the nine

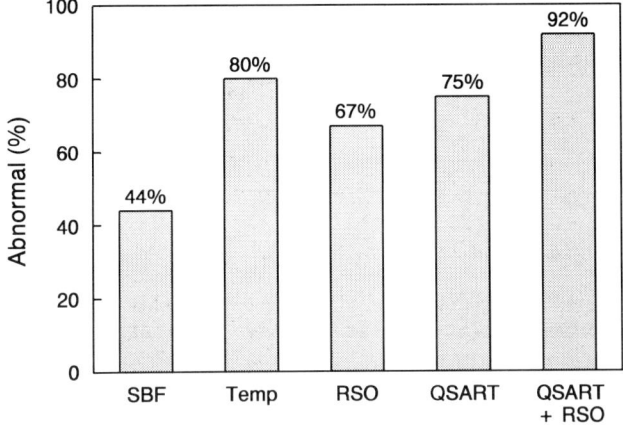

Fig. 2. Frequency of abnormalities expressed as percentage of abnormal responses detected by measurements of skin blood flow (SBF), temperature differences (Temp), unstimulated sweat output (RSO), quantitative sudomotor axon reflex (QSART), and a combination of RSO and QSART. (Low et al. 1994)

affected sides showed a reduced latency. An increased RSO was usually associated with an increase in QSART volume. A warmer affected limb was associated with either increased (two cases) or reduced (two cases) sudomotor responses. A cooler limb was associated with no change in sudomotor function (one case), increase (two), or reduction (one).

CONCLUSION

We concluded that vasomotor and sudomotor indices can be quantitated accurately and that patients with RSD/SMP had concomitant abnormalities. The RSD/SMP screen was considered a satisfactory laboratory test to supplement the clinical examination.

PERIOD II: REVIEW OF MAYO EXPERIENCE, 1982-1991

The second phase of our studies was conducted from December 1982 to 1991. To determine the clinical utility of laboratory testing, Chelimsky et al. (in press) did a blinded retrospective analysis of the medical record and laboratory data on patients referred to the Mayo Autonomic Reflex laboratory to "rule out RSD/SMP." The main objectives of the study were to: (1) relate indices of autonomic testing to the clinical diagnosis of RSD/SMP, and (2) to evaluate the predictive value of tests of autonomic function, using the endpoint of response to sympathetic block.

CHANGES IN METHODOLOGY

The following changes occurred. We abandoned recordings of skin blood flow, substituting instead infrared telethermography. Mean temperatures were derived by an averaging algorithm and recorded to nearest 0.1°C.

CHARACTERISTICS OF THE PATIENTS

We evaluated 407 patients; the median age was 41 years (range 9–81 years) and 67% were female. An initiating injury occurred in 79% of patients.

We developed an RSD/SMP probability scale, based on the presence of allodynia, protopathia (dull diffuse pain of unpleasant quality with significant after-pain), vasomotor changes, and swelling (Table III). A definite diagnosis of RSD/SMP required the presence of both allodynia and protopathia, and the presence of swelling and vasomotor alterations on examination.

Table III
Reflex sympathetic dystrophy clinical probability scale
used in the retrospective study of 407 patients

Clinical Feature	Definite	Probable	Possible	Unlikely	Not RSD/SMP
Protopathia (a)	Yes	a or b	a or b	a or b	a or b
Allodynia (b)	Yes				
Vasomotor	Yes				
history (a)	Yes	a or b	a or b	a or b	a or b
exam (b)					
Swelling		a or b	a or b	a or b	a or b
history (a)					
swelling (b)					
Total Required	All	3/3	2/3	1/3	0/3

CHARACTERISTICS OF THE PAIN

Patients on average had a duration of pain for about one year, equally distributed between diffuse and localized pain. Upper extremity was most common, followed by lower extremity pain and then combined pain (Table IV). There was no significant overrepresentation of left versus right-sided pain. Pain, allodynia, and protopathia were most commonly moderate in severity, and abnormalities on examination were less frequently found than by history.

Table IV
Characteristics of pain in retrospective study of 407 patients

Duration	Median: 13 months	
	Range: 1 week to >10 years	
Location	Diffuse:	51%
	Localized:	48%
Upper Limb	Right:	114 (29%)
	Left:	82 (21%)
Lower Limb	Right:	63 (16%)
	Left:	84 (22%)
Bilateral	Upper:	7 (7%)
	Lower:	17 (4%)

DIAGNOSIS OF RSD/SMP

A clinical diagnosis of RSD/SMP was definite in 5% of patients, probable in 26%, and possible in 32%. RSD/SMP was ruled out or doubtful in 36%. Laboratory evaluation confirmed a diagnosis of RSD/SMP in 49% of patients and indicated a possible diagnosis in 29%; 22% had normal values. The best correlate of the clinical diagnosis of RSD/SMP was a reduced QSART response, which can be ipsilateral, contralateral, or bilateral. A combination of four factors (QSART reduction, diffuse pain, increased RSO, X-ray demineralization) has a sensitivity of 100% and a specificity of 77%. For the leg the combination of three factors (diffuse pain, QSART reduction, X-ray demineralization) has a sensitivity and specificity of 90% each.

PREDICTIVE VALUE OF RESPONSE TO SYMPATHETIC BLOCK

Logistic regression analysis showed that four factors were independently predictive of a positive response to sympathetic block for the leg. The factors, in descending order of importance, were QSART response ($P < 0.001$), ipsilateral increase in skin temperature ($P < 0.001$), allodynia ($P = 0.025$), and psychiatric diagnosis ($P = 0.048$). If QSART was not bilaterally reduced and skin was warmer, or allodynia prominent, response rate was 100%. If QSART was reduced bilaterally and skin was not warmer, response rate was 0%. The presence of psychiatric diagnosis reduced the response rate. For the upper extremity, the best predictor of response to sympathetic block was a short duration of pain (less than six months).

CONCLUSIONS

We made the following preliminary conclusions. First, in the absence of a diagnostic gold standard, the most reasonable approach was to use a clinical probability scale, which can be modified or weighted with the availability of new information. Second, among the clinical indices, the three most important from the diagnostic and predictive (of response to sympathetic block) standpoint, are allodynia, severity of pain, and short duration (less than six months) of pain. Third, not all laboratory indices are in equally good agreement with the clinical diagnosis of RSD/SMP. Unilateral reduction in QSART and increased RSO have the best agreement. Fourth, clusters of clinical tests are able to generate sensitivity and specificity of 90% each. Fifth, the best predictors of a response to sympathetic block are QSART response, allodynia, a unilateral warmer extremity, and to a lesser extent, psychiatric factors. It was possible to develop an algorithm to predict a 0% response or a 100% response to block.

PERIOD III: PROSPECTIVE STUDY, 1994

This study differed from our retrospective study in several ways. First it was a prospective study with defined endpoints. Second, based on our results from the earlier study, we modified our clinical probability scale. Third, the laboratory indices had become better standardized. All vasomotor studies were done with infrared telethermography. We did a prospective evaluation of 102 consecutive patients referred to the Mayo Autonomic Reflex Laboratory and posed two questions. First, what are the demographic and clinical features of the condition? Second, how do the clinical features relate to laboratory indices, which are based on the recognition of asymmetric vasomotor and sudomotor effector function? We are continuing to use response to sympathetic block to study the predictive value of autonomic function tests (Willner et al., in preparation).

DEFINITION OF RSD/SMP

We generated a clinical RSD/SMP probability scale and a laboratory RSD/SMP probability scale. The clinical scoring of RSD/SMP is shown in Table V. We modified this RSD/SMP probability scoring scale (RSD/SMPPSS) from our earlier scale to place a greater emphasis on allodynia, and a slight deemphasis on clinical autonomic indices, because we assumed that these latter indices are more accurately evaluated in the laboratory. RSD/SMPPSS diagnoses RSD/SMP by a combination of symptoms and signs of allodynia,

Table V
Reflex sympathetic dystrophy
probability scoring system (prospective study)*

Parameter	Definite	Probable	Possible	Not RSD/SMP
Allodynia touch (a) pressure (b) movement (c)	3/3	2/3	1/3	0/3
Vasomotor history (a) exam (b) Swelling history (a) exam (b)	4/4	≥2/4	≤1/4	0/4

*Grading is dependent on a combination of a and b.

vasomotor changes, and swelling. The scale can be subdivided into two major subdivisions, the allodynia component (RSD/SMPPSS-allo), and vasomotor component (RSD/SMPPSS-VM). The clinical diagnosis of RSD/SMP is based on RSD/SMPPSS score (0-7) as follows:

Score	Diagnosis
7	Definite RSD/SMP
4-6	Probable RSD/SMP
2-3	Possible RSD/SMP
0-1	Not RSD/SMP

The laboratory diagnosis of RSD/SMP is based on the following:

Score	Diagnosis
>6	Definite RSD/SMP
4-6	Probable RSD/SMP
2-3	Possible RSD/SMP
0-1	Doubtful

The laboratory scoring scale for RSD/SMP (RSD/SMPLAB) has been refined and a quantitative score that corrects for the compounding effects of age and gender is shown in Table VI. RSD/SMPLAB incorporates a composite score of QSART, RSO, and telethermography (vasomotor). Each subset is separately evaluated and graded according to reduction or increase of the respective autonomic change on the affected side when compared to the healthy contralateral side.

Table VI
Autonomic laboratory grading of RSD/SMP (RSD/SMPLAB; prospective study)

Autonomic Scoring Scale		
QSART	RSO	Vasomotor
Reduction-1 or Increase-1	Reduction-1 or Increase-1	Reduction-1 or Increase-1
Reduction-2 or Increase-2	Reduction-2 or Increase-2	Reduction-2 or Increase-2
Reduction-3 or Increase-3	Reduction-3 or Increase-3	Reduction-3 or Increase-3

An additional point is provided if the variation in temperatures over the toe pads or finger pads between two sets of thermographic recordings are ≥2°C.

QSART, RSO, and vasomotor indices were scored from 0 to 3 depending on the degree of side-to-side asymmetry and distribution of abnormalities. For QSART and RSO, which are measurements of volume, the difference in volume between the affected side and the unaffected side is divided by the volume of the unaffected side and expressed as a percentage. A score of 1 refers to 25–50% asymmetry, 2 to greater than 50% involving any pair of recording sites, and 3 to greater than 50% asymmetry for all recording pairs. For the vasomotor index, a score of 1 indicates a difference of greater than 0.5 but less than 1°C affecting fewer than four sites, or >1° for any site. A score of 2 indicates a difference of 0.5–1° affecting more than four sites or >1° affecting two to four sites. A score of 3 is assigned when the difference of >1° affects more than 50% of the recording sites. An additional point is provided if the variation in temperature difference between left and right, over the toe pads or finger pads between the two sets of thermographic recording, is greater than 2°C. In this way the scores of RSD/SMPLAB have a range of 0 to 10.

RESULTS

Demography, type of injury, and effect of chronic pain

As in the retrospective study, females were overrepresented and comprised approximately three-fourths of the patients seen (76/102). The mean age was 45 years (SD 16). All patients had an antecedent injury. The most common injury was a sprain or strain type injury. The causes listed under "other injuries" were numerous, including soft tissue injury, joint trauma, surgical operation, and repetitive trauma.

Pain

Duration of limb pain was slightly longer than in our earlier study. The number of patients who had the condition for less than one year (45%) was

Table VII
Characteristics of pain in 102 patients (prospective study)

Type of Pain	%	Severity of Pain (%)			
		Severe	Moderate	Mild	Absent
Dull	53	17	23	5	7
Burning	25	5	6	4	10
Shooting/stabbing	22	9	7	2	4

Duration of Pain (months)	%	Severity of Pain	
		VAS	%
<6	26	<4	9
6–12	19	4–7	27
>12	55	>7	64

slightly less than those who had the condition for more than one year (55%), and most of these latter patients (44% of total) had the pain for one to five years. These patients were either severely impaired (55%) or at least moderately impaired (35%) in their ability to perform activities of daily living, such as work in their occupations or at home.

Patients typically had several types of pain, but when asked for the most dominant or common pain, about one-half (53%) had a dull pain, one-fourth had burning, and 22% had sharp pain. The severity of the pain (verbal) was similar to those that reported in the second study, being most commonly moderate (Table VII). By visual analog scale of pain severity, the majority had severe (64%) pain, defined as a score greater than 7 on a 10-point scale (Table VII).

Clinical autonomic changes

By history, swelling was noted in 75% of patients, although this was confirmed on examination at the time of evaluation in slightly less than half the patients (44%), and was most commonly mild. An alteration in sweating was less common; 67% reported no change and 84% were considered normal on clinical examination. Vasomotor alterations, most commonly described as excessive redness or bluish discoloration, either at rest or more commonly with the limb dependent, were reported in 49% of patients, and unilateral coldness was reported in 21%. On examination, these alterations were seen in only 31% of patients. This pattern of alterations was similar to that found in phase 2. Trophic changes were less common, seen in 20%, and consisted of either an increase or reduction in hair, skin, or nail thickness. Contractures were seen in 13% of patients.

Table VIII
Summary of autonomic function tests in 102 patients the prospective study

Test	QSART (%)	RSO (%)	Vasomotor (%)
Normal	41	71	42
Abnormal	59	29	58
reduced	37	22	39
increased	22	7	19

Neurologic function

Strength was intact in 60% of patients and reduced to varying degrees in the remainder. A tremor was seen in 4% and dystonia was also uncommon, seen in only 4%.

Autonomic function tests

QSART was abnormal in 59% and normal in 41% of patients; with 37% showing a reduction and 22% an increase. RSO was abnormal in 29% of subjects and normal in 71%, most of the abnormalities being a reduction (Table VIII). Skin temperature distribution was abnormal in almost identical numbers (58%), being twice as commonly reduced than increased on the affected side.

Correlation of clinical with laboratory indices

To evaluate the reliability of the questionnaire, we correlated symptoms with the relevant neurological examinations, using Pearson correlation analysis with Bonferroni-adjusted probabilities. We first analyzed clusters of symptoms and signs within RSD/SMPPSS. For each category (1–4), correlation was excellent with $P < 0.001$.

1. Vasomotor cluster: skin color and temperature, swelling by history and examination, sweating by history and by examination
2. Pain cluster: shooting pain, dull pain, burning pain, type of injury
3. Motor function: motor strength, joint movement, contractures, activities of daily living
4. Allodynia to: light touch, pressure, movement, cold

Within RSD/SMPLAB scores, good concordance was also generally found. RSO reduction correlated significantly with QSART reduction $P < 0.001$, and significantly but somewhat less precisely with temperature reduction (0.032).

Similarly, QSART reduction correlated significantly with temperature reduction (0.02).

We next correlated clinical (RSD/SMPPSS) with laboratory RSD/SMP scores, and did the following subanalysis using Bonferroni-adjusted probabilities. RSD/SMPPSS correlated significantly with RSD/SMPLAB ($P = 0.035$). It correlated even better with the combination of RSO+QSART ($P = 0.009$). It also correlated with QSART reduction ($P = 0.025$) and RSO (0.049).

Within the RSD/SMPPSS, the allodynia component (RSD/SMPPSS-allo) (Table V) correlated with the vasomotor component (RSD/SMPPSS-VM; $P = 0.000$). The best correlation was with the triad of reductions in QSART, RSO, and temperature ($P = 0.000$). There was no significant correlation with increments of these indices. RSD/SMPPSS-allo also correlated with QSART reduction ($P = 0.04$), RSO reduction ($P = 0.01$), and temperature reduction ($P = 0.007$). RSD/SMPPSS-VM also correlated significantly ($P = < 0.001$) with the triad of reductions in QSART, RSO and temperature, but not with their increments. Table IX compares the percentage of abnormal results using symptoms (RSD/SMPPS) versus laboratory evaluation (RSD/SMPLAB).

Table IX
Comparison of RSD/SMP probability scoring scales using clinical (RSD/SMPPSS) and laboratory (RSD/SMPLAB) indices

RSD/SMPPSS	%	RSD/SMPLAB	%
<2	31	<2	29
2–3	45	2–3	29
4	8	4	20
>4	15	>4	22

DISCUSSION

We gained several insights from our three studies. Despite extensive publications on RSD/SMP, information is scant on the frequency distribution of the clinical features, and controversy exists on the prevalence of motor deficits, tremor, and dystonia. In this prospective study, the frequency of motor involvement is common but the frequency of dystonia is lower than in recent reports (Schwartzman and Kerrigan 1990). The changes likely relate in part to diagnostic criteria. What might be diagnosed as dystonia by some investigators might be recognized as pain-related bracing of muscles by others.

Several attempts have been made to define the clinical diagnosis of RSD/SMP. There is good general agreement that RSD/SMP is characterized by diffuse pain, typically distal, developing following injury, with superficial and deep allodynia, and commonly associated with vasomotor, sudomotor, swelling, and trophic changes (Bonica 1973; Willner 1993). There is good agreement that chronic diffuse limb pain is mandatory, associated with allodynia and autonomic dysfunction. The latter is manifested as unilateral vasomotor or sudomotor alterations and the related manifestation of swelling.

Several findings implicate sympathetic involvement in pain. First, allodynia, a key criterion of RSD/SMP, and predictive of response to sympathetic block (Chelimsky et al., in press) is significantly correlated with the RSD/SMPPSS cluster, with vasoconstriction, and with sudomotor dysfunction (RSO, QSART). The two limbs of the clinical scale—RSD/SMPPSS-allo and RSD/SMPPSS-VM—are highly correlated. The severity of pain is also significantly correlated with indices of sympathetic dysfunction.

Of interest is the apparent paradox of the correlation of RSD/SMPPSS with a reduction in RSO and QSART but not with an increment. Indeed the best correlation of both RSD/SMPPSS-allo and RSD/SMPPSS-VM was with the gestalt of reductions in RSO, QSART, and skin temperature. This finding is identical to an earlier retrospective study where the best agreement of swelling on examination, the clinical diagnosis RSD/SMP, severe pain, and vasomotor alterations on examination correlated best with a reduction in QSART (Chelimsky et al., in press). The mechanism of these changes is uncertain. Sudomotor activity is dependent on skin temperature (Low et al. 1994), and these reductions may be due in part to the lower temperature. The reduction in temperature is relatively small; the more likely possibility is the reduction in blood flow to the eccrine sweat gland, or other microenvironmental changes as part of the disease process.

Several features in the present study lend support to the notion of clinical and laboratory RSD/SMP probability scoring systems. First, there is the close correlation of indices within clusters assumed to have the same underlying mechanisms. These include pain and vasomotor and allodynia clusters. Second, there is good correlation among clinical symptoms, signs, and laboratory measurements of the same indices. Third, there is good correlation between the two major limbs of the RSD/SMPPSS scoring scale (the allodynia and vasomotor components). Finally, there is good correlation between the clinical (RSD/SMPPSS) and laboratory (RSD/SMPLAB) scales. Based on these findings, we propose a modified scoring system and a combined scale. RSD/SMPPSS-allo can be combined with RSD/SMPLAB: (1) Definite = RSD/SMPPSS-allo (2–3/3) + RSD/SMPLAB showing reduction in temperature + reduction in either RSO or QSART. (2) Probable = RSD/SMPPSS-allo (1–2) + RSD/SMPLAB showing reduction in temperature + reduction in either RSO or QSART. (3) Possible = RSD/SMPPSS-allo (1/3) + RSD/SMPLAB showing reduction in temperature, RSO, or QSART. This scale combines the strengths of both approaches. RSD/SMPLAB is more accurate, sensitive, and specific in detecting side-by-side and absolute changes in autonomic indices, thereby enhancing the clinical evaluation of vasomotor and sudomotor alterations. RSD/SMPPSS provides the unique historical aspects of the patient's symptoms and essential information on allodynia. The two approaches should not be viewed as competitive but complementary. Finally, irrespective of whether sympathetic dysfunction is etiologically related to RSD/SMP, sympathetic dysfunction is an integral component in making the clinical diagnosis, and the combined approach sharpens the clinical diagnosis of RSD/SMP.

RECOMMENDATIONS

Irrespective of etiopathogenetic considerations, the best current clinical approach to the diagnosis of RSD/SMP is to use a combined clinical and laboratory approach, with particular emphasis on: (1) severity of pain, (2) distribution of pain (diffuse), and (3) allodynia on the RSD/SMPPSS and combining this with RSD/SMPLAB, which focuses on QSART asymmetry, RSO, and possibly skin vasomotor alterations. This approach results in the following modification of our current scale:

I. Definite RSD/SMP: allodynia to touch, pressure, and movement plus unilateral asymmetry of QSART (grade 3) or RSO (grade 3 asymmetry)

II. Probable RSD/SMP: RSD/SMPPSS (probable) plus any of the following on RSD/SMPLAB:

a. QSART3 or RSO3
b. QSART2 + RSO2 or VM2

III. Possible RSD/SMP: chronic limb pain plus QSART1 or RSO1 or VM1

REFERENCES

Bonica, J.J., Causalgia and other reflex sympathetic dystrophies, Postgrad. Med., 53 (1973) 143–148.
Chelimsky, T.C., Low, P.A., Naessens, J.M., Wilson, P.R., Amadio, P.C. and O'Brien, P.C., The value of autonomic testing in reflex sympathetic dystrophy, Mayo Clin. Proc. (in press)
Low, P.A., Laboratory evaluation of autonomic failure. In: P.A. Low (Ed.), Clinical Autonomic Disorders: Evaluation and Management, Little, Brown and Company, Boston, 1993a, pp. 169–195.

Low, P.A., Pitfalls in autonomic testing. In: P.A. Low (Ed.), Clinical Autonomic Disorders: Evaluation and Management, Chapter 28, Little, Brown and Company, Boston, 1993b, pp. 355-354.
Low, P.A. and Zimmerman, I.R., Development of an autonomic laboratory. In: P.A. Low (Ed.), Clinical Autonomic Disorders: Evaluation and Management, Little, Brown and Company, Boston, 1993, pp. 345–354.
Low, P.A., Caskey, P.E., Tuck, R.R., Fealey, R.D. and Dyck, P.J., Quantitative sudomotor axon reflex test in normal and neuropathic subjects, Ann. Neurol., 14 (1983) 573–580.
Low, P.A., Opfer-Gehrking, T.L., Proper, C.J. and Zimmerman, I., The effect of aging on cardiac autonomic and postganglionic sudomotor function, Muscle Nerve, 13 (1990) 152–157.
Low, P.A., Kihara, M. and Cardone, C., Pharmacology and morphometry of the eccrine sweat gland in vivo. In: P.A. Low (Ed.), Clinical Autonomic Disorders: Evaluation and Management, Little, Brown and Company, Boston, 1993, pp. 367–373.
Low, P.A., Amadio, P.C., Wilson, P.R., McManis, P.G. and Willner, C.L., Laboratory findings in reflex sympathetic dystrophy: a preliminary report, Clin. J. Pain, 10 (1994).
Raja, S.N., Treede, R.D., Davis, K.D. and Campbell, J.N., Systemic alpha-adrenergic blockade with phentolamine: a diagnostic test for sympathetically maintained pain, Anesthesiology, 74 (1991) 691–698.
Sato, A. and Schmidt, R.F., Somatosympathetic reflexes: afferent fibers, central pathways, discharge charateristics, Physiol. Rev., 53 (1973) 916–947.
Schwartzman, R.J. and Kerrigan, J., The movement disorder of reflex sympathetic dystrophy (Abstract), Neurology, 40 (1990) 57.
Shahani, B.T., Halperin, J.J., Boulu, P. and Cohen, J., Sympathetic skin response—a method of assessing unmyelinated axon dysfunction in peripheral neuropathies, J. Neurol. Neurosurg. Psychiatry, 47 (1984) 536–542.
Verdugo, R.J. and Ochoa, J.L., 'Sympathetically maintained pain,' I. Phentolamine block questions the concept, Neurology, 44 (1994) 1003–1010.
Verdugo, R.J., Campero, M. and Ochoa, J.L., Phentolamine sympathetic block in the painful polyneuropathies. II. Further questioning of the concept of 'sympathetically maintained pain,' Neurology, 44 (1994) 1010–1014.
Willner, C.L., Pain and the sympathetic nervous system: clinical considerations. In: P.A. Low (Ed.), Clinical Autonomic Disorders: Evaluation and Management, Little, Brown and Company, Boston, 1993, pp. 493–503.

Correspondence to: Phillip A. Low, MD, Autonomic Disorders Research Center, Department of Neurology, Mayo Clinic, Rochester, MN 55905, USA. Tel: 507- 284-3375; Fax: 507-284-1814.

4

Reflex Sympathetic Dystrophy in Children and Adolescents: Differences from Adults

Robert T. Wilder

Department of Anesthesia, Children's Hospital, and Department of Anaesthesia, Harvard Medical School, Boston, Massachusetts, USA

CLINICAL ASPECTS OF RSD IN CHILDREN

Until the mid-1980s, it was not recognized that reflex sympathetic dystrophy (RSD) occurred in children or adolescents. Indeed, series published to that point found no incidence in children younger than 16 years of age. Occasional case reports of RSD in children appeared during the 1970s (Matles 1971; Carron and McCue 1972; Fermaglich 1977; Kozin et al. 1977; Stilz et al. 1977; Richlin et al. 1978; Wettrell et al. 1979), but as these reports totaled only eight patients, the condition was still thought to be exceedingly rare in this age group.

Over the last decade, however, it has become apparent that RSD can occur in children. Several series ranging from five to 70 patients now have been published describing cases in children younger than 18 years of age (Ruggeri et al. 1982; Laxer et al. 1985; Aftimos 1986; Doury et al. 1986; Kesler et al. 1988; Sherry and Weisman 1988; Silber and Majd 1988; Schiller 1989; Dietz et al. 1990; Touzet et al. 1991; Wilder et al. 1992; Stanton et al. 1993), and individual case reports abound.

More than 395 pediatric patients aged 18 or younger have been reported with this syndrome. There is a marked predominance of females: 316 females to 79 males, a ratio of 4:1. There is also a marked predominance of lower extremity involvement: 332 lower extremity versus 63 upper extremity, a ratio of 5.3:1. Average age of onset in this group is 12.5 years, with a range of 3 to 18 years. Two three-year-olds suffered causalgia (complex regional pain syndrome [CRPS] type II) resulting from intraneural injection of antibiotics into the sciatic nerve. In this chapter I will analyze these reports to determine aspects of the presentation and treatment of RSD that may differ in children and adults (Table I).

As defined above, RSD is a clinical syndrome (Chapters 2, 3, and 5, this volume). RSD "is a syndrome with variable sensory and autonomic symptoms which develops after a noxious event. Leading symptoms are spontaneous and evoked pain, swelling, and weakness. Its symptoms and signs are disproportionate to the inciting event and are distally generalized irrespective of the site and type of the provoking lesion. This diagnosis is excluded by the coexistence of another condition or identifiable pathology proportionate to the degree of pain and dysfunction." The name does not imply a specific etiology or pathophysiology. Some children with this constellation of signs and symptoms

Table I
Contrasts in pediatric and adult RSD

	Children	Adults
Site	Marked lower extremity predominance (5.3:1)	Upper extremity commonly involved
Spontaneous pain	Common	Common
Mechanical allodynia	Most patients	Most patients
Sex ratio	Marked female predominance (4:1)	Studies mixed
Psychological aspects	Psychiatric pathology not well documented. Possible increased tendency to RSD with psychosocial stressors	Psychiatric pathology not well documented
Three-phase bone scan	Mixed results: use to rule out other pathology	Increased uptake of radionucleotide in the affected extremity
Treatment strategy	Resolution often possible with PT, TENS, and CBPMT	Early sympathetic block strongly advocated (Bonica 1990)
Timing of treatment	Duration of disease of little consequence in success of treatment	Early sympathetic block strongly advocated (Bonica 1990)
Technique for sympathetic block	Place catheter, run continuous infusion as inpatient	Multiple outpatient "single shot" blocks

RSD = reflex sympathetic dystrophy (CRPS Type I); PT = physical therapy; TENS = transcutaneous electrical nerve stimulation; CBPMT = cognitive and behavioral pain management techniques.

will have sympathetically mediated pain, but some will not. Emphasis on the sympathetic component of etiology and treatment may not always be in the patient's best interest.

The primary component of the work-up and differential diagnosis of RSD is thus the history and physical examination. Most pediatric patients present a history of minor trauma or repeat stress injury, although many are unable to define any precipitating event leading to the onset of their pain (Olsson et al. 1990; Wilder et al. 1992). The magnitude of the pain (usually rated as eight out of 10 or above on a visual analog scale) and disability far exceed the inciting event, which often leads practitioners unfamiliar with the disease to suspect malingering, conversion reaction, or other psychological disturbance. Most pediatric patients bear little or no weight on their affected leg at the time of referral. Allodynia is extremely common on physical examination. The extremity by definition exhibits signs of autonomic dysfunction, most commonly edema (77%), decreased temperature (77%), or color changes (54%) (Wilder et al. 1992).

DIAGNOSTIC STUDIES

Diagnostic studies have limited usefulness in the diagnosis of RSD in children. Plain radiographs are necessary to rule out fractures or other pathology, but will typically only show demineralization in long-standing RSD.

Bone scintigraphy, when performed as part of the work-up of children with RSD, most commonly reveals diffusely decreased uptake in the affected extremity (Doury et al. 1986; Le Loet et al. 1987; Goldsmith et al. 1989), although normal scans as well as those with increased uptake have also been reported (Laxer et al. 1985; Stanton et al. 1993). These observations contrast to the findings in adults with RSD, who show increased uptake of radionucleotide (Atkins et al. 1993; O'Donoghue et al. 1993). Pediatric patients have increased radionucleotide uptake relative to adults at baseline (Eissner and Wolf 1980) due to normal growth and remodeling. Presumably, the decrease in uptake with RSD reflects decreased blood flow to and demineralization of the bone caused by immobilization of the limb secondary to pain. Although the three-phase bone scan is felt to have prognostic value for adults with RSD (Weiss et al. 1993), results are sufficiently variable with pediatric patients to make this test of little value. Given this variability, I believe the primary role of the three-phase bone scan should be to rule out other pathology that might be causing the pain and other symptoms rather than to "rule in" RSD.

The phentolamine test has been recommended in the diagnosis of RSD (Arnér 1991), but I rarely perform this test. As a predictor of which patients will respond to sympathetic block, Olsson et al. (1990) reported that the phentolamine test had a positive predictive value of 100%. All 28 patients who responded to the phentolamine test also responded with resolution or improvement to sympathetic block; however, the negative predictive value was only 53%. Seven of 15 patients not responding to the phentolamine test nonetheless had a positive response to sympathetic block. Given that the phentolamine serves only for diagnosis, whereas performance of a sympathetic block may be therapeutic, I prefer simply to perform a block when this is clinically indicated.

Lightman et al. (1987) suggested that thermography is useful in the diagnosis of RSD in children. Although this test does quantify the observed temperature differences between extremities, our study reported that 23% of patients who otherwise fitted the criteria for RSD did not have asymmetrical temperature between limbs (Wilder et al. 1992). Among those patients who do, the temperature difference is usually dramatic enough to be detectable with the examiner's hand or a crystalline thermometer. The additional benefit of formal thermography remains undocumented (Awerbuch 1991).

PSYCHOLOGICAL ASPECTS

Patients with chronic pain are often felt to have psychological disturbances underlying their pain syndromes. The evidence supporting such a view is remarkably scant. Sherry and Weisman (1988) reported no major psychopathology among their 21 patients, although they found a significant incidence of family dysfunction. Twelve of 21 families had problems with marital discord. All families demonstrated a high incidence of "parental enmeshment," defined as "inappropriate closeness and involvement of the child in parental affairs and vice versa." Although this finding was prominent in the study, no comparison was made to control groups of either healthy adolescents or other patients with chronic disease.

In her doctoral dissertation, Vieyra (1990) did not find major differences when she compared patients with RSD with children suffering from arthritis or with normal controls ($N = 30$ patients in each group). Olsson et al. (1990), however, reported that 15 of 85 children referred to his clinic with the presumptive diagnosis of RSD had "evident psychosocial stress factors;" several received the diagnosis of conversion reaction by a psychiatrist on the team. These patients, although clinically indistinguishable from the whole group by signs and symptoms, were unlikely to respond to sympathectomy. In contrast, we reported (Wilder et al. 1992) that "in our study population, there were no cases of major psychosis, and evidence for somatoform or factitious disorders was generally lacking. For certain patients, it appeared to all clinicians involved that pressures of academics or organized sports or significant family stress such as divorce, marital conflict, sibling rivalry or concurrent illness amplified both the severity of symptoms and the reaction of the family to the symptoms of reflex sympathetic dystrophy. The high incidence of involvement of our patients in organized individual sports and dance was striking, and this association is underemphasized in many previous reports. While psychological antecedents and consequences of reflex sympathetic dystrophy are difficult to quantify, 60% of our patients did involve themselves in psychological treatment including biofeedback, relaxation training, cognitive-behavioral therapy, and individual or family psychotherapy. Many of these patients had favorable results. This supports our belief that such techniques should be an integral part of the care of these patients."

When treating pediatric patients with RSD, clinicians should remember that this disease process effects the entire family, not just the patient. Although "treating the family" is a truism throughout pediatric medicine, it is of utmost importance in families dealing with chronic, and especially painful, disease. Family counseling may be of benefit to prevent secondary breakdown of family dynamics during this time of increased stress. Such counseling may also help identify issues of secondary gain that might serve to prolong pain behavior.

Although RSD is not primarily a psychological disorder, it is worth emphasizing to patients and their families that living with chronic pain or illness of any sort is stressful and may produce secondary feelings of anxiety or depression. These feelings are normal and can be treated effectively with appropriate individual and family counseling. Stress may also exacerbate the symptoms of RSD by increasing sympathetic tone. Relaxation training and biofeedback may be extremely effective in reducing the pain of RSD. Psychoanalytical counseling may also be appropriate for some patients with significant stressors such as a history of sexual or physical abuse, school phobia, or recent significant loss.

Disability in pediatric patients with chronic pain such as RSD is defined in terms of school days missed. In the United States, the typical school year through high school is 180 days. In evaluating our first 70 patients with RSD, we found that the average patient had missed more than 40 days of school in the year following the injury, nearly one-fourth of the academic year. With treatment, school loss secondary to pain dropped on average to less than five days per year.

At the time of the initial interview, the clinician should emphasize that the treatment of RSD involves not only relief of pain, but also return of function. The latter aspect is at least as important as the former. Return to school with gradual reintegration into physical education and sports should be a primary goal of the treatment program. At-home tutoring should not be regarded as an acceptable alternative because school teaches children much more than what is found in textbooks. Social skills, including increased independence from the family, learning respect for authority, and dealing with issues of sexuality are important tasks of the junior high and high school student. These tasks are not addressed when the patient is isolated in the home. For those patients hospitalized for sympathetic catheter blockade, behavioral and psychological pain management, and physical therapy, a daily schedule should include tutoring on schoolwork and activities with other children the same age. Such a schedule may be more typical for an adolescent than the experience at home and may provide a smoother transition back to school.

THERAPEUTIC APPROACH TO RSD IN CHILDREN

Several authors have suggested that RSD in children is a relatively benign, easily treated disease (Stilz et al. 1977; Richlin et al. 1978; Bétend et al. 1981; Fourastier et al. 1986; Paulson 1987; Ashwal et al. 1988; Kesler et al. 1988; Dietz et al. 1990; Gedalia et al. 1990). Physical therapy is the primary treatment modality for this condition, and many children can be effectively treated with physical therapy alone. For this strategy to be successful it is necessary to emphasize to both the patient and the physical therapist the nonprotective nature of neuropathic pain. It is necessary to work through some level of pain to make progress, and doing so will not further injure the limb. The therapy for RSD needs to emphasize the return of function as a primary goal with importance equal to or greater than the decrease in pain. Movement of the affected extremity is expected to lead eventually to a decrease in pain (Kakigi et al. 1993), whereas immobilization will worsen pain by decreasing pain thresholds.

Many patients will be unable to work through the pain of their RSD. Some will require only simple noninvasive measures to provide analgesia during the initial treatment period. These measures include transcutaneous electrical nerve stimulation (TENS) (Richlin et al. 1978), biofeedback, or other cognitive and behavioral approaches to pain management (Barowsky et al. 1987; Kawano et al. 1989; or acupuncture, Fialka et al. 1993). These measures form our first line of attack in treating the pain of RSD in pediatric patients. It must be stressed that no one therapy is universally successful (Wilder et al. 1992; Stanton et al. 1993) in reducing the pain associated with RSD. Although Richlin et al. (1978) cited excellent results in treating patients with TENS, our study found it useful in only half of the patients treated, and fully 10% felt TENS worsened their pain (Wilder et al. 1992).

Other patients will need the addition of an analgesic medication such as the nonsteroidal anti-inflammatory drugs or amitriptyline or another tricyclic antidepressant. Our study (Wilder et al. 1992) and a report by Stanton et al. (1993) suggest that nonsteroidal anti-inflammatory medications are not highly effective for RSD, but occasional patients will respond quite favorably. Although we lack controlled prospective data to show that tricyclic antidepressants are effective analgesics in patients with RSD per se, well-controlled studies demonstrate analgesic efficacy in other forms of neuropathic pain (Max et al. 1987). Our prospective but unblinded and uncontrolled study (Wilder et al. 1992) demonstrated that 56% of patients receiving tricyclic antidepressants for the pain of RSD attributed some of the improvement in their pain to the antidepressant medication.

Differences in analgesic efficacy among the tricyclic antidepressants are not well documented. I thus choose a specific medication based on the side-effect profile. Amitriptyline and nortriptyline are useful for patients who are having difficulty sleeping or who are awakened by pain during the night. We prefer nortriptyline both because it is less sedating and has been associated with fewer cases of cardiac arrhythmias than has amitriptyline. Desipramine is the least sedating of the tricyclic antidepressants. Trazodone may be better for patients who are bothered by the anticholinergic side effects. Strategies to minimize daytime sleepiness include using only a single nighttime dose, taking the medication two to three hours before the hour of sleep, and starting with low doses that are gradually increased as tolerated. Among children who are seen early in the course of their RSD, more than half will respond to such simple measures. Many will have complete resolution of their symptoms.

Sympathetic nerve blocks do play an important role in the treatment of the child with RSD. I do not recommend using nerve blocks as the initial therapy for the child with RSD, because in many children the pain and symptoms will resolve without the need for this invasive procedure. Nerve blocks are used for the patient who is suffering from pain sufficient to prevent participation in any form of physical therapy, and for the patient who is working at physical therapy but is still experiencing significant pain not relieved by other, noninvasive modalities. Sympathetic nerve blocks should not be used in isolation or as the primary treatment modality. Rather, they need to be viewed as a means of providing a period of analgesia during which physical therapy can commence. Contrary to Bonica's recommendation that sympathetic blocks should be performed early and aggressively in adult patients with RSD to maximize the chance of complete recovery (Bonica 1990), Olsson et al. (1990) and Wilder et al. (1992) found that in pediatric patients the duration of the disease process made no difference in the success rate of sympathetic blockade.

In adult patients, many authors recommend performing repeated sympathetic nerve blocks every other day or twice weekly (Bonica 1990). For pediatric patients requiring lumbar sympathetic blocks, we recommend placing a catheter into the sympathetic chain and running a continuous infusion of local anesthetic. We believe this procedure is safer in this age group for two reasons: first, to ensure optimal placement we prefer to use fluoroscopy guidance for lumbar sympathetic blocks; second, most children and adolescents are rather phobic of needles, especially 5-inch long needles, no matter how thin. We have found that sedation, sometimes to the point of a brief general anesthetic, is required to achieve cooperation from these patients. By placing a single catheter we can minimize both the total need for anesthetics as well as radiation exposure. In young women nearing childbearing age, minimizing the radiation dose to the ovaries is appropriate. During the time that the sympathetic block is working, it is important to maximize active physical therapy. We admit the patient to the hospital for the block and schedule physical therapy sessions twice daily. We prefer not to place epidural blocks, although they are technically simpler, because the sensory and motor blocks interfere with the patient's ability to participate actively in physical therapy. For the patient with sympathetically mediated pain, a specific sympathetic block is indicated.

In the minority of pediatric patients with upper extremity RSD, several choices exist for performing sympathetic blocks. Repeated stellate blocks are better tolerated than are repeated lumbar sympathetic blocks and do not require radiation to ensure accurate placement. Some children will nonetheless be sufficiently frightened of the procedure that they will not lie completely still as is required for safe placement of a stellate block. Alternatives include placement of a cervical epidural catheter, a interpleural catheter, or intravenous regional bretylium blocks. The cervical epidural provides an excellent sympathectomy, but also causes sensory and motor block that may interfere with active participation in physical therapy. Most practitioners also prefer fluoroscopic guidance in placing cervical epidurals, which is an additional disadvantage. An interpleural catheter can also provide a good sympathetic block for treatment of upper extremity RSD (Reiestad et al. 1989). In pediatric patients, however, continuous interpleural infusions causing clinically useful levels of analgesia may be associated with levels of local anesthetics high enough to cause seizures (McIlvaine et al. 1988; Berde 1992). We thus have tended to dose these catheters intermittently. This technique has proven useful primarily in patients who have obtained sympathectomy to the face, but not the upper extremity, from a stellate block.

Finally, intravenous regional (Bier) blocks with bretylium provide effective pain relief through sympathetic blockade for an average of 20 days (Hord et al. 1992). This alternative is an excellent one, especially for the upper extremity, which requires lower total volumes than does the lower extremity. Olsson et al. (1990) reported that i.v. regional blocks with guanethidine also had a high success rate (47 of 55 patients recovered or improved). Unfortunately, guanethidine is not readily available in the United States, which makes bretylium a more attractive alternative in this country.

SUMMARY

In conclusion, children with RSD present with many of same issues as do adults with this syndrome, although the expression may differ in an age-appropriate manner. Although causalgia (CRPS type II) has been well described in three-year olds, and RSD in children as young as five, the incidence definitely increases at about the time of puberty. Thus, most pediatric patients with RSD are young, adolescent females. Many pediatric patients are appropriately treated with only conservative measures such as physical therapy and TENS; however, in the larger series and in some individual cases reports, a subset of patients have pain and symptoms that are resistant to all forms of therapy including aggressive use of nerve blocks and other invasive techniques. Only about half of our patient population had complete resolution of all signs and symptoms (Wilder et al. 1992). The remainder had some degree of residual difficulty ranging from mild, intermittent pain in times of stress to severe unremitting pain with complete disability. These patients require long-term pain treatment to learn to how to live the highest quality life possible with their pain.

REFERENCES

Aftimos, S., Reflex neurovascular dystrophy in children, New Zealand Medical Journal, 99 (1986) 761–763.

Arnér, S., Intravenous phentolamine test: diagnostic and prognostic use in reflex sympathetic dystrophy, Pain, 46 (1991) 17–22.

Ashwal, S., Tomasi, L., Neumann, M. and Schneider, S., Reflex sympathetic dystrophy syndrome in children, Pediatr. Neurol., 4 (1988) 38–42.

Atkins, R.M., Tindale, W., Bickerstaff, D. and Kanis, J.A., Quantitative bone scintigraphy in reflex sympathetic dystrophy, Br. J. Rheumatol., 32 (1993) 41–45.

Awerbuch, M.S., Thermography—its current diagnostic status in musculoskeletal medicine [see comments], Med. J. Aust., 154 (1991) 441–444.

Barowsky, E.I., Zweig, J.B. and Moskowitz, J., Thermal biofeedback in the treatment of symptoms associated with reflex sympathetic dystrophy, J. Child Neurol., 2 (1987) 229–232.

Berde, C.B., Convulsions associated with pediatric regional anesthesia [editorial; comment], Anesth. Analg., 75 (1992) 164–166.

Bétend, B., Lebacq, E., Kohler, R. and David, L., Metaphyseal osteolysis: unusual aspect of reflex algodystrophy in children, Archives Francaises de Pediatrie, 38 (1981) 121–123.

Bonica, J.J., Causalgia and other reflex sympathetic dystrophies. In: J.J. Bonica (Ed.), The

Management of Pain, Vol. 1, 2nd ed., Lea & Febiger, Philadelphia, 1990, pp. 230–243.
Carron, H. and McCue, F., Reflex sympathetic dystrophy in a ten-year old, South. Med. J., 65 (1972) 631–632.
Dietz, F.R., Mathews, K.D. and Montgomery, W.J., Reflex sympathetic dystrophy in children, Clin. Orthop., 258 (1990) pp. 225–231.
Doury, P., Pattin, S., Eulry, F., Granier, R. and Gaillard, F., Algodystrophy in children and young adults with low isotope retention in the bones: apropos of 5 cases, Revue du Rhumatisme et des Maladies Osteo-Articulaires, 53 (1986) 681–684.
Eissner, D. and Wolf, R., The radiation dose to children from bone scintigraphy with 99mTc-phosphate compounds, ROFO: Fortschritte auf dem Gebiete der Rontgenstrahlen und der Nuklearmedizin, 132 (1980) 331–335.
Fermaglich, D.R., Reflex sympathetic dystrophy in children, Pediatrics, 60 (1977) 881–883.
Fialka, V., Resch, K.L., Ritter-Dietrich, D., Alacamlioglu, Y., Chen, O., Leitha, T., Kluger, R. and Ernst, E., Acupuncture for reflex sympathetic dystrophy [letter], Arch. Intern. Med., 153 (1993) 661, 665.
Fourastier, J., Pialoux, B., Bracq, H., Fares, A. and Guibert, L., Post-traumatic algodystrophy in children, Chirurgie Pediatrique, 27 (1986) 313–317.
Gedalia, A., Adar, A. and Kornmehl, P., Reflex sympathetic dystrophy in children, Harefuah, 119 (1990) 197–198.
Goldsmith, D.P., Vivino, F.B., Eichenfield, A.H., Athreya, B.H. and Heyman, S., Nuclear imaging and clinical features of childhood reflex neurovascular dystrophy: comparison with adults, Arthritis Rheum., 32 (1989) 480–485.
Hord, A.H., Rooks, M.D., Stephens, B.O., Rogers, H.G. and Fleming, L.L., Intravenous regional bretylium and lidocaine for treatment of reflex sympathetic dystrophy: a randomized, double-blind study, Anesth. Analg., 74 (1992) 818–821.
Kakigi, R., Matsuda, Y. and Kuroda, Y., Effects of movement-related cortical activities on pain-related somatosensory evoked potentials following CO_2 laser stimulation in normal subjects, Acta. Neurol. Scand., 88 (1993) 376–380.
Kawano, M., Matsuoka, M., Kurokawa, T., Tomita, S., Mizuno, Y. and Ueda, K., Autogenic training as an effective treatment for reflex neurovascular dystrophy: a case report, Acta Paediatr. Jpn., Overseas Edition, 31 (1989) 500–503.
Kesler, R.W., Saulsbury, F.T., Miller, L.T. and Rowlingson, J.C., Reflex sympathetic dystrophy in children: treatment with transcutaneous electric nerve stimulation, Pediatrics, 82 (1988) 728–732.
Kozin, F., Haughton, V. and Ryan, L., The reflex sympathetic dystrophy syndrome in a child, J. Pediatr., 90 (1977) 417–419.
Laxer, R.M., Allen, R.C., Malleson, P.N., Morrison, R.T. and Petty, R.E., Technetium 99m-methylene diphosphonate bone scans in children with reflex neurovascular dystrophy, J. Pediatr., 106 (1985) 437–440.
Le Loet, X., Lefort, J., Daragon, A., Derumeaux, B. and Deshayes, P., Bone isotope hypofixation in algodystrophy in children, Revue du Rhumatisme et des Maladies Osteo-Articulaires, 54 (1987) 53.
Lightman, H.I., Pochaczevsky, R., Aprin, H. and Ilowite, N.T., Thermography in childhood reflex sympathetic dystrophy, J. Pediatr., 111 (1987) 551–555.
Matles, A.I., Reflex sympathetic dystrophy in a child, a case report, Bull. Hosp. Jt. Dis., 32 (1971) 193–197.
Max, M.B., Culnane, M., Schafer, S.C., Gracely, R.H., Walther, D.J., Smoller, B. and Dubner, R., Amitriptyline relieves diabetic neuropathy pain in patients with normal or depressed mood, Neurology, 37 (1987) 589–596.
McIlvaine, W.B., Knox, R.F., Fennessey, P.V. and Goldstein, M., Continuous infusion of bupivacaine via intrapleural catheter for analgesia after thoracotomy in children, Anesthesiology, 69 (1988) 261–264.
O'Donoghue, J.P., Powe, J.E., Mattar, A.G., Hurwitz, G.A. and Laurin, N.R., Three-phase bone

scintigraphy: asymmetric patterns in the upper extremities of asymptomatic normals and reflex sympathetic dystrophy patients, Clin. Nucl. Med., 18 (1993) 829–836.

Olsson, G.L., Arnér, S. and Hirsch, G., Reflex sympathetic dystrophy in children. In: D. C. Tyler and E. J. Krane (Eds.), Pediatric Pain, Vol. 15, Raven Press, New York, 1990, pp. 323–331

Paulson, R.R., Reflex sympathetic dystrophy in a teenaged girl, Postgrad. Med., 81 (1987) 66–67.

Reiestad, F., McIlvaine, W.B., Kvalheim, L., Stokke, T. and Pettersen, B., Interpleural analgesia in treatment of upper extremity reflex sympathetic dystrophy, Anesth. Analg., 69 (1989) 671–673.

Richlin, D.M., Carron, H., Rowlingson, J.C., Sussman, M.D., Baugher, W.H. and Goldner, R.D., Reflex sympathetic dystrophy: successful treatment by transcutaneous nerve stimulation, J. Pediatr., 93 (1978) 84–86.

Ruggeri, S.B., Athreya, B.H., Doughty, R., Gregg, J.R. and Das, M.M., Reflex sympathetic dystrophy in children, Clin. Orthop., 163 (1982) 225–230.

Schiller, J.E., Reflex sympathetic dystrophy of the foot and ankle in children and adolescents, J. Am. Podiatr. Med. Assoc., 79 (1989) 545–551.

Sherry, D.D. and Weisman, R., Psychologic aspects of childhood reflex neurovascular dystrophy, Pediatrics, 81 (1988) 572–578.

Silber, T.J. and Majd, M., Reflex sympathetic dystrophy syndrome in children and adolescents. Report of 18 cases and review of the literature, Am. J. Dis. Child., 142 (1988) 1325–1330.

Stanton, R.P., Malcolm, J.R., Wesdock, K.A. and Singsen, B.H., Reflex sympathetic dystrophy in children: an orthopedic perspective, Orthopedics, 16 (1993) 773–779.

Stilz, R.J., Carron, H. and Sanders, D.B., Reflex sympathetic dystrophy in a 6-year-old: successful treatment by transcutaneous nerve stimulation, Anesth. Analg., 56 (1977) 438–443.

Touzet, P., D'Ornano, P., Chaumien, J.P., Prieur, A.M. and Rigault, P., Misleading forms of algoneurodystrophy in children and adolescents: apropos of 19 cases, Annales de Pediatrie, 38 (1991) 673–681.

Vieyra, M.A., Children's pain and family functioning: a comparative analysis, doctural dissertation, University of Connecticut, Storrs, CT, 1990.

Weiss, L., Alfano, A., Bardfeld, P., Weiss, J. and Friedmann, L.W., Prognostic value of triple phase bone scanning for reflex sympathetic dystrophy in hemiplegia, Arch. Phys. Med. Rehabil., 74 (1993) 716–719.

Wettrell, G., Hallbook, T. and Hultquist, C., Reflex sympathetic dystrophy in two young females, Acta Pædiatr. Scand., 68 (1979) 923–924.

Wilder, R.T., Berde, C.B., Wolohan, M., Vieyra, M.A., Masek, B.J. and Micheli, L.J., Reflex sympathetic dystrophy in children. Clinical characteristics and follow-up of seventy patients, J. Bone Joint Surg. Am., 74 (1992) 910–919.

Correspondence to: Robert T. Wilder, MD, PhD, 99 Pond Ave., #505, Brookline, MA 02146-7117, USA. Tel: 617-734-1663; Fax: 617-355-7887.

5

Complex Regional Pain Syndromes: Symptoms, Signs, and Differential Diagnosis

Robert A. Boas

Pain Clinic, Auckland Hospital, Auckland, New Zealand

Two groups from the 1993 Orlando workshop discussed the two important clinical foundations of diagnosis of complex regional pain syndrome (CRPS): signs and symptoms and differential diagnosis.* Both spent much of their time seeking a consensus on what constituted a traditional diagnosis for reflex sympathetic dystrophy (RSD). Each group felt that the classical presentation occurred in those cases precipitated by injury and with spontaneous pain, allodynia/hyperalgesia, motor dysfunction, abnormal sweating and abnormal vascular reactivity, plus trophic changes in later stages of the disorder, all in a distal nondermatomal distribution of a limb. Such patients were the foundation from which arose the concepts of the pathophysiology and use of the term. Consequently, emphasis on therapy was directed to interruption of supposed overactive sympathetic function. However, there was agreement that not all patients referred under this RSD banner met the classical case scenario, and many of those who met diagnostic criteria responded poorly to long-term treatment. Variability in symptoms and signs over time, a lack of consistency in supportive diagnostic testing, and lack of responsiveness to sympathetic blockade belied the simplistic elements inherent in the mechanistic label of RSD. Participants agreed that use of the term RSD had lost its usefulness as a clinical designation and had also become an indiscriminate diagnosis for patients showing elements of neuropathic pain or resistance to therapy. Therefore, the need to develop alternative concepts and nomenclature was accepted.

---

*The members of these groups were: R. Baron, H. Blumberg, R.A. Boas, J.N. Campbell, J.D. Haddox, S.J. Hassenbusch, M. Koltzenburg, H. Merskey, P.P. Raj, M. Stanton-Hicks, and R.T. Wilder.

NOMENCLATURE

The two "diagnosis" and "symptoms and signs" groups, after extensive grappling with their respective responsibilities, returned to the entire workshop with proposals directed to two main issues. First, they addressed questions as to why it has taken so long and been so difficult to develop an agreed set of diagnostic criteria. The reasons given were:

1. Until the establishment of pain clinics, specialists, and their professional bodies, diverse disciplines have been involved in caring for CRPS/RSD patients, with an associated lack of communication.
2. Sympathetic nervous system excitation has proven difficult to identify in clinical and laboratory research.
3. Treatment based on interruption of sympathetic function has failed to provide lasting benefit for many apparently typical CRPS patients.
4. Lack of animal models has limited basic research.
5. Absence of a "gold standard" for testing and diagnosis focused attention to diagnostic procedures such as thermography, three-phase scanning, sweat testing, quantitative sensory testing and phentolamine infusions, which have helped promote more extensive critical examination of the syndrome.

Against this background, the workshop members felt that the vicious cycle hypothesis, so well propounded by Livingstone (1943) and continued by Bonica (1953, 1979, 1990), though still conceptually valid in many respects, was no longer sufficiently robust to sustain the RSD terminology or the therapeutic emphasis this imparted.

The groups then proposed the following principles to be followed in revising the relevant nomenclature:

1. Nomenclature should not have mechanistic connotations.
2. Durability for any new nomenclature was important.
3. An acronym was thought desirable.
4. A single, semi-descriptive word, with definition, was also acceptable.

Various of the options considered under these principles were regional (or reactive) sensitization disorder (discarded because of its mechanistic connotations, but attractive for its retention of the old acronym), peripheral autonomous pain syndrome (PAPS; also smeared because of its restricted designation), and peripheral edema vascular abnormality (PEVA; closer to a pathological inflammatory state than a pain syndrome). A new, semidescriptive functional term, *dysalgia,* somewhat analogous to causalgia, was also offered, but generated only muted support. Perhaps the term PAMS syndrome, projecting a disorder with pain, autonomic, motor, and sensory abnormalities would bear more utility? However, it could be argued that "autonomic" does convey a mechanistic element in mediation of the edema, swelling, temperature, and vascular changes, which could just as readily be due to local inflammatory mediators.

In the final analysis, descriptive clinical symptoms and signs were used to form the basis for this terminology. They allow for evolutionary change as improved clinical studies and specific testing methods become available.

CLASSIFICATION

The umbrella term for all disorders falling within the domain of causalgia and reflex sympathetic dystrophy was now designated as a complex regional pain syndrome (CRPS). *Complex* denoted the varied and dynamic nature of the clinical presentation within a single person over time, and among persons with seemingly similar disorders. It also included the features of inflammation, autonomic, cutaneous, motor, and dystrophic changes, which distinguish this from other forms of neuropathic pain. *Regional*—as in the wider distribution of symptoms and findings beyond the area of the original lesion—is a hallmark of these disorders. Such symptoms and signs usually affect the distal part of a limb but occasionally can involve discrete regions or spread to other body areas (Bentley 1980).

Pain is the *sine qua non* for the CRPS syndrome—pain that is disproportionate to the inciting event. This is not just burning pain, but includes spontaneous pain and thermal or mechanically induced allodynia. As a *syndrome*, the constellation of symptoms and signs of CRPS represents a series of correlated events that are sufficient to be designated as a distinctive entity, even though we are not sure what constitutes each of these events, or which are essential, nor the nature of the pathological changes that ensue.

Within the CRPS designation are three subsets proposed as types I, II, and III, depending on their cause and presentation (Table I). Though CRPS type I is essentially the old RSD and type II causalgia, a major departure is the separation of sympathetic elements from the definitions. This issue has been addressed under a category of its own, namely sympathetically maintained pain (SMP) or sympathetically independent pain (SIP) (Table I), as first suggested by Roberts (1986). Under this classification almost any type of pain disorder, including CRPS, could manifest either with an element of SMP or

Table I
Classification: chronic regional pain syndrome (CRPS)

CRPS describes a variety of painful conditions that usually follow injury, occur regionally, have a distal predominance of abnormal findings, exceed in both magnitude and duration the expected clinical course of the inciting event, often result in significant impairment of motor function, and show variable progression over time.

CRPS Type 1 (RSD)

1. Follows an initiating noxious event.
2. Spontaneous pain or allodynia/hyperalgesia occurs beyond the territory of a single peripheral nerve(s), and is disproportionate to the inciting event.
3. There is or has been evidence of edema, skin blood flow abnormality, or abnormal sudomotor activity, in the region of the pain since the inciting event.
4. This diagnosis is excluded by the existence of conditions that would otherwise account for the degree of pain and dysfunction.

CRPS Type II (Causalgia)

This syndrome follows nerve injury. It is similar in all other respects to type I.

1. Is a more regionally confined presentation about a joint (e.g., ankle, knee, wrist) or area (e.g., face, eye, penis), associated with a noxious event.
2. Spontaneous pain or allodynia/hyperalgesia is usually limited to the area involved but may spread variably distal or proximal to the area, not in the territory of a dermatomal or peripheral nerve distribution.
3. Intermittent and variable edema, skin blood flow change, temperature change, abnormal sudomotor activity, and motor dysfunction, disproportionate to the inciting event, are present about the area involved.

Sympathetically Maintained Pain

Pain that is maintained by sympathetic efferent activity or neurochemical or circulating catecholamine action, as determined by pharmacological or sympathetic nerve blockade. SMP may be a feature of several types of pain disorder, and is not an essential component of any one condition. Conditions without any response to sympathetic block are, by contrast, designated as having sympathetic independent pain states (SIP).

without, that is, SIP (Fig. 1). At the same time there is provision for some conditions to be present in several variants, such as a nerve injury plus CRPS type II, or a nerve injury with SMP, where sympathetic block alleviated some part of the pain but the presentation did not contain sufficient features to comply with a full CRPS diagnosis, or simply a nerve injury without additional moderating features.

A category of CRPS type III was allowed for those difficult cases that contained pain and sensory changes, with either motor or tissue changes, but did not comply fully with the more classical forms. This category was seen as a point for later development, but until more precise quantification of diagnostic

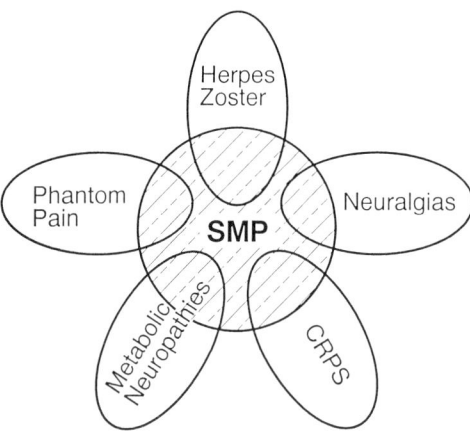

Fig. 1. Relationship between sympathetically maintained pain (SMP) and some selected painful conditions. This illustration is intended as a conceptual framework without indication of quantitative relationships between the inter-sections. Many varied pain disorders may have a component of sympathetically maintained pain.

criteria could be established, this "not otherwise specified" category was felt appropriate. Once this separation had been accepted, the classification allowed for identification of a sympathetic component to many varied forms of acute and chronic pain, as evidenced by the improvement achieved following sympathetic block in these disorders (Fig. 2). The clinicians felt, based on their observations of RSD patients, that many of the phenomena seen could be generated by sympathetic overactivity or hyperresponsiveness, but that this construct did not lead to diagnosis.

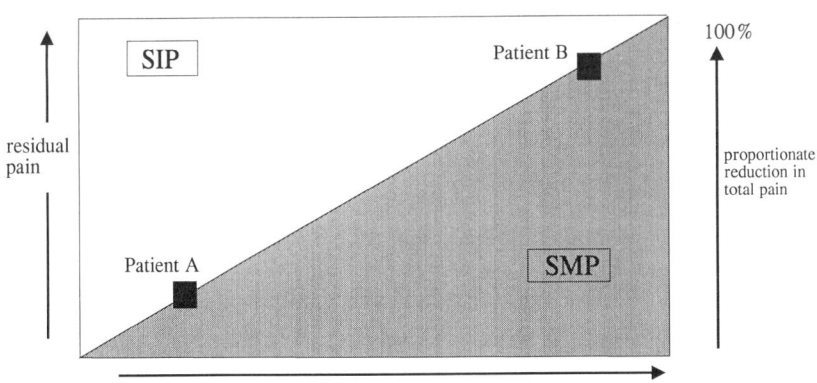

Fig. 2. The relative contribution that SMP may have to the overall pain: **A:** a person whose pain is predominantly unresponsive to sympatholysis; **B:** a patient with pain that is almost totally sympathetically maintained. Points A and B may represent different patients or the same patient at different times.

The neutrality and nonmechanistic assignment to this nomenclature was seen as positive designation, rather than as a compromise between differing views. A contrary argument might suggest that the lack of specificity in this definition defeats the value of any change it promotes. Until good evidence allows further review, the consensus achieved at this workshop was to accept terms that were at least consistent with current understanding, despite the wider interpretations that might follow. Evolutionary changes were accepted as inevitable, but it was hoped, as extensions of CRPS rather than replacements.

UNANSWERED QUESTIONS ON CLASSIFICATION

Several rhetorical questions arose in pondering the elements of diagnosis and the implications of functional disturbances. Do the changes in CRPS disorders represent a disease or are they an exaggeration of normal protective processes? Is the expanded sensitization state and functional impairment of CRPS a means of promoting rest? Is there an exaggeration and prolongation of such changes in some persons compared to others? If such a process exists for limb injuries, is it confined only to these regions, or can other areas, visceral organs, or even the whole body become subject to similar changes? Can conditioning factors accentuate such changes?

Behavioral changes encountered in many CRPS patients have led to instances of *post hoc (ergo) propter hoc* deductions applied to possible psychiatric diagnoses for these cases. Members of the workshop were in general agreement with the review by Lynch (1992) that the very frequent psychiatric and psychological features of CRPS (RSD) are consequences rather than causes of the disorder, as further detailed by Covington (Chapter 11, this volume). Genetic predisposition to such disorders is another fascinating proposal (Mailis and Wade 1994), with many implications.

Neither staging nor grading of different clinical presentations were seen as having utility from a descriptive, diagnostic, or therapeutic standpoint at this time. Insufficient data were available to make valid distinctions, though consideration could be given to this matter again when further clinical studies such as those by Blumberg et al. (1994), Ochoa et al. (1994), and Veldman et al. (1993) are published. Not until reproducible quantitative measures of symptomatic and functional disturbance are developed can there also be a universally accepted standard of grading. Even simple designations of mild, moderate, or severe forms require a minimum of inclusion criteria, time elements, symptom intensities, sensory disturbances, distribution, inflammatory changes, etc., which were beyond current knowledge levels.

SYMPTOMS AND SIGNS

Neither of the two groups nor the full workshop was able to arrive at a list of individual symptoms or signs that would provide a "gold standard" for the diagnosis of CRPS. Instead, clinical presentations from the experiences of group members and from reported studies were collated and assembled for features of short- and long-term characteristics and responses to testing, which are critical to diagnosis. A grading of importance for these diagnostic criteria was considered, but felt inappropriate given the lack of critical knowledge at this time. One of the important distinguishing characteristics for all CRPS cases is that both pain and other somatosensory abnormalities extend outside the distribution of peripheral nerves, even if the inciting injury involved a peripheral nerve, thereby separating CRPS from other more specific neuropathic pain disorders.

SPONTANEOUS PAIN

After extensive discussion, workshop participants agreed that pain is an absolute requirement for CRPS diagnosis, as the name implies. Pain follows an initiating noxious event that usually involves tissue injury in a limb, but is disproportionate in duration, severity, and distribution to that expected from the clinical course of the inciting event. Sometimes the syndrome occurs following central nervous system, visceral, or psychological or psychiatric disorders. Several case reports of regional pains involving the trunk, face, body quadrants, or hemilateral distributions, are also accepted as fulfilling current criteria for CRPS diagnosis. The pain itself is deep and aching in quality, with orthostatic aggravation as seen in type I CRPS, but often with an added superficial burning element in type II. These pains tend to be worse in the evening and can be aggravated by cold or in some cases by heat. More than 75% of patients have pain that is spontaneous and constant, and the remainder have movement or touch-evoked pains that probably are consequences of increased mechanical receptivity.

ALLODYNIA AND HYPERALGESIA

Either mechanical or thermal allodynia is a feature of CRPS, occurring in 70–80% of patients, although these symptoms were much less evident in the report by Blumberg and Jänig (1994). Movement-induced pain is probably a reflection of mechanical allodynia. The classical presentation of a patient with a well-wrapped, elevated, supported arm reflects the attempt to protect the limb from extraneously induced pain. Clearly, pain provoked by usually innocuous touch or cold provides a clear basis for applying the term allodynia to the clinical description for CRPS. However, the distinction between hyperalgesia and pressure-, cold-, or heat-induced allodynia, is not sufficiently distinctive to make a separation for routine use. Quantitative sensory testing provides the appropriate investigative tool for better delineation of these sensory changes, though it may be sufficient for clinical purposes to merely record reduced threshold levels of pain response to each of the physical stimuli.

OTHER SOMATOSENSORY CHANGES

Diffuse sensory changes in addition to pain and allodynia are similarly reported in more than 70% of cases. These changes are less specific, however, and manifest as variable degrees of hypoesthesia, hyperesthesia, and a sense of diffuse numbness or heaviness. These symptoms are subjective, variable, and sometimes difficult to validate with clinical testing, a problem that sometimes leads to misinterpretation. In this context these symptoms may be misconstrued as representing psychosomatic responses, especially when they extend in a glove or stocking, quadrantic or hemilateral distribution, defying conventional wisdom because the changes are inconsistent with known patterns of dermatomal or peripheral nerve distributions. Perhaps more surprising, in the sense of conventional sensory neurophysiology, is the almost immediate relief of these symptoms following successful sympathetic or other focal block, applied remote from the site of abnormal sensation.

SWELLING

Patients describe swelling of limbs in nearly all instances, though objective testing may confirm this in less than 50% of cases, suggesting that some abnormal sensory or body image processing forms part of the somatosensory disturbance of the syndrome (Ochoa et al. 1994), although the incidence of swelling also declines over time (Veldman et al. 1993). Tissue swelling (and pain) may result from neuromediators such as nerve growth factor, released from sympathetic postganglionic neurons (Kinmann and Levine 1995; Woolf et al. 1994), but other mechanisms can be involved, as included in the 1994 paper from Blumberg et al. from the 7th World Congress on Pain. Another example, with neuropeptide release from primary afferent nociceptors as a cause for edema, is suggested by Heller et al. (1994). Nonneurally based inflammation is similarly possible in CRPS cases, part of the so-called autonomic component to CRPS/RSD, with inflammation involving a diffuse regional distribution outside of any peripheral nerve distribution.

TEMPERATURE AND COLOR CHANGE

In the three studies with specific testing of clinical features, 75–98% of cases report altered limb temperature and color, usually warmer in the early phase and cold in later stages of the syndrome, with increased vasomotor lability reported by Veldman et al. (1993). The vasoconstrictive component and its reversal with sympathetic block has long been the justification for intervention with pharmacolotherapy, regional blockade, or surgical techniques of sympathectomy for reversal of this component and, it is hoped, the pain also. While sympathetic overactivity is not necessarily required for this vascular reactivity in CRPS, there is no doubt that sympathetic block can be dramatically effective in reversing, even if only temporarily, the cold, blue, painful limb. Conversely, those with warm, vasodilated, painful limbs can be worsened with the same treatments. As discussed with features of swelling and edema, changes in vascular reactivity and temperature may similarly reflect the response to one or more of several neural or tissue mediators, in contrast to those that are due to a predominant sympathetically generated change. Thermography has proven helpful in demonstrating cutaneous temperature changes and in following these over time and through treatment responses.

MOTOR CHANGES

Weakness, tremor, and reduced movement are often present in CRPS, to the extent that some members of the workshop felt it should be an inclusion criterion in definition of the disorder. Dystonia and incoordination is also expressed by some patients but is less well verified. Lack of simple objective clinical measures hamper quantitative documentation of such dysfunction, but to the patient these changes can be as limiting as the pain. Vocational tasks, writing, even simple domestic tasks and self-care, can be impaired. Some felt that lack of movement and limb activation contributed to the development of CRPS and to failures of therapy, though this observation was purely anecdotal.

SYMPATHETIC OUTFLOW CHANGES

Vascular and sweating abnormalities have been considered one of the hallmarks of RSD, supporting evidence for the "sympathetic" overactivity in its pathophysiology. Although their diagnostic importance under the new CRPS umbrella is retained, their mechanistic relevance may be decreased if they represent consequences of locally mediated responses. The incidence of these features seems to decrease over time to about 50% prevalence. Still unanswered is an explanation for the clinical benefit derived in many of these patients from various forms of sympathetic interruption.

TROPHIC CHANGES

There was some agreement that trophic changes were a late stage of the disorder and that local cutaneous changes were also part of the syndrome, though rarely described (Webster et al. 1993). Skin, nail, and hair growth changes are more evident in the presence of severe mechanical allodynia when touch or slight movement precipitate pain. Grooming and washing are so painful that the limb becomes unkempt and is held in a neutral protective posture that allows the joints and tendons to become fixed and immobilized. Osteoporosis is often dramatic, but can also accompany disuse of the limb, whether CRPS induced or otherwise. Delayed uptake and retention in three-phase bone scans reveal altered blood flow and active bone resorption, but there is some contention whether these observations offer further diagnostic sensitivity or specificity beyond the basic clinical symptoms and signs. Atrophic, shiny skin and contracted, atrophic muscles with stiffened joints are seen in advanced and more intractable forms of the syndrome.

INCLUSION CRITERIA

It proved difficult to establish the point at which inclusion of a minimum level of clinical features reached the threshold for a CRPS diagnosis. The overall concept was one of a constellation of clinical changes as depicted in Fig. 3, with varying levels of functional disturbance in each of the elements shown, in addition to regional pain. However, it was felt that sensory, autonomic/inflammatory, and probably motor dysfunction were essential minimum diagnostic criteria for inclusion under the CRPS umbrella. Wilson

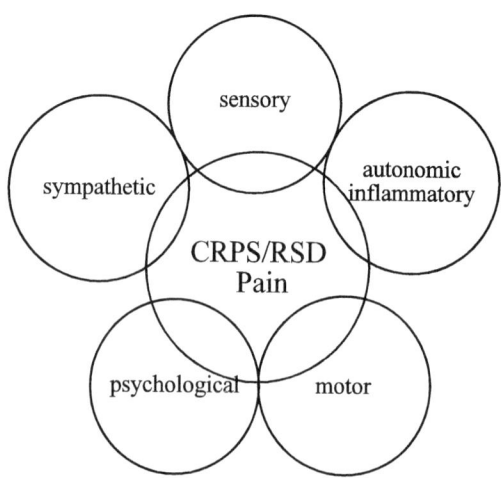

Fig. 3. The elements that constitute the primary clinical components of CRPS. Neither the magnitude of each element nor the degree of intersection are intended to have quantitative relationship.

and colleagues (Chapter 6, this volume) address the same issues in their algorithm discussion. Those cases demonstrating such changes in well-confined regional patterns with day-by-day fluctuations, as in patellofemoral knee pain and posttraumatic foot and wrist pains, where only two features dominate but where others are present to a minor degree, may represent CRPS type III cases, at least until a more definitive diagnostic test is available. As the diagnostic definitions improve, so too will future grading of inclusion criteria for each of the CRPS divisions allow for more graded ratings of each of the symptoms, signs, and diagnostic tests.

CONTRIBUTING FACTORS

Several clinical factors may predispose persons to the development of CRPS. These factors have not yet be subjected to rigorous controlled trial, but form important material for future clinical research.

Genetic predisposition. Experimental sciatic neuropathies in rats (Devor and Rabor 1990) have demonstrated genetic traits to autotomy, while familial frequency is also reported for reflex sympathetic dystrophy (Griepp and Thomas 1991). More important are the HLA antigen profiles reported by Mailis and Wade (1994), which suggest a possible genetic susceptibility profile in those patients with refractory RSD.

Disuse. Anecdotal statements from clinical reports suggest that the association of inactivity with passive posture contributes either to the onset of the syndrome or its persistence once developed. Many treatment programs focus on aggressive reactivation as the mainstay to therapy. In some instances the use of sympathetic or neural blockade may not specifically treat the underlying pathology so much as facilitate the reactivation during symptomatic relief and help sustain patient compliance with physical therapy and exercise.

Fear/anxiety. High profiles of anxiety and depression in patients with CRPS are consistent with profiles encountered in most forms of chronic pain, but where inactivation is a prominent feature of the syndrome, the distinction between neurogenic and psychosomatic inhibition of function might be crucial in setting appropriate treatment modules (Chapter 11, this volume).

CNS injury. The association of CRPS with central nervous system injury, deafferentation disorders, and neuropathies may signal plasticity or sensitization changes in the central nervous system that predispose to the development of CRPS disorders. Prior traumatic bodily injury may similarly induce CNS changes that more readily lead to sensitization and CRPS with a subsequent noxious event.

Repetitive noxious stimulation. Dickenson (1994) has reviewed increasing evidence for spinal sensitization of NMDA receptors leading to induction of second-messenger systems from repetitive C-fiber stimulation. This evidence gives strong pointers to mechanistic processes that might develop in chronic pain states, including the induction of possible long-term trophic changes with CNS plasticity.

DIFFERENTIAL DIAGNOSIS

The neuropathic pain disorders have provided difficulties in the past in differential diagnosis of CRPS/RSD syndromes. A definition of CRPS that excludes patients with an identifiable nerve injury should now allow a clearer distinction to be made. The exclusion of cases responding positively to sympathetic block, but otherwise manifesting as identifiable neuropathic pains, i.e., postherpetic neuralgia or diabetic peripheral neuropathy, should more narrowly define those cases as sympathetically maintained pains, not within a CRPS category.

Perhaps the most difficult and conceptually challenging patients are those with a diversity of clinical findings consistent with CRPS, who have repetitive episodes of pain, but who do not meet sufficient severity, duration, or distribution criteria to provide a confident CRPS diagnosis. Some of those who have only pain, mechanical hyperalgesia, and temperature change may represent type III CRPS or a myofascial pain syndrome. Where widespread tenderness/hyperalgesia is evident, but perhaps more readily identified about the epicondyles or classical muscle groups, the diagnosis of occupational overuse syndrome, tennis elbow, bursitis, nerve entrapment, or similar is often made, though the distinction between one diagnosis and another may depend more on the specialty of the physician than on the presenting findings. It is also common to find patients with concurrent or sequential chronic pains, which suggests a common factor is involved in many of these other regional pain disorders. Patterns of pain hyperresponsiveness have been identified in patients with fibromyalgia (Lautenbacher et al. 1994), with associated presentations of stiffness, headache, fatigue, sleeplessness, swelling, depression, irritable bowel, as might similarly occur with CRPS. The challenge is to conduct prospective studies of CRPS patients and similarly determine their global and regional sensory threshold and pain sensitivities, together with an inventory of past and present pain states. The strongly female predisposition to many of these pain syndromes, and the apparent genetic predisposition in some, coupled with common clinical elements across several similar disorders, suggest that the same or similar underlying mechanisms may be involved.

SUMMARY

Participants in the workshop on reflex sympathetic dystrophy felt the term and its descriptors were no longer appropriate in the light of current knowledge. Instead, a new classification under the umbrella term complex regional pain syndrome (CRPS) is proposed. This classification is based on clinical symptoms and signs without mechanistic connotations, comprising three categories: type I analogous to the old RSD, type II analogous to causalgia, and type III representing a group with two or three primary elements but not fulfilling all of the clinical criteria. The previously sympathetic basis to this syndrome has been confined to a group of pain disorders that respond positively to sympathetic block, but that may be independent of those with CRPS. Thus, patients may have sympathetically maintained pain in a variety of painful conditions, including or independent of CRPS. Similarly, CRPS disorders may have sympathetically maintained pain (SMP), or sympathetic independent pain (SIP). Clinical presentations are varied and dynamic, within a person over time and among persons, and may include spontaneous pain, allodynia or hyperalgesia, swelling, variable sensory and motor changes, vascular and temperature changes, abnormal responses from sympathetic influences in skin, and possibly trophic changes. Such features must be in a distribution beyond the confines of the original initiating lesion, usually distally in a limb and disproportionate to the inciting event.

REFERENCES

Bentley, J.B. and Hameroff, S.R., Diffuse reflex sympathetic dystrophy, Anesthesiology, 53 (1980) 256–257.

Blumberg, H. and Jänig, W., Clinical manifestations of reflex sympathetic dystrophy and sympathetically maintained pain. In: R. Melzack and P.D. Wall (Eds.), Textbook of Pain, 3rd ed., Churchill Livingstone, Edinburgh, 1994, pp. 685–698.

Blumberg, H., Hoffman, U., Mohadjer, M., and Scheremet, R., Clinical phenomenology and mechanisms of reflex sympathetic dystrophy: emphasis on edema. In: G.F. Gebhart, D.L. Hammond and T.S. Jensen (Eds.), Proceedings of the 7th World Congress on Pain, Progress in Pain Research and Management, Vol. 2, IASP Press, Seattle, 1994, pp. 455–481.

Bonica, J.J., Causalgia and other reflex sympathetic dystrophies. In: J.J. Bonica (Ed.), The Management of Pain, Lea & Febiger, Philadelphia, 1953, pp. 913–978.

Bonica, J.J., Causalgia and other reflex sympathetic dystrophies. In: J.J. Bonica, J.C. Liebeskind and D.G. Albe-Fessard (Eds.), Advances in Pain Research and Therapy, Raven Press, New York, 1979, pp. 141–166.

Bonica, J.J., Causalgia and other reflex sympathetic dystrophies. In: J.J. Bonica (Ed.), The Management of Pain, 2nd ed., Lea & Febiger, Philadelphia, 1990, pp. 220–243.

Devor, M. and Rabor, P., Heritability of symptoms in an experimental model of neuropathic pain, Pain, 42 (1990) 51–67.

Dickenson, A.H., NMDA receptor antagonists as analgesics. In: H.L. Fields and J.G. Liebeskind (Eds.), Pharmacological Approaches to the Treatment of Pain: New Concepts and Critical

Issues, Progress in Pain Research and Management, Vol. 1, IASP Press, Seattle, 1994, pp. 173–187.
Drummond, P.D., Noradrenaline increases hyperalgesia to heat in skin sensitised by capsaicin, Pain, 60 (1995) 311–315.
Griepp, M.E. and Thomas, A.F., Familial occurrences of reflex sympathetic dystrophy, Clin. J. Pain, 7 (1991) 48.
Hedergen, T., Rudiger, S., Mayer, B., Bravo, R. and Zimmerman, M., Expression of nitric oxide synthase and co-localisation with Jun, Fos and Krox transcription factors in spinal cord neurones following noxious stimulation of the rat hindpaw, Brain Res. Mol. Brain Res., 22 (1994) 245–258.
Heller, P.H., Green, P.G., Tanner, K.D., Miao, F.J-P. and Levine, J.D., Peripheral neural contributions to inflammation. In: H.L. Fields and J.C. Liebeskind (Eds.), Pharmacological Approaches to the Treatment of Pain: New Concepts and Critical Issues, Progress in Pain Research and Management, Vol. 1, IASP Press, Seattle, 1994, pp. 31–42.
Kinnman, E. and Levine, J.D., Sensory and sympathetic contributions to nerve injury induced sensory abnormalities in the rat, Neuroscience, 64 (1995) 751–767.
Lautenbacher, S., Rollman, G.B. and McCain, G.A., Multi-method assessment of experimental and clinical pain in patients with fibromyalgia, Pain, 59 (1994) 45–53.
Livingstone, W.K., Pain Mechanisms: A Physiological Interpretation of Causalgia and its Related Symptoms, Macmillan & Co., London, 1943.
Lynch, M.E., Psychological aspects of reflex sympathetic dystrophy: a review of the adult and pediatric literature, Pain, 49 (1992) 337–347.
Mailis, A. and Wade, J., Profile of caucasian women with possible genetic predisposition to reflex sympathetic dystrophy: a pilot study, Clin. J. Pain, 10 (1994) 210–217.
McLachlan, E.M., Jänig, W., Devor, M. and Michaelis, M., Peripheral nerve injury triggers noradrenergic sprouting within dorsal root ganglia, Nature, 363 (1993) 543–546.
Merskey, H. and Bogduk, N., Classification of Chronic Pain: Descriptions of Chronic Pain Syndromes and Definitions of Pain Terms, 2nd ed., IASP Press, Seattle, 1994.
Ochoa, J.L., Verdugo, R.J. and Campero, M., Pathophysiological spectrum of organic and psychogenic disorders in neuropathic pain patients fitting the description of causalgia or reflex sympathetic dystrophy. In: G.F. Gebhart, D.L. Hammond and T.S. Jensen (Eds.), Proceedings of the 7th World Congress on Pain, Progress in Pain Research and Management, Vol. 2, IASP Press, Seattle, 1994, pp. 483–494.
Roberts, W.J., A hypothesis on the physiological basis for causalgia and related pain, Pain, 24 (1986) 297–311.
Tracey, D.J., Cunningham, J.E. and Romm, M.A., Peripheral hyperalgesia in experimental neuropathy: mediation by alpha-2-adrenoreceptors on post-ganglionic sympathetic terminals, Pain, 60 (1995) 317–327.
Veldman, P.H.J.M., Reynen, H.M., Arntz, I.E. and Goris, R.J.A., Signs and symptoms of reflex sympathetic dystrophy: prospective study of 829 patients, Lancet, 342 (1993) 1012–1016.
Webster, G.F., Iozzo, R.V., Schwartzman, R.J., Tahmoush, A.J., Knobler, R.L. and Jacoby, R.A., Reflex sympathetic dystrophy: occurrence of chronic edema and nonimmune bullous skin lesions, J. Am. Acad. Dermatol., 28 (1993) 29–32.
Woolf, C.J., Safieh-Garabedian, B., Ma, Q.P., Crilly, P. and Winter, J., Nerve growth factor contributes to the generation of inflammatory sensory hypersensitivity, Neuroscience, 62 (1994) 327–331.
Zhang, X., Bao, I., Xu, Z.Q., Kopp, J., Arvidsson, U., Elde, R. and Hokefelt, T., Localisation of neuropeptide Y Y1 receptors in the rat nervous system with special reference to somatic receptors on small dorsal root ganglion neurons, Proc. Natl. Acad. Sci. USA, 91 (1994) 11738–11742.

Correspondence to: Robert A. Boas, MB BCh, Pain Clinic, Auckland Hospital, Auckland, New Zealand. Tel: 64-9-373-7599; Fax: 64-9-373-7556.

6

Diagnostic Algorithm for Complex Regional Pain Syndromes

Peter R. Wilson,[a] Phillip A. Low,[a]
Marshall D. Bedder,[b] Edward C. Covington,[c]
and Richard L. Rauck[d]

[a]*Mayo Clinic, Rochester, Minnesota,* [b]*St. Vincent Medical Center, Portland Oregon,* [c]*Cleveland Clinic, Cleveland, Ohio,* [d]*Bowman Gray School of Medicine, Winston-Salem, North Carolina, USA*

Reflex sympathetic dystrophy (RSD) is a venerable diagnosis of a heterogenous clinical condition. Many causes and many therapies have been reported in the literature in the last 130 years. However, most published information is in the form of case reports and clinical series. Meta-analysis of the literature does not appear to be possible at present because of a lack of consensus on diagnostic criteria and lack of controlled studies and objective outcome measures. RSD is thus a descriptive diagnostic term that implicates the sympathetic nervous system in a reflex response to injury, with consequent dystrophic changes.

Exaggerated responses to injury occur in these cases, with involvement of autonomic, sensory, and motor systems (Willner 1993; Chapters 2 and 3, this volume). Many authors have focused on the sympathetic component of RSD, and have regarded it as a specific syndrome of autonomic dysfunction. However, this may not be the case. Ochoa and Verdugo (1993) indicated numerous problems with interpretation of the literature relating to pain syndromes that have any component of autonomic involvement. They point out that the nonspecific state of RSD can be generated by a variety of neurologic mechanisms ranging from cutaneous receptor dysfunction through peripheral nerve, spinal cord, and brain dysfunction to psychologic dysfunction. They also addressed the difficulties in the diagnosis of sympathetically maintained pain, and suggested that the precise effects of the sympathetic nervous system cannot be reliably predicted. Both up- and down-regulation of activity is possible at different anatomic sites and at different times in the course of the condition, but the controlling factors have not yet been fully elucidated.

Willner (1993) presented an overview of the clinical diagnostic dilemmas. She indicated a lack of adequate information about the roles and interactions of the somatic and autonomic nervous systems, and local tissue factors in RSD or other pain states. This lack necessarily leads to diagnostic difficulties in any pain state that involves these three components. Furthermore, an avenue of research that does not appear to have been exploited is the use of autonomic changes to measure progress of the condition. Available evidence indicates that the autonomic changes may return to normal after recovery from the condition, with associated return of normal function. Additional difficulties in the definition of robust diagnostic criteria lie in the disputed assumption of three phases of RSD—acute, dystrophic, and atrophic (e.g., Romanoff 1993). There do not appear to be substantial published data supporting this view.

This chapter will develop a diagnostic algorithm for the complex regional pain syndromes. This algorithm should be a working operational model containing a minimum of subjective nodes. It should be useful and practical for clinicians and researchers. Diagnosis should be based on multiple criteria, and still be a probability model. The algorithm should be based on criteria that can be measured and quantified rather than on clinical impressions and opinions. However, in the absence of adequate scientific evidence to construct a probability model, the Delphi method may be applied. This technique relies on a consensus achieved in group discussion by experienced clinicians and researchers. It is essential that all participants be equally familiar with the clinical problems and the basic and clinical scientific literature.

HISTORICAL DIAGNOSTIC CRITERIA

Many proposed definitions of RSD have been based on "clinical impressions," and many were peculiar to the clinician or institution. However, three recent formal attempts have been made to define RSD.

Kozin et al. (1976a,b) evaluated the role of the radioactive three-phase bone scan in RSD and established the diagnostic criteria shown in Table I. It was apparent that this particular classification was too broad, and included cases that did not behave clinically like RSD. For example, many clinicians described cases that appeared to be RSD, but did not respond to sympathetic interventions.

In an attempt to clarify this situation, Gibbons et al. (1992) proposed an empiric scale for RSD (Table II). This arbitrary scale was based on a series of patients who had not responded to local anesthetic sympathetic ganglion

Table I
Diagnostic criteria for RSD proposed by Rosen et al. (1976)

Definite RSD
  Pain and tenderness in the distal extremity
  Signs or symptoms of vasomotor instability
  Swelling in the extremity (often with periarticular prominence)
  Dystrophic skin changes usually present

Probable RSD
  Pain and tenderness and vasomotor instability or swelling
  No pain, but mild to moderate tenderness may be present
  Dystrophic skin changes occasionally present

Doubtful RSD
  Unexplained pain and tenderness in an extremity

blockade, but who responded favorably to somatic local anesthetic peripheral nerve block. The scale was based on clinical history and examination and results of laboratory testing. It must be stressed, however, that these criteria were based on clinical impressions, as no objective outcome criteria were specified in this (or any previous) study. Also, the presence of sympathetically maintained pain was not essential to the diagnosis in this scheme. It became

Table II
Diagnostic scale for RSD proposed by Gibbons et al. (1992)

Clinical symptoms and signs
  Burning pain
  Hyperpathia and allodynia
  Temperature and color changes
  Edema
  Hair and nail changes

Laboratory results
  Thermometry and thermography >1°C asymmetry
  X-ray demineralization of affected extremity
  Three-phase bone scan consistent with RSD
  Quantitative sweat test asymmetry
  Response to sympathetic blockade

Interpretation
  Score 1 for each criterion, maximum score 10
   >6 probable RSD
   3–5 possible RSD
   <3 unlikely RSD

clear that this scheme was inadequate in some cases, particularly in the presence of sympathetically independent pain.

The attempt had been made to deemphasize sympathetically maintained pain by only assigning one point of the possible 10. Consequently, Blumberg et al. (1994) proposed a numeric grading scheme for RSD based on the autonomic-motor-sensory triad (Table III). This system allows a "full RSD syndrome" to have a maximum score of 18. The system was illustrated in a group of 24 patients with acute RSD (duration 0.1 ± 0.1 months), and 157 patients with long-standing RSD (duration 6 ± 16 months). Each group had a mean RSD score of 14 (± 3). In common with the other schemes, this one was based on the authors' clinical experience, and could possibly represent selection bias. Also in common with the other schemes, it contains both subjective and objective criteria, and has not been used to follow progress or outcome. Interestingly, Blumberg and colleagues consider allodynia to be rare and give equal weight to the motor disorders, whereas other clinicians consider allodynia to be common and the motor disturbances to be secondary to the pain.

We are dimayed by the absence of published validated diagnostic criteria for complex regional pain syndromes, and the absence of long-term controlled outcome studies with objective functional measures. We also note that the diagnosis of complex regional pain syndrome is one of exclusion at this time. For example, a hot, red, painful, swollen hand might be the result of a septic arthritis, acute trauma, insect bite, local allergy, a factitious situation, or "RSD." A cold, blue, sweaty, atrophic, painful extremity might be the result

Table III
Numeric grading scale for RSD proposed by Blumberg et al. (1994)

Autonomic symptoms

    Distally generalized swelling (3)
    Warm or cold affected extremity (2)
    Hypohidrosis or hyperhidrosis (1)

Motor symptoms

    Active movement reduced (3)
    Muscular strength diminished (2)
    Tremor (postural or action) (1)

Sensory symptoms

    Deep spontaneous pain (3)
    Hypoalgesia or hyperalgesia (2)
    Hypoesthesia or hyperesthesia (1)
    Mechanical allodynia (rare, not scored)

Maximum score 18

of chronic vascular insufficiency (e.g., Raynaud's, scleroderma), disuse (from any cause, including stroke or other neurologic pathology), immobilization, or "RSD." We could not address all possible differential diagnoses of complex regional pain syndrome.

DEFINITION

Complex regional pain syndromes represent a group of disorders in which the pain and dysfunction are disproportionate in severity or duration to those expected from the initiating event. Two main categories appear to be distinguished according to the presence or absence of major peripheral nerve injury.

COMPLEX REGIONAL PAIN SYNDROME, TYPE I (REFLEX SYMPATHETIC DYSTROPHY)

Clinical presentation

This pain syndrome usually has an initiating noxious event in the periphery and evidence of sympathetic dysfunction in the affected extremity at some stage. There are associated sensory, motor, and functional changes. A single extremity is involved initially, and symptoms may spread proximally and to other extremities. The onset of symptoms is usually within a month of the initiating incident. Exclusion criteria include identifiable major nerve injury or dysfunction or any other medical, surgical, or psychiatric cause of the symptoms and signs.

Symptoms

Pain is reported in the affected extremity. The pain may be spontaneous or evoked, and is usually reported as diffuse burning, in an area not consistent with the distribution of a peripheral nerve. The pain may also be reported as aching or throbbing. It may be intermittent or continuous, exacerbated by physical or emotional stressors. The patient often adopts a protective posture.

Sensory changes are reported at some stage, and include hyperesthesia and allodynia in the region of the pain. Hyperesthesia may occur to any modality. Allodynia may occur to light touch, thermal stimulation (cold, warm), deep pressure, or to joint movement.

Sympathetic dysfunction is reported as vasomotor or sudomotor instability in the affected limb when compared with an unaffected limb. Fluctuations may occur from time to time in both vasomotor and sudomotor function. The patient may report that the extremity is warm and red or cold and blue/purple or mottled. The temperature and color of the digits (pads) appear to be more significant than that of more central parts of the limb. Sweating, particularly of the palms or soles, may be reported as unchanged, increased, or decreased. There may be periods of apparently normal sympathetic function.

Swelling may be reported at any stage of the condition. Edema is typically peripheral, and may be intermittent or permanent. It may be exacerbated by the dependent position of the limb, and may be of the pitting or brawny type. Swelling may be improved by elevation of the affected limb.

Trophic changes of the skin and appendages may be reported later in the course of the condition. The nails may be hypertrophic or atrophic, hair growth and texture may be increased or decreased, and the skin may become atrophic.

Motor dysfunction may be reported, and may include tremor, dystonia, and loss of strength and endurance of the affected muscle groups. Joint stiffness and swelling may be reported, particularly of the digits.

Psychological changes are reviewed by Covington (Chapter 11, this volume).

Signs

Sensory examination. Hyperalgesia may be evaluated by comparing sensory reports from nonpainful stimulation between the painful area and a normal area (ideally symmetrically). Allodynia may be evaluated in the usual modalities by applying nonnoxious stimuli to the affected limb (cold, warm, light touch, deep pressure, joint movement), again comparing with a normal extremity.

Vasomotor examination. Temperature of the affected extremity (digit pads, palm/sole, forearm/calf) should be measured with noncontact thermometry (inexpensive infrared thermometers are available) or thermography. Simultaneous measurements must be made with symmetrical points on the unaffected extremity. Serial measurements should be made, as peripheral temperature fluctuates widely (but usually symmetrically) under normal circumstances. Skin color can be estimated visually or by pulse oximetry.

Sudomotor examination. Resting sweat output may be estimated by skin impedance (Schondorf 1993), or cobalt blue or quinizarin testing (Fealey 1993). It can be estimated directly as part of the quantitative sudomotor reflex test (QSART) (Low and Pfeiffer 1993). The QSART measures resting sweat output by hygrometry, and changes evoked by iontophoresis of acetylcholine into the skin, as discussed by Low et al. (Chapter 3, this volume).

Edema. Volume displacement methods provide quantitative estimates of the extent of edema, and allow objective measurement of treatment. However, many find the method cumbersome, and rely on clinical impressions. In either case, comparison must be made with the unaffected side.

Trophic changes. Compare hair, skin, and nails of the affected side with the unaffected side. Clinical photography might be helpful in following progress.

Motor dysfunction. The presence of tremor, dystonia, and changes in strength are measured clinically. Where possible, objective measurements should be made (grip, apposition and opposition pinch strength, weight-bearing on lower extremity).

Psychological changes. No psychometric instrument has been validated in the treatment of RSD or CRPS. The psychiatrist or psychologist should use familiar instruments as part of the initial assessment and in follow-up.

Laboratory testing

Testing may be by invasive or noninvasive methods. Unfortunately, data are not available for sensitivity or specificity of any of the tests listed below. Tests thus must be interpreted within the clinical context. These tests may also be used to monitor progress of treatment. They are intended to estimate the degree of autonomic and somatic dysfunction, and of physical and psychologic impairment.

Surface temperature. Skin temperature fluctuates widely with changes in sympathetic tone. The digit pads are capable of a range from ambient temperature to core temperature. The digit pads thus are the most sensitive indicators of peripheral perfusion. However, temperature tends to change symmetrically, with a gradient from head and trunk to the digit tips. Skin temperature differences >1°C (measured on all digit pads symmetrically and simultaneously) between the affected and normal extremity (measured symmetrically) indicate unilateral sympathetic dysfunction (over- or underactivity). The patient must have acclimatized to a thermoneutral environment (room temperature 20°C) with minimal physical or emotional distractions before measurements are made. Measurements should be by noncontact thermometry (infrared) or thermography, and must be repeated over a suitable period of time. Exaggerated responses may be seen with provocative testing, for example, the cold pressor test.

Sudomotor activity. Resting sweat output is determined by cholinergic sympathetic activity, and is not necessarily related to adrenergic (vasoconstrictor) activity. The quantitative sudomotor axon reflex test (QSART) measures both resting cholinergic sympathetic tone (resting sweat output) and sudomotor activity evoked by iontophoresed acetylcholine. High sympathetic activity is indicated by a high resting sweat output. Sympathetic overactivity is associated with an increased sweat output in response to iontophoresed acetyl choline with a decreased latency and prolonged duration when compared to the control site.

Three-phase bone scan. Delayed views of the technetium bone scan that indicate increased periarticular uptake are said to be indicative of RSD (Kozin et al. 1976b). However, the same appearance has been described following sympathetic blockade in patients without RSD, indicating that this investigation should be reevaluated.

Tourniquet ischemia test. Temporary ischemia of a limb appears to produce progressive blockade of nerve transmission in a predictable order, with mechanical hyperalgesia being more sensitive than cold sensation (and A-delta or C-fiber pain). However, the interpretation of this test is under intense scrutiny, and conclusions are difficult to justify.

Radiographic demineralization. X-rays comparing the affected and normal extremities may demonstrate bony demineralization, sometimes very early in the course of the condition (Sudeck's atrophy). These changes may be identical to those of disuse or immobilization, and their diagnostic utility in CRPS has not been defined.

Miscellaneous testing. The following procedures have not yet proven their utility in the diagnosis of CRPS/RSD: EMG, somatosensory-evoked potentials, transcutaneous oxygen tension, laser Doppler measurements of cutaneous blood flow, computer-assisted sensory testing, and microneuronographic measurement of peripheral sympathetic function.

Sympathetic blockade. The diagnosis of sympathetically maintained pain (SMP) is made when the pain is relieved by appropriately controlled sympathetic blockade. The role of the placebo response is discussed elsewhere in this volume (Chapter 10). All sympathetic block techniques have technical difficulties, and successful blockade can only be assumed if signs of sympathetic activity are absent. Skin temperature must increase to near core temperature, and sweating must be absent before the results can be correctly interpreted. The sympathetic efferent system can be blocked at the peripheral adrenoceptor, peripheral nerve, ganglion, spinal cord, or brainstem. Techniques of sympathetic blockade are discussed by Stanton-Hicks et al. (Chapter 12, this volume). The diagnosis of sympathetically independent pain (SIP) is one of exclusion, as both peripheral and central somatic nerve blocks also block peripheral sympathetic fibers. Pain relief following such a diagnostic somatic block might therefore represent SMP, SIP, or a combination of the two.

Pitfalls of autonomic testing (Low 1993). It is accepted that CRPS has a component of autonomic (sympathetic) dysfunction. Demonstration of such dysfunction is necessary for the diagnosis of CRPS. Although many noninvasive tests of autonomic function may be performed simply, interpretation of the results, like the interpretation of the results of neural blockade, is usually difficult and unreliable. Test of autonomic function should be sensitive, specific, and reliable. They should examine the appropriate component of the autonomic reflex (afferent limb, central components, efferent limb and receptor/end organ function). Low (1993) summarized the problems (without considering the general problems of placebo, conditioning, and learning):

1. Noninvasive tests of autonomic function are easy to do but difficult to interpret.
2. Noninvasiveness is often associated with suboptimal instrumentation and the monitoring of an inadequate number of parameters.
3. The applied stimulus may be several steps removed from the stimulus recognized by the receptor.
4. The response is usually an indirect effector response. The underlying reflex is often complex and modulated by multiple confounding inputs.
5. In a clinical laboratory environment, extraneous patient variables may also affect the test results.
6. These facts allow for test results that allow for a valid interpretation only within a narrow range of conditions: extrapolations are hazardous.
7. Some popular tests have been poorly validated for general use, and suggested normal ranges are of doubtful value. Criteria based on sensitivity, specificity, reproducibility, and relevance are suggested as a means of evaluating new tests of autonomic function.
8. To define the site of the lesion, the tests compared must have similar sensitivity and specificity.

We therefore did not attempt to adjudicate between competing tests of autonomic function, or make recommendations regarding their use.

COMPLEX REGIONAL PAIN SYNDROME, TYPE II (CAUSALGIA)

The principal difference between type I and type II is that type II occurs after partial injury of a nerve or one of its branches (Chapter 5, this volume). Onset usually occurs immediately after the injury, but may be delayed for months. Impairment of motor function is common. Pain may be sympathetically maintained, sympathetically independent (neuropathic), or both. The clinical characteristics are similar in both types of CRPS.

DIAGNOSTIC ALGORITHM FOR CRPS

The lack of generally accepted diagnostic criteria is one of the factors that contribute to the difficulties surrounding CRPS/RSD. Numerical schemes are superficially attractive, but may be difficult to implement, particularly if any of the laboratory tests or clinical data are not available. The empiric assignment of values for each item, and arbitrary weighting of the clinical importance of each item, reduces the robustness of these diagnostic schemes. There might be more clinical relevance if an algorithm such as proposed in Table IV could be formulated to guide the diagnostic process.

It must be emphasized that the algorithm should be used to evaluate a patient for the presence or absence of CRPS. No attempt is made to determine the stage of the condition (if stages do, in fact, exist) or the severity. In addition, the algorithm is not involved in the diagnosis of sympathetically maintained pain. It is also not used to direct or monitor therapy.

As can be seen from the initial discussions, the algorithm represents expert opinion rather than validated scientific fact. It is therefore open to testing as a hypothesis, to be confirmed or refuted with additional scientific facts when they become available.

Symptoms are subjective phenomena reported by the patient. These may include pain, increased sensitivity to cutaneous or other superficial stimulation, perceived changes in color or temperature of the skin, perceived changes in sweating, hair and nail growth, and changes in muscle strength and joint mobility.

Signs, on the other hand, are phenomena or variables that can be observed by an examiner. These may be subjective or objective. For example, hyperesthesia and allodynia may be expressed verbally or nonverbally during the sensory examination. They are rarely quantitated in clinical practice. However, skin temperature can be measured with great precision by infrared techniques, and sweat output can be accurately measured.

SUMMARY

Complex regional pain syndromes (CRPS) present as amplified somatic, motor, and sympathetic responses to injury or immobilization. Type I CRPS does not have identifiable major nerve injury, while Type II has identifiable major peripheral nerve injury. Spontaneous or evoked pain is out of proportion to the inciting event. Sensory changes include hyperesthesia, hyperalgesia, and allodynia. Motor changes include tremor, dystonia, and weakness. Sympathetic dysfunction causes changes in skin blood flow and sweating. Pain may be sympathetically maintained, sympathetically independent, or both. Associated signs include changes in bone mineralization and blood flow, and dystrophic changes of skin and integuments, joints and muscles. The criteria proposed for the diagnosis are a history of spontaneous or evoked pain out of proportion to the inciting injury, sensory changes in the affected extremity, and at least two signs of sympathetic dysfunction, in the absence of other anatomic, physiologic, or psychiatric pathology.

Table IV
Algorithm for diagnosis of CRPS

Pain

The diagnosis of CRPS cannot be made in the absence of pain; it is a pain syndrome. However, the characteristics of the pain may vary with the initiating event and other factors. The pain is often described as burning, and might be spontaneous or evoked in the context of hyperalgesia or allodynia. Both spontaneous and evoked pain may occur together.

History

Develops after an initiating noxious event or immobilization
Unilateral extremity onset (rarely may spread to another extremity)
Symptom onset usually within a month

Exclusion criteria

Identifiable major nerve lesion (CRPS II)
Existence of anatomic, physiologic, or psychological conditions that would otherwise account for the degree of pain and dysfunction

Symptoms (Patient Report)

A. Pain (spontaneous or evoked)
   Burning
   Aching, throbbing

B. Hyperalgesia or allodynia (at some time in the disease course) to mechanical stimuli (light touch or deep pressure), to thermal stimulation, or to joint motion

C. Associated symptoms (minor)
   Swelling
   Temperature or color: asymmetry and instability
   Sweating: asymmetry and instability
   Trophic changes: hair, nails, skin

Signs (Observed)

Hyperalgesia or allodynia (light touch, deep pressure, joint movement, cold)
Edema (if unilateral and other causes excluded)
Vasomotor changes: color, temperature instability, asymmetry
Sudomotor changes
Trophic changes in skin, joint, nail, hair
Impaired motor function (may include components of dystonia and tremor)

Criteria Required for Diagnosis of CRPS I

History of pain
   plus allodynia, hyperalgesia, or hyperesthesia
   plus two other signs from the above list

Characteristics of spontaneous pain
   Sympathetically maintained pain (SMP)
   Sympathetically independent pain (SIP)
   Combined SMP + SIP

(continued on next page)

Table IV (continued)

Criteria for Diagnosis of Sympathetic Dysfunction

Noninvasive tests
    Surface temperature asymmetry by $\geq 1°$ C, either spontaneous or in response to provocative testing
    Resting or evoked sudomotor asymmetry

Invasive tests
    Sympathetic ganglion block (if equivocal, up to three may be required); will usually be considered adequate only if there is demonstrated inhibition of sympathetic mediated vasoconstriction of the involved extremity.
    Systemic alpha adrenergic antagonists, placebo controlled
    Neuraxial blockade above the lesion may provide useful information.

Tests of unknown pathophysiologic significance
    Three-phase bone scan
    Radiographic patchy demineralization
    Tourniquet ischemia test
    Measurements of cutaneous blood flow with laser Doppler, percutaneous oxygen partial pressure differences, and computer-assisted sensory examination are interesting but evolving technologies that require further study.
    Somatosensory-evoked potential measurement is not of demonstrated utility.
    Regional sympathetic blockade is not recommended for diagnostic use due to multiple physiologic actions that confound interpretation.

REFERENCES

Blumberg, H., A new clinical approach for diagnosing reflex sympathetic dystrophy. In: M.R. Bond, J.E. Charlton and C.J. Woolf (Eds.), Proceedings of the VIth World Congress on Pain, Pain Research and Clinical Management, Vol. 4, Elsevier, Amsterdam, 1991, pp. 399–407.

Blumberg, H., Hoffmann, U., Mohadjer, M. and Scheremet, R., Clinical phenomenology and mechanisms of reflex sympathetic dystrophy: emphasis on edema. In: G.E. Gebhart, D.L. Hammond, and T.S. Jensen (Eds.), Proceedings of the 7th World Congress on Pain, Progress in Pain Research and Management, Vol. 2, IASP Press, Seattle, 1994, pp. 455–481.

Fealey, R.D., The thermoregulatory sweat test. In: P.A. Low (Ed.), Clinical Autonomic Disorders, Little, Brown & Co., Boston, 1993, pp. 217–229.

Gibbons, J. and Wilson, P.R., RSD score: criteria for the diagnosis of reflex sympathetic dystrophy and causalgia, Clin. J. Pain, 8 (1992) 260–263.

Kozin, F., McCarty, D.J., Sims, J. and Genant, H.K., The reflex sympathetic dystrophy syndrome. I. Clinical and historical studies: evidence for bilaterality, response to corticosteroids and articular involvement, Am. J. Med., 60 (1976a) 321–331.

Kozin, F., Genant, H.K., Bekerman, C. and McCarty, D.J., The reflex sympathetic dystrophy syndrome. II. Roentgenographic and scintigraphic evidence of bilaterality and of periarticular accentuation, Am. J. Med., 60 (1976b) 332–338.

Low, P.A., Pitfalls in autonomic testing. In: P.A. Low (Ed.), Clinical Autonomic Disorders, Little, Brown & Co., Boston, 1993, pp. 355–365.

Low, P.A. and Pfeifer, M.D., Standardization of clinical tests for practice and clinical trials. In: P.A. Low (Ed.), Clinical Autonomic Disorders, Little, Brown & Co., Boston, 1993, pp. 287–296.

Ochoa, J.L. and Verdugo, R., Reflex sympathetic dystrophy: definitions and history of the ideas with a critical review of human studies. In: P.A. Low (Ed.), Clinical Autonomic Disorders, Little, Brown & Co., Boston, 1993, pp. 473–492.

Romanoff, M.E., Reflex sympathetic dystrophy. In: S. Ramamurthy and J.N. Rogers (Eds.), Decision Making in Pain Management, Mosby-Year Book, St. Louis, 1993, pp. 50–53.

Schondorf, R., The role of the sympathetic skin response in the assessment of autonomic function. In: P.A. Low (Ed.), Clinical Autonomic Disorders, Little, Brown & Co., Boston, 1993, pp. 231–241.

Willner, C.L., Pain and the sympathetic nervous system: clinical considerations. In: P.A. Low (Ed.), Clinical Autonomic Disorders, Little, Brown & Co., Boston, 1993, pp. 493–503.

Correspondence to: Peter R. Wilson, MB BS, PhD, Department of Anesthesiology, Mayo Clinic, Rochester, MN 55905, USA. Tel: 507-284-2511; Fax: 507-266-7732.

7

Animal Models and Their Contribution to Our Understanding of Complex Regional Pain Syndromes I and II

Gary J. Bennett[a] and William J. Roberts[b]

[a]*Neurobiology and Anesthesiology Branch, National Institute of Dental Research, National Institutes of Health, Bethesda, Maryland, and* [b]*R.S. Dow Neurological Sciences Institute, Portland, Oregon, USA*

Over the last 50 years, animal experimentation has taught us much about the neural mechanisms of normal pain sensation and about the pharmacological control of pain. No one interested in pain research would believe that animal experiments will tell us all there is to know about human pain conditions, but it is reasonable to accept the results of animal experiments as of at least potential benefit in understanding human problems. There is much less history of animal experimentation related specifically to neuropathic pain. With the exception of the pioneering work by Wall and his colleagues (Wall et al. 1979) on experimental anesthesia dolorosa, animal models of painful peripheral neuropathies have appeared only in the last eight years. Despite the relative recency of this work, there is now a considerable body of evidence that is likely to be relevant to the human pain conditions that have been designated complex regional pain syndrome (CRPS) types I and II, and sympathetically maintained pain.

The major difference between CRPS I and II is that type II (causalgia) has a subtotal nerve lesion verified by inspection or traditional electrodiagnostic methods. While suspicion of a nerve lesion is not uncommon in patients diagnosed as CRPS I (RSD), definite evidence of nerve damage is, by definition, lacking. Most of the animal work reviewed below involves a frank nerve lesion and thus relates most closely to CRPS II (causalgia); its relevance to CRPS I (RSD) depends on whether or not CRPS I and II share similar or overlapping pathophysiologic mechanisms (a suspected, but not proven proposition). SMP, which in the newly proposed classification is not a necessary component of either CRPS I or II, is nevertheless often believed to be present in both conditions (and perhaps other conditions as well). Evidence from animal experimentation concerning SMP is thus emphasized in the material that follows.

EXPERIMENTAL PAINFUL PERIPHERAL NEUROPATHIES DUE TO SUBTOTAL NERVE DAMAGE

There are three widely used animal models of neuropathic pain following partial peripheral nerve damage:

1. The chronic constriction injury (CCI) model of Bennett and Xie (1988) is produced by tying loosely constrictive ligatures around the rat's sciatic nerve at mid-thigh level. This evokes intraneural edema; the swelling is opposed by the ligatures, and the nerve self-strangulates. The CCI produces a differential deafferentation: almost all the large myelinated (A-beta) afferents and a preponderance of the small, thinly myelinated (A-delta) afferents are interrupted at the site of nerve injury, but a large percentage of the unmyelinated (C-fiber) afferents survive. Thus, the sciatic nerve territory is innervated by a reduced population of C fibers and a very small remnant of the A-delta fibers; all or almost all of the A-beta low-threshold mechanoreceptors (Aβ-LTM) are disconnected from their peripheral receptors. A neuroma-in-continuity forms at the site of constriction.

2. The partial nerve transection (PNT) model of Seltzer and his colleagues (Seltzer et al. 1990) is produced by piercing the rat's sciatic nerve (upper thigh level) with a small needle and suture and tightly ligating (and thus transecting) about one-third to one-half of the nerve's volume. The PNT thus produces a partial, but not a differential, deafferentation. The sciatic nerve territory is innervated by a reduced (one-half to two-thirds) population of all fiber types. A neuroma-in-continuity is formed at the site of partial transection.

3. The spinal nerve transection (SNT) model developed by Kim and Chung (1992) involves tight ligation (and hence transection) of the L5 and L6 spinal nerves close to their respective ganglia. It is not known whether neuromas-in-continuity form at the transection sites. This procedure produces a partial, but not a differential, deafferentation of the nerves that compose the L5 and L6 roots—chiefly the sciatic and saphenous nerves. The hindpaw is innervated by a reduced (approximately 50%) population of all fiber types.

All three models produce signs of abnormal pain that resemble those found in patients (Bennett and Xie 1988; Attal et al. 1990; Seltzer et al. 1990; Kim and Chung 1991, 1992; Choi et al. 1994; Tal and Bennett 1994). Heat-hyperalgesia, mechano-hyperalgesia, mechano-allodynia, and cold-allodynia are all present. Signs of spontaneous or ongoing pain (e.g., limping and guarding the affected hindpaw) are also present, as are some of the nonpain symptoms traditionally associated with RSD and causalgia: hypertrophic nail (claw) growth and abnormal cutaneous temperature regulation. Edema, even in the early postinjury stage, is minor or absent in all three models, which is notably different than what is seen in early-stage CRPS patients. Hyperhydrosis is also absent, but this is probably a function of the small number of sweat glands in rat skin.

These models were originally developed in highly inbred strains of laboratory rats (the Sprague-Dawley strain for the CCI and SNT models and the Wistar-derived Sabra strain for the PNT model). In the original strains, abnormal pain appears in almost every animal that receives the lesion. But there is evidence that the incidence and perhaps the severity of the pain syndromes may vary in different strains (e.g., Kupers et al. 1992). No sex differences have been noted.

The onset of abnormal pain in the SNT and PNT models appears to be within hours of surgery, but abnormal pain in the CCI model is not detected until two or more days postsurgery. This difference may be of little significance because the actual nerve injury (i.e., the constriction) in the CCI case is not created at the time of surgery; it develops over the course of a day or so as the nerve swells. Abnormal pains are present in the CCI model for two to three months (Bennett and Xie 1988; Attal et al. 1990; for unknown reasons, other laboratories report a significantly shorter duration). The abnormal pain syndrome produced by the SNT model lasts for one to two months, and that of the PNT model lasts for six months or more. These are all relatively long durations, considering that the rat's life span is about 2.5 years.

It is important to note that these models are not redundant. For example, contralateral ("mirror-image") pain abnormalities are prominent in the SNT and PNT models, but minor or absent in the CCI model. Moreover, the evidence suggests that the mechano-allodynia seen in the PNT and SNT models is evoked by afferent input from Aβ-LTMs (Shir and Seltzer 1990; Na et al. 1993). This can not be the case in the CCI model, where the rats have a total or near total loss of Aβ-LTM cutaneous innervation. Most notably, and as reviewed below, the SNT and PNT models appear to be completely SMP, whereas the role of the sympathetic efferents in the CCI model appears to be limited and evident only during the early (about one week) postsurgery stage.

WHAT HAVE THE MODELS TAUGHT US?

It is not our purpose here to review exhaustively the large body of experimental evidence that has come from work on the animal models. Instead, we have selected certain findings that we believe have an obvious relevance to understanding patients with CRPS type I and II.

THE EXTRATERRITORIAL DISTRIBUTION OF NEUROPATHIC PAIN

CRPS type I and II are defined as regional pain syndromes because the abnormal pain sensations are not necessarily confined to the territory of a nerve(s) or root(s). These two conditions often affect the extremities, and patients commonly present with a glove-like or stocking-like distribution of pain. A regional pain distribution recalls the glove- or stocking-like pattern of paralysis in Charcot's classical description of hysteria (conversion disorder), and supports continuing suspicion of a possible underlying (partial or complete) psychogenic mechanism. This suspicion has been especially common in CRPS type I patients because of the absence of concrete signs of relevant organic pathology. Clinicians have reported that the pain of CRPS I and II sometimes spreads unilaterally or "jumps" to a homologous region contralaterally (mirror-image pain) at some time after its presence has become established ipsilaterally. These phenomena have no known organic mechanism and they are also sometimes advanced as presumptive evidence of psychogenic causation, or even of deliberate self-inflicted injury.

The distribution of abnormal evoked pain sensations has been mapped in CCI rats (Kingery et al. 1993; Tal and Bennett 1994). As in the human foot, a narrow strip of skin on the medial edge of the rat's hindpaw is innervated by a branch of the femoral nerve, the saphenous; this nerve is not injured in CCI rats. Clear signs of heat-hyperalgesia, mechano-hyperalgesia, and mechano-allodynia develop in the saphenous nerve's territory. No responses can be evoked from the saphenous territory after an acute transection of the saphenous, but the hyperalgesic and allodynic sensations remain after acute transection of the remnant of the sciatic nerve. Thus, the abnormal responses from the saphenous territory are almost certainly due to impulses traveling to the spinal cord via the saphenous nerve. Tal and Bennett found that the onset and severity of mechano-hyperalgesia and mechano-allodynia were the same in the saphenous and sciatic nerve territories.

There is no evidence from any of the three animal models for the unilateral spread of neuropathic pain anomalies, but careful tests for this have not been reported. In addition, there is no evidence in the animals of pain "jumping" to the other side after a long-standing ipsilateral presence. However, several studies of rat models report that neuropathic pain (of lesser severity) appears in the contralateral hindpaw at about the same time as it appears ipsilaterally (Attal et al. 1990; Seltzer et al. 1990; Kim and Chung 1992), an observation also noted in a version of the PNT model produced in monkey (Carlton et al. 1994).

Extraterritorial pain is explicable if somatosensory processing regions of the central nervous system are at least partly involved in the pathogenesis of the pain. The body is represented in several CNS somatotopic maps (e.g., in the ventrobasal thalamus and first and second somatosensory cortices). In the spinal cord dorsal horn, for example, neurons with receptive fields on the foot lie next to those with receptive fields on the lower leg and these, in turn, lie next to neurons with receptive fields on the thigh. These receptive fields are often not coincident with the territory of a nerve or root because many neurons are excited by input from more than one nerve or root. It therefore follows that pain due to a dysfunction of dorsal horn neurons will be felt in a portion of the somatotopic map, and this will not necessarily coincide with the anatomical borders of the peripheral nerves or dorsal roots. The animal data thus teach us that regional pain in humans may have an explicable organic basis in CNS dysfunction, and that psychogenic mechanisms are not the only logical explanation for pain with a regional distribution.

CNS CONTRIBUTIONS TO PAIN SYNDROMES EVOKED BY PERIPHERAL NERVE DAMAGE

There is an old debate about whether the cause of neuropathic pain following nerve injury resides in the peripheral or central nervous system. Work with the animal models has shown us that the answer to the question is, in at least some cases, that both PNS and CNS mechanisms are of great importance, as is their interaction.

The presence of extraterritorial pain is not the only evidence indicating a CNS component to the neuropathic pain models. For example, many laboratories have shown that centrally acting drugs that block glutaminergic receptors of the N-methyl-D-aspartate (NMDA) subtype are effective in the animal models, and there are several reports confirming a spinal site of action for this effect (for review, see Bennett 1994). Importantly, NMDA receptor blockers have a specific effect on the abnormal pain sensations, with little or no effect on pain sensitivity in normal regions. They are thus antihyperalgesics rather than morphine-like analgesics. The animal experiments with NMDA receptor blockers directed our attention to an entirely new class of drugs for the treatment of painful peripheral neuropathy.

Clinicians have long noted that a local anesthetic block of the painful region may give the patient relief for a period that is greatly in excess of the duration of the block of impulse conduction. This finding has sometimes been cited as presumptive evidence of hysteria, malingering, or exaggerated placebo responding, especially in CRPS type I patients. It is thus of note that rats also obtain long-duration relief from a local anesthetic block. In the experiments reported by Mao et al. (1992), a bolus injection of bupivacaine onto the sciatic nerve of CCI rats (proximal to the injury site and with a dose that blocks impulse conduction for no more than a few hours) significantly reduced heat-hyperalgesia for at least 24 hours after the block. An intrathecal injection of an NMDA receptor blocker, again at a dose whose pharmacological action lasts for only a few hours, also gave at least 24 hours of relief. Combining the local anesthetic block with the intrathecal NMDA receptor blocker gave at least 72 hours of relief.

How can a drug or drug combination with a brief duration of pharmacological action produce pain relief of long duration? Based on clinical experiments, Gracely et al. (1992) have proposed that the abnormal pains of peripheral neuropathy patients are at least partly due to a source of ongoing nociceptor input that dynamically maintains the central hyperexcitable state that is known to be produced by C-nociceptor input and NMDA receptor activation (Woolf and Thompson 1991). Temporary suppression of the maintaining input allows the central hyperexcitable state to gradually return toward normal; resumption of the maintaining drive reestablishes central hyperexcitability. The results obtained by Mao et al. in CCI rats are consistent with this hypothesis: suppression of a maintaining afferent input via local anesthetic nerve block, or by NMDA receptor blockade in the spinal dorsal horn, temporarily allowed the central hyperexcitable state to wane. The source of maintaining afferent input in the CCI case is believed to be spontaneous ectopic discharge in damaged sciatic afferents (Kajander and Bennett 1992).

Additional evidence for a central contribution to pain following nerve injury comes from work on rats with transection neuromas of the sciatic nerve (Wall et al. 1979). These rats self-mutilate the denervated hindpaw. This behavior is called autotomy and is believed to reflect the animal's response to a phantom pain state like that which develops in humans. Seltzer et al. (1991) have shown that electrical stimulation of the sciatic nerve at intensities that activate C nociceptors reduced the average day of onset of autotomy to 10 days from the control value of about 29 days, and increased the incidence of severe autotomy to about 80% from a control value of about 20%. Systemic injections of pharmacological doses of magnesium (an anticonvulsant and, perhaps, an inhibitor of the NMDA receptor-gated ion channel) has the opposite effect: it prolonged the onset of autotomy and lessened its severity (Feria et al.

1993). The most remarkable thing about these two experiments is that the effects of these short-acting manipulations are not manifested until days afterwards.

In summary, work with the animal models has clearly demonstrated pathogenic mechanisms in the CNS. Previous work in animals with transection neuromas has demonstrated several abnormalities in damaged primary afferents: spontaneous discharge, ephaptic cross-talk, an acquired sensitivity to cold and norepinephrine, etc. We have thus learned that both the PNS and the CNS contribute to neuropathic pain following nerve injury, and work such as that by Mao et al. (1992) and Gracely et al. (1992) highlight the importance of the interaction between these two sites of pathophysiology.

OCCULT INJURY AND "NEUROPATHIC" PAIN

CRPS type I is often precipitated by a deep tissue injury such as a sprain or orthopedic surgery. Soreness at the injury site is often present in addition to the more florid symptoms of allodynia and hyperalgesia. As Gracely et al. (1992) have pointed out, an unresolved tissue injury might serve as the source of maintaining nociceptor input for the central hyperexcitable state.

Maves and his colleagues (1993a,b) have shown that an inflammation of the rat's sciatic nerve sheath (a neuritis) at mid-thigh level can produce hyperalgesia in the ipsilateral hindpaw that lasts for about a week. The neuritis was produced by applying the pro-inflammatory chemical, pyrogallol, or an irritant (acidified saline) to the surface of the nerve; electron microscopy confirmed that actual damage to the axons within the nerve was not necessary for the effect. It is possible to imagine that an undetected neuritis in a patient might have the same effect, and that it might be expressed chronically if the neuritis was recurrent or prolonged for some reason. We can also imagine that any occult injury (e.g., an undetected stress fracture, nerve irritation from traction from operative scar tissue, a poorly healed ligament tear) might also serve as a maintaining drive for central hyperexcitability. We might also speculate that the appearance of the florid signs of central hyperexcitability, allodynia and hyperalgesia, would mask the pain of the unhealed injury from both patient and physician.

In the strict sense, the pain found in the condition produced by Maves et al. is not "neuropathic." It demonstrates, instead, that central hyperexcitability and its symptoms appear after C-nociceptor input from whatever source, be it ordinary nociception, as from an ongoing injury process, or neuropathic, as from the spontaneous discharge of damaged C-nociceptor axons. The animal models thus have taught us that there is considerable overlap in the mechanisms that produce postinjury pain and tenderness and those that are generally considered neuropathic. More specifically, animal data like that provided by Maves et al. suggest that at least some CRPS type I patients may suffer from symptoms of central hyperexcitability that are the product of ongoing nociception from the lack of resolution of the precipitating injury. It is of interest that NMDA receptor blockers are expected to block the symptoms of central hyperexcitability but not those of ongoing nociception. NMDA receptor blockers might thus allow the detection of a source of ongoing nociception by removing the florid overlay of allodynia and hyperalgesia that makes a thorough examination of the patient so difficult.

DIFFERENT PAINS, DIFFERENT MEDICINES?

Clinical trials of drugs to treat painful peripheral neuropathies typically ask the patient to rate the pain intensity before and after the drug. However, many patients have several distinct pain abnormalities, and these can occur in several combinations (Price et al. 1989), e.g., spontaneous burning pain, mechano-allodynia evoked by activation of intact Aβ-LTMs (Chapter 9, this volume), paroxysmal lancinating pains, and cold allodynia. Animal and clinical research have identified several possible pathological mechanisms for the different kinds of abnormal sensations and there is no logical reason why such different mechanisms can not coexist. For example, the preceding sections have discussed two mechanisms that almost certainly do coexist in at least some cases: spontaneous discharge from damaged C-nociceptor axons and NMDA receptor-mediated central hyperexcitability. Spontaneous discharge from damaged C nociceptors is expected to produce spontaneous burning pain, central hyperexcitability is expected to produce several symptoms, including Aβ-LTM-mediated mechano-allodynia. It is easy to imagine that these two mechanisms might respond differently to a drug. For example, an NMDA receptor blocker would be expected to reverse central hyperexcitability without affecting spontaneously discharging nociceptors. If this occurred in a patient, we would expect mechano-allodynia to decrease, but spontaneous burning pain to continue. Could we know that this had happened by asking the patient to rate *the* pain?

A considerable body of evidence from the animal models indicates that different kinds of abnormal pain respond differently to different drugs. For example, in CCI rats, Lee et al. (1994) have shown that doses of morphine and mu, delta, and kappa-opioid receptor subtype-specific agonists that powerfully suppress abnormal responses to mechanical stimulation (the Randall-Silleto paw pressure test) have little or no effect on the abnormal responses evoked by warm, hot, and cold stimuli. Tal and Bennett (1994) have shown, also in CCI rats, that a dose of the NMDA receptor blocker dextrorphan, which almost completely suppresses heat-hyperalgesia, has not even a hint of an effect against mechano-allodynia (which is not Aβ-LTM-mediated in CCI rats) in the same animals. Differential symptom sensitivity in CCI rats has been reported for several other drug treatments: systemic injections of clonidine (Kayser et al. 1995), systemic magnesium (Xiao and Bennett 1994), application of an N-type calcium channel blocker to the site of nerve injury (Xiao and Bennett 1995a), systemic and intrathecal administration of the antiepiletic, gabapentin (Xiao and Bennett 1995b), and systemic injections of a mechanistically different antiepileptic, felbamate (Imamura and Bennett 1995).

At present, there is very little evidence for differential drug sensitivity to different kinds of neuropathic pain sensations in humans. However, case reports that may demonstrate a specific reduction of central hyperexcitability by NMDA receptor blockade have appeared recently (e.g., Persson et al. 1995). In addition, there is a commonly held (but not scientifically demonstrated) clinical belief that carbamezepine is specific for paroxysmal lancinating pain in conditions other than trigeminal neuralgia. However, studies expressly designed to detect differential symptom sensitivity have only recently been started. If the phenomenon is found in humans, then the animal studies will have alerted us to the need for drug cocktails in the treatment of painful peripheral neuropathy.

THE SYMPATHETIC NERVOUS SYSTEM AND PAINFUL PERIPHERAL NEUROPATHY

The last 10 years of animal experimentation have contributed greatly to our knowledge of interactions between the sympathetic nervous system and pain mechanisms. Much of this data is likely to be relevant to understanding sympathetically maintained pain (SMP) and its contribution to CRPS type I and II, as well as other conditions.

SMP IN ANIMAL MODELS OF PAINFUL PERIPHERAL NEUROPATHY

There is no question whatsoever that SMP exists in animals. In the PNT and SNT models (Kim and Chung 1991; Shir and Seltzer 1991; Kim et al. 1993), sympathectomy (surgical, or chemically with guanethidine or 6-hydroxydopamine) or pharmacological sympathetic block (systemic injections of phentolamine and other alpha-adrenergic blockers) appears to completely eliminate the abnormal pain sensations. The pain relief occurs within 30 minutes, which is as soon as it is practical to make the examination in the animals (Kim et al. 1993). Application of alpha-2 adrenoceptor agonists intensifies the heat-hyperalgesia seen in the PNT model (Tracey et al. 1995). There is considerable debate about how to interpret the results of diagnostic (and therapeutic) sympathectomies in patients (Chapter 10, this volume) and this, in turn, has raised the question of whether SMP exists in humans. Of course, data from rats can not give the definitive answer to the clinical question, but the animal work has taught us clearly that SMP is a real organic phenomenon.

In contrast to what is found in the PNT and SNT models, the role of the sympathetic nervous system in the CCI model appears to be much more complex. First, CCI rats have the same warm-to-cold progression of abnormal skin temperature that is seen in many CRPS I and II patients. However, the cold skin of CCI rats is not due to hyperactivity of the sympathetic vasoconstrictor innervation. In fact, the sympathetic vasoconstrictor innervation to the affected hind paw of these animals disappears, perhaps due to a die-off of the postganglionic neurons as a result of absent or decreased retrograde axoplasmic transport of nerve growth factor (Wakisaka et al. 1991). As might be expected, sympathectomy during the cold phase (ca. 15 days postinjury) has no effect on the animals' abnormal pain (Wakisaka et al. 1991). These observations are of considerable importance because they contradict the common clinical assumption that cold skin is indicative of sympathetic vasoconstrictor hyperactivity and is thus prognostic for a therapeutic sympathectomy. Indeed, considerable clinical evidence now shows that the sympathetic vasoconstrictor hyperactivity hypothesis is wrong (e.g., Drummond et al. 1991). The cause of the rats' cold skin is not known, but it may reflect the vasculature's denervation supersensitivity to circulating catecholamines, as has been shown for CRPS type I patients (Arnold et al. 1993).

However, the pain syndrome seen in CCI rats does respond to sympathectomy during the first few days postinjury, but even this effect is partial: abnormal sensitivity to heat and cold were strongly suppressed but mechano-hyperalgesia was only slightly affected (Neil et al. 1991; Perrot et al. 1993). In summary, it appears that the pain syndrome produced in the CCI model is mixed SMP and SIP (sympathetically independent pain) during its early phase and entirely SIP during its later stage. This observation contrasts markedly to the apparently total and persistent SMP character of the syndromes produced in the PNT and SNT models.

If nerve injuries in rats can produce such strikingly diverse "clinical" pictures, then we should not be surprised if nerve injuries in humans produce a complex mixture of pathophysiologies. How many different conditions are we describing under the CRPS type I and II categories?

ARE FAILED SYMPATHECTOMIES REALLY FAILURES?

There are many clinical reports of CRPS type I and II patients returning to the clinic with a recurrence of pain a few weeks or months after an apparently successful sympathectomy. In such cases it is commonly assumed that the original sympathectomy was incomplete (especially if it was done at another hospital!), or that a new sympathetic innervation has arrived via ganglia rostral or caudal to those excised or from the other side. Animal experiments suggest another cause: sympathectomy itself induces SMP; specifically, sympathectomy induces acquisition of responsiveness to norepinephrine (NE) in intact C nociceptors, a phenomenon that might better be called "adrenoceptor-mediated pain (AMP)."

The initial evidence for this came from rabbits with partial lesions of the greater auricular nerve (Sato and Perl 1991). C nociceptors that survived the lesion were excited by norepinephrine (NE) applied via close arterial injection, by electrical stimulation of the sympathetic chain, or by intracutaneous injection into the nociceptor's cutaneous receptive field. Similar changes do not occur in the A-delta nociceptors (Perl 1994).

Recent work shows that nerve lesions evoke the de novo expression of alpha-2 adrenoceptors in a subset of dorsal root ganglion cells (Nishiyama et al. 1993). In addition, it has been shown that the sympathetic efferents that normally innervate the blood vessels within the dorsal root ganglia sprout and functionally innervate primary afferent cell bodies following a nerve lesion (McLachlan et al. 1993).

The rabbit's ear is a thermoregulatory organ and thus the greater auricular nerve contains a high percentage of sympathetic postganglionic fibers. Subsequent work has shown that selective damage to these fibers, by destruction of the superior cervical ganglion, is sufficient to induce NE responsiveness in C nociceptors (Perl 1994).

The relevance of this animal data to SMP and CRPS type I and II is obvious. First, partial nerve lesions that damage sympathetic postganglionic fibers may induce a situation where intact C nociceptors begin to discharge in the presence of NE, which may come from the circulation or from nearby intact sympathetic postganglionic terminals. Second, sympathectomy induces the same phenomenon. It is thus possible that an initial low incidence of NE-responsive C nociceptors is rendered asymptomatic by sympathectomy, but that symptoms (pain) reappear as a greater percentage of C nociceptors acquire NE responsiveness. If such were the case, then we can speculate that the pain-producing source of NE might change: nearby sympathetic terminals prior to sympathectomy and circulating NE (spill over from intact sympathetic terminals and, perhaps, from the adrenal glands) following sympathectomy.

The delayed development of pain after sympathectomy may also be misperceived as a recurrence of the presurgical syndrome when, in fact, it represents a new syndrome, namely postsympathectomy neuralgia. The quality of the pain in this condition may be similar to that of CRPS type I, but the locus of pain in postsympathectomy neuralgia is typically proximal to the original pain (Tracy and Cockett 1957). Knowledge gained from animal and human studies has led to the hypothesis that postsympathectomy neuralgia results from hyperexcitability of central pain pathways, due partly to preexisting, nociceptor-induced effects and partly to deafferentation-induced changes consequent to surgical transection of primary afferents projecting through the sympathetic trunk and white rami (Kramis et al. 1995). Sympathetic activation of primary afferents in the more proximal tissues also appears to play a role in postsympathectomy neuralgia, just as it does in CRPS types I and II.

SMP IN THE ABSENCE OF NERVE INJURY

The foregoing section focused on the nerve-lesioned case and it is thus most relevant to CRPS type II (causalgia). However, animal experimentation has begun to teach us a great deal about interactions between the sympathetic efferents and primary afferents in the absence of nerve injury; this work is particularly relevant to our understanding of CRPS type I (RSD).

The initial work in this area showed that the hyperalgesia that occurs in inflamed skin is made worse by NE, made better by adrenoceptor blockers, and can be partially prevented by prior sympathectomy (for review see Levine et al. 1986). It is reasonable to ascribe, at least in part, the behavioral evidence for hyperalgesia in these studies to sensitization of C nociceptors. Indeed, it has been shown that some C nociceptors with receptive fields in inflamed skin acquire an excitatory response to stimulation of the sympathetic chain or close arterial NE injections (Hu and Zhu 1989). In the absence of inflammation, the sympathetic outflow does not excite C nociceptors; in fact, it tends to suppress C-nociceptor responses to brief noxious stimuli.

Sympathetic discharge per se does not appear to be important for the induction of C-nociceptor sensitization, instead it is the presence of the sympathetic terminal that appears to be critical. Levine and his colleagues (Levine et al. 1986; Gonzales et al. 1991) have presented data that indicate that activation of the alpha-2 adrenergic autoreceptors on the sympathetic terminal evokes the synthesis of prostaglandin which, in turn, is responsible (directly or, perhaps, via intermediary steps) for sensitization of the nociceptor terminal. In addition, there is now evidence to suggest that sensitized nociceptor terminals in inflamed skin acquire NE responsiveness like that described above in the nerve-injured case (Sato et al. 1993).

The relevance of these data for patients with SMP in general, and for CRPS type I patients in particular, is not yet proven, but the implications are obvious. First, it appears that C-nociceptor sensitization may be at least partly dependent on chemical signals derived from the sympathetic terminal and that once sensitized in conjunction with ongoing inflammation, C nociceptors acquire NE responsiveness. These are normal physiological responses to injury and inflammation. Recent evidence from experiments in normal humans supports this hypothesis (Drummond 1995). We must presume that in the normal case NE responsiveness disappears when the inflammation subsides. The pathology (SMP) would appear if either the inflammation persisted for some reason, or the C-nociceptor NE responsiveness did not disappear with healing.

Sympathetic effects on non-nociceptive afferents may also contribute to pain in CRPS type I. This conclusion is derived partly from clinical demonstrations that suggest that central pain pathways that receive input from both nociceptive and non-nociceptive afferents are hyperexcitable (Price et al. 1989). Furthermore, animal studies have shown that many classes of non-nociceptive afferents can be sympathetically activated (Roberts and Foglesong 1988a,b). The concept of SMP in response to activity in non-nociceptive afferents (Roberts 1986) is consistent with the finding that most patients with CRPS type I have mechanical allodynia and that in some persons the first sensation elicited by electrical stimulation of A-beta afferents is pain and dysesthesia (Price et al. 1989).

Although animal studies have provided important leads toward an understanding of CRPS type I, the varied signs and symptoms in humans and their progression over time suggest that multiple processes contribute to the syndrome(s). It remains to be seen whether the currently available animal models of nerve-injury-evoked neuropathic pain are relevant to the human condition, especially for late-stage CRPS I.

REFERENCES

Arnold, J.M.O., Teasell, R.W., MacLeod, A.P., Brown, J.E. and Carruthers, S.G., Increased venous alpha-adrenoceptor responsiveness in patients with reflex sympathetic dystrophy, Ann. Intern. Med., 118 (1993) 619–621.

Attal, N., Jazat, F., Kayser, V. and Guilbaud, G., Further evidence for "pain-related" behaviours in a model of unilateral peripheral mononeuropathy, Pain, 41 (1990) 235–251.

Bennett, G.J., Animal models of neuropathic pain. In: G.F. Gebhart, D.L.Hammond and T.S. Jensen (Eds.), Proceedings of the 7th World Congress on Pain, Progress in Pain Research and Management, Vol. 2, IASP Press, Seattle, 1994, pp. 495–510.

Bennett, G.J. and Xie, Y.-K., A peripheral mononeuropathy in rat that produces disorders of pain sensation like those seen in man, Pain, 33 (1988) 87–107.

Carlton, S.M., Lekan, H.A., Kim, S.H. and Chung, J.M., Behavioral manifestations of an experimental model for peripheral neuropathy produced by spinal nerve ligation in the primate, Pain, 56 (1994) 155–166.

Choi, Y., Yoon, Y.W., Na, H.S., Kim, S.H. and Chung, J.M., Behavioral signs of ongoing pain and cold allodynia in a rat model of neuropathic pain, Pain, 59 (1994) 369–376.

Desmeules, J.A., Kayser, V. and Guilbaud, G., Selective opioid receptor agonists modulate mechanical allodynia in an animal model of neuropathic pain, Pain, 53 (1993) 277–285.

Drummond, P.D., Noradrenaline increases hyperalgesia to heat in skin sensitized by capsaicin, Pain, 60 (1995) 311–315.

Drummond, P.D., Finch, P.M. and Smythe, G.A., Reflex sympathetic dystrophy: the significance of differing plasma catecholamine concentrations in affected and unaffected limbs, Brain, 114 (1991) 2025–2036.

Feria, M., Abad, F., Sanchez, A. and Abreu, P., Magnesium sulphate injected subcutaneously suppresses autotomy in peripherally deafferented rats, Pain, 53 (1993) 287–293.

Gonzales, R., Sherbourne, C.D., Goldyne, M.E. and Levine, J.D., Noradrenaline-induced prostaglandin production by sympathetic postganglionic neurons is mediated by α2-adrenergic receptors, J. Neurochem., 57 (1991) 1145–1150.

Gracely, R.H., Lynch, S. and Bennett, G.J., Painful neuropathy: altered central processing, maintained dynamically by peripheral input, Pain, 51 (1992) 175–194.

Hu, S., and Zhu, J., Sympathetic facilitation of sustained discharges for polymodal nociceptors, Pain, 38 (1989) 85–90.

Imamura, Y. and Bennett, G.J., Relief of experimental painful peripheral neuropathy with felbamate, J. Pharmacol. Exp. Ther., in press.

Kajander, K.C. and Bennett, G.J., The onset of a painful peripheral neuropathy in rat: a partial and differential deafferentation and spontaneous discharge in Aβ and Aδ primary afferent neurons, J. Neurophysiol., 68 (1992) 734–744.

Kayser, V., Desmeules, J. and Guilbaud, G., Systemic clonidine differentially modulates the abnormal reactions to mechanical and thermal stimuli in rats with peripheral mononeuropathy, Pain, 60 (1995) 275–285.

Kim, S.H. and Chung, J.M., Sympathectomy alleviates mechanical allodynia in an experimental animal model for neuropathy in the rat, Neurosci. Lett., 134 (1991) 131–134.

Kim, S.H. and Chung, J.M., An experimental model for peripheral neuropathy produced by segmental spinal nerve ligation in the rat, Pain, 50 (1992) 355–363.

Kim, S.H., Na, H.S., Sheen, K. and Chung, J.M., Effects of sympathectomy on a rat model of peripheral neuropathy, Pain, 55 (1993) 85–92.

Kingery, W.S., Castellote, J.M. and Wang, E.E., A loose ligature-induced mononeuropathy produces hyperalgesia mediated by both the injured sciatic nerve and the adjacent saphenous nerve, Pain, 55 (1993) 297–304.

Kramis, R.C., Roberts, W.J. and Gillette, R.G., Postsympathectomy neuralgia: hypotheses on peripheral and central neuronal mechanisms, Pain, in press.

Kupers, R.C., Nuytten, D., De Castro-Costa, M. and Gybels, J.M., A time course study of the changes in spontaneous and evoked behaviour in a rat model of neuropathic pain, Pain, 50 (1992) 101–112.

Lee, S.H., Kayser, V., Desmeules, J. and Guilbaud, G., Differential action of morphine and various opioid agonists on thermal allodynia and hyperalgesia in mononeuropathic rats, Pain, 57 (1994) 233–240.

Levine, J.D., Taiwo, Y.O., Collins, S.D. and Tam, J.K., Noradrenaline hyperalgesia is mediated through interaction with sympathetic postganglionic neurone terminals rather than activation of primary afferent nociceptors, Nature, 323 (1986) 158–160.

Mao, J., Price, D.D., Mayer, D.J., Lu, J. and Hayes, R.L., Intrathecal MK 801 and local nerve anesthesia synergistically reduce nociceptive behaviors in rats with experimental peripheral mononeuropathy, Brain Res., 576 (1992) 254–262.

Maves, T.J., Pechman, P.S., Gebhart, G.F. and Meller, S.T., Possible chemical contribution from chronic gut sutures produces disorders of pain sensation like those seen in man, Pain, 54 (1993a) 57–69.

Maves, T.J., Pechman, P.S., Gebhart, G.F. and Meller, S.T., Continuous infusion of acidified saline around the rat sciatic nerve produces a reversible thermal hyperalgesia. In: Abstracts, 7th World Congress on Pain, IASP Publications, Seattle, 1993b, p. 31.

McLachlan, E.M., Jänig, W., Devor, M., and Michaelis, M., Peripheral nerve injury triggers noradrenergic sprouting within dorsal root ganglion, Nature, 363 (1993) 543–546.

Na, H.S., Leem, J.W. and Chung, J.M., Abnormalities of mechanoreceptors in a rat model of neuropathic pain: possible involvement in mediating mechanical allodynia, J. Neurophysiol., 70 (1993) 522–528.

Neil, A., Attal, N. and Guilbaud, G., Effects of guanethidine on sensitization to natural stimuli and self-mutilating behaviour in rats with a peripheral neuropathy, Brain Res., 565 (1991) 237–246.

Nishiyama, K., Brighton, B.W., Bossut, D.F. and Perl, E.R., Peripheral nerve injury enhances $\alpha 2$-adrenergic receptor expression by some DRG neurons, Soc. Neurosci. Abstr., 19 (1993) 499.

Perl, E.R., A reevaluation of mechanisms leading to sympathetically related pain. In: H.L. Fields and J.C. Liebeskind (Eds.), Pharmacological Approaches to the Treatment of Chronic Pain: New Concepts and Critical Issues, Progress in Pain Research and Management, Vol. 1, IASP Press, Seattle, 1994, pp. 129–150.

Perrot, S., Attal, N., Ardid, D. and Guilbaud, G., Are mechanical and cold allodynia in mononeuropathic and arthritic rats relieved by systemic treatment with calcitonin or guanethidine? Pain, 52 (1993) 41–47.

Persson, J., Axelsson, G., Hallin, R.G. and Gustafsson, L.L., Beneficial effects of ketamine in a chronic pain state with allodynia, possibly due to central sensitization, Pain, 60 (1995) 217–222.

Price, D.D., Bennett, G.J. and Rafii, A., Psychophysical observations on patients with neuropathic pain relieved by a sympathetic block, Pain, 36 (1989) 273–288.

Roberts, W.J., A hypothesis on the physiological basis for causalgia and related pains, Pain, 24 (1986) 297–311.

Roberts, W.J. and Foglesong, M.E., I. Spinal recordings suggest that wide-dynamic-range neurons mediate sympathetically maintained pain, Pain, 34 (1988a) 289–304.

Roberts, W.J. and Foglesong, M.E., II. Identification of afferents contributing to sympathetically evoked activity in wide-dynamic-range neurons, Pain, 34 (1988b) 305–314.

Sato, J. and Perl, E.R., Adrenergic excitation of cutaneous pain receptors induced by peripheral nerve injury, Science, 251 (1991) 1608–1610.

Sato, J., Suzuki, S., Iseki, T. and Kumazawa, T., Adrenergic excitation of cutaneous nociceptors in chronically inflamed rats, Neurosci. Lett., 164 (1993) 225–228.

Seltzer, Z., Dubner, R. and Shir, Y., A novel behavioral model of neuropathic pain disorders produced in rats by partial sciatic nerve injury, Pain, 43 (1990) 205–218.

Shir, Y. and Seltzer, Z., A-fibers mediate touch-evoked allodynia and hyperesthesia and C-fibers mediate thermal hyperalgesia in a rat model of sympathetically-maintained neuropathic pain, Neurosci. Lett., 115 (1990) 62–67.

Shir, Y. and Seltzer, Z., Effects of sympathectomy in a model of causalgiaform pain produced by partial sciatic nerve injury in rats, Pain, 45 (1991) 309–320.

Tal, M. and Bennett, G.J., Extra-territorial pain in rats with a peripheral mononeuropathy: mechano-hyperalgesia and mechano-allodynia in the territory of an uninjured nerve, Pain, 57 (1994) 375–382.

Tracey, D.J., Cunningham, J.E. and Romm, M.A., Peripheral hyperalgesia in experimental neuropathy: mediation by $\alpha 2$-adrenoreceptors on post-ganglionic sympathetic terminals, Pain, 60 (1995) 317–327.

Tracy, G.D. and Cockett, F.B., Pain in the lower limb after sympathectomy, Lancet, 1 (1957) 12–14.

Wakisaka, S., Kajander, K.C. and Bennett, G.J., Abnormal skin temperature and abnormal sympathetic vasomotor innervation in an experimental painful peripheral neuropathy, Pain, 45 (1991) 299–313.

Wall, P.D., Devor, M., Inbal, R., Scadding, J.W., Schonfeld, D., Seltzer, Z. and Tomkiewicz, M.M., Autotomy following peripheral nerve lesions: experimental anesthesia dolorosa, Pain, 7 (1979) 103–113.

Woolf, C.J. and Thompson, S.W.N., The induction and maintenance of central sensitization is dependent on N-methyl-D-aspartic acid receptor activation: implications for the treatment of post-injury pain hypersensitivity states, Pain, 44 (1991) 293–299.

Xiao, W.-H. and Bennett, G.J., Magnesium suppresses abnormal pain responses via a spinal site of action in rats with an experimental peripheral neuropathy, Brain Res., 666 (1994) 168–172.

Xiao, W.-H. and Bennett, G.J., Synthetic omega-conopeptides applied to the site of nerve injury suppress neuropathic pains in rats, J. Pharmacol. Exp. Ther., 274 (1995a) 666–672.

Xiao, W.-H. and Bennett, G.J., Gabapentin relieves abnormal pains in a rat model of painful peripheral neuropathy, Soc. Neurosci. Abstr., 21 (1995b) 897.

Correspondence to: Gary J. Bennett, PhD, Neurobiology and Anesthesiology Branch, National Institute of Dental Research, National Institutes of Health, Building 49/1A11, 49 Convent Dr., Bethesda, MD 20892-4410, USA. Tel: 301-496-2807; Fax: 301-402-0667.

8

Afferent Mechanisms Mediating Pain and Hyperalgesias in Neuralgia

Martin Koltzenburg

Department of Neurology, University of Würzburg, Würzburg, Germany

Patients in neuropathic pain are considerably heterogeneous and often present with a wide range of enigmatic sensory abnormalities. These usually include stimulus-independent persistent pain or dysaesthesias and a wide range of stimulus-induced hyperalgesias. Traditionally, an attempt is made to classify the condition according to the presumptive cause, such as posttraumatic neuropathic pain, painful diabetic neuropathy, or postherpetic neuralgia. However, it has been difficult to identify a common determinant for the pains in such diverse diseases. Moreover, it is unclear why only a small fraction of patients suffering from a particular disease, such as herpes zoster, develop neuralgia and why the symptoms within an etiologically defined population of patients can be extremely diverse. Furthermore, the use of a wide range of ornate, but ill-defined terms, such as reflex sympathetic dystrophy, has done little but camouflage our ignorance and even has been positively misleading in implying pathophysiological mechanisms without adequate experimental support. Finally, present treatment options are limited and even if the underlying cause of the disease is understood and can be effectively treated, such as in diabetes mellitus, there is often little corresponding pain relief. Therefore, the traditional classification of neuropathic pain states is often only of limited usefulness in the clinical management of patients in neuropathic pain.

This chapter will focus on a different approach to neuropathic pain conditions. Its rationale is based on the view that clinically distinct pain symptoms can be linked to adaptive changes of the nervous system that occur following peripheral nerve injury. For example, nociceptive afferents that develop ongoing activity after axon injury would mediate persistent pain regardless of the precipitating event. Moreover, as most patients suffer from a variable number of pain symptoms, it is possible that separate neuropathic mechanisms can coexist. It is also becoming clear that one common clinical feature of neuropathy, namely hypersensitivity to mechanical stimuli, can be mediated by several neural mechanisms and these may be simultaneously found in an individual patient.

This chapter describes the different types of hyperalgesia that can be found in humans and discusses possible underlying primary afferent mechanisms. A symptom-centered approach to neuralgia may also have clear practical advantages for targeting underlying pathophysiological mechanisms for the treatment of pain. For example, a drug preventing the sensitization of nociceptors to heat may be beneficial for those suffering from heat hyperalgesia, but may be rather ineffective in ameliorating other aspects of the pain. If multiple pathophysiological events are operating in an individual patient, a single treatment regimen may not be sufficient for obtaining global pain relief. A symptom-orientated approach to neuralgia does not negate that different painful neuropathies show clearly different clinical presentations and that some diseases may predispose to a certain constellation of pain symptoms.

Recent years have seen a surge of major discoveries on neuropathic pain mechanisms based on animal models, patient studies, and experimental skin injury in normal human volunteers. In this chapter I will focus on mechanisms that have been identified in humans as contributing to pain and hyperalgesia with special emphasis on changes affecting the primary afferent pathway. Although it is clear that changes of central nervous properties are crucial for the development of painful symptoms, notably brush-evoked pain, several lines of evidence indicate that changes in the excitability of primary nociceptive afferents may be the single most important factor in the generation and maintenance of acute inflammatory or chronic neuropathic pain in humans.

ACUTE PAIN SIGNALED BY NOCICEPTORS IN NORMAL SUBJECTS

There is broad consensus that acute pains as studied under laboratory conditions are evoked by excitation of nociceptors with thin myelinated or unmyelinated axons (Treede et al. 1992b; Handwerker and Kobal 1993; Meyer et al. 1994). In studies of concious subjects, simultaneous microneurographic recordings of primary afferents and psychophysical magnitude estimation techniques have shown that cutaneous nociceptors can encode the intensity of painful heat (Gybels et al. 1979; Van Hees and Gybels 1981; Robinson et al. 1983; LaMotte et al. 1984; Torebjörk et al. 1984b) or mechanical (Koltzenburg and Handwerker 1994) stimuli lasting few seconds (Fig. 1). However, it is also agreed that firing of a single nociceptor cannot necessarily be equated with the perception of pain. In human microneurographic experiments, it is not uncommon to activate individual nociceptors with painless stimuli. Moreover, mechano-heat-sensitive C fibers (CMH units, also known as polymodal nocicptors) innervating the hairy skin have thresholds around 41–43° C, but the psychophysical heat-pain threshold of individuals is often considerably higher (LaMotte et al. 1984; Torebjörk et al. 1984b). Increases of skin temperature that evoke an average discharge of less than 0.3 impulses per second over a 15-second period are usually painless (Van Hees and Gybels 1981). Brief mechanical impact stimuli can elicit bursts of activity with instantaneous frequencies exceeding 10 Hz without being called painful (Koltzenburg and Handwerker 1994) (Fig. 1). There is also often a considerable time lag between the firing of nociceptors and the appearance of pain following application of algesic chemicals (Adriaensen et al. 1980). In aggregate, these results led to the conclusion that both temporal and spatial summation in a population of nociceptors is important for encoding the magnitude of pain.

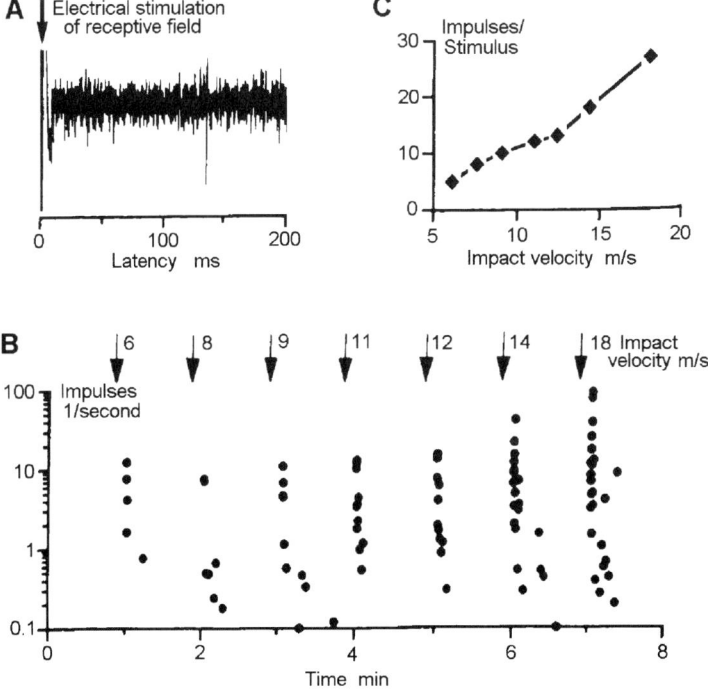

Fig. 1. A: Unmyelinated human nociceptor innervating the hairy skin and responding to transcutaneous electrical stimulation of its receptive field. B: Painless or painful mechanical stimulation was applied by graded mechanical impact stimuli (shooting a light metal probe at different impact velocities perpendicularly against the skin). Velocities below 11 m/s were not painful, despite the vigorous discharge of the nociceptor at these stimulus intensities. C: Stimulus-response function of the unit. (Koltzenburg and Handwerker 1994)

THE STIMULUS-INDEPENDENT PAIN OF NEURALGIA IS SIGNALED BY SPONTANEOUSLY ACTIVE NOCICEPTORS

Several lines of evidence converge to indicate that stimulus-independent pain in neuralgia is also mediated by nociceptive primary afferents in most patients. First, pain is often abolished or at least significantly reduced by local anesthetic block of damaged peripheral nerves (Kibler and Nathan 1960; Arnér et al. 1990; Nurmikko et al. 1991; Torebjörk et al. 1995) or affected skin (Rowbotham and Fields 1989; Gracely et al. 1992; Rowbotham et al. 1995), indicating that neural activity arising in the nerve or possibly even in the receptive endings, contributes to the pain. Second, background pain and some forms of stimulus-induced pain sensations persist during a differential nerve fiber block that eliminates conduction in myelinated nonnociceptive afferents (Campbell et al. 1988, 1992; Ochoa and Yarnitzky 1993; Koltzenburg et al. 1994b, Torebjörk et al. 1995). Third, psychophysical experiments suggest that different levels of ongoing nociceptor activity correlate with different magnitudes of pain (Gracely et al. 1992; Koltzenburg et al. 1994b). Finally, animal experiments have shown that thin myelinated or unmyelinated afferents projecting into a damaged nerve can develop ongoing activity (Devor and Jänig 1981; Häbler et al. 1987; Jänig 1988; Devor 1994; Devor et al. 1994b; Koltzenburg et al. 1994b).

The exact mechanisms contributing to the ectopic discharge are not fully understood. One possible explanation is the novel expression or upregulation of sodium channels; alternatively, a depression of potassium conductances could produce increased excitability (Devor 1994; Devor et al. 1994b). Thus, the crucial element mediating persistent pain in neuropathic conditions is the continuous discharge of nociceptors. This stereotypic reaction of nociceptors is also found in inflammatory conditions (Handwerker and Reeh 1991; Meyer et al. 1994) where the magnitude of chemogenic pain in psychophysical experiments correlates with the intensity of the discharge observed in human microneurographic recordings (Handwerker et al. 1991; LaMotte et al. 1992). The continuous discharge of nociceptors supplying damaged tissue is probably moderated by a combinations of inflammatory mediators that can directly depolarize the receptive terminals (Handwerker and Reeh 1991; Meyer et al. 1994). Although the mechanisms leading to continuous nociceptor discharge are probably different in neuropathic or inflammatory conditions, they entail similar psychophysical consequences. This is the reason why virtually all inflammatory pains and probably most neuropathic pain states can be abolished by local anesthesia of affected nerves. As the mechanisms causing persisting discharges of nociceptors are different, it is not surprising that drugs often are not equally effective in both conditions.

Nonetheless, commonalties in acute inflammatory and chronic neuropathic conditions also have been observed for a variety of stimulus-induced hyperalgesias. In fact, progress on the understanding of some enigmatic symptoms of neuralgia has been provided by the comparison between patients with neuropathic pain and normal human volunteers subjected to experimental skin lesions. Dating back to the pioneering studies of Lewis (1942), Hardy (1952), and their colleagues, two zones of increased pain sensitivity (hyperalgesia) can be distinguished following experimental injury (Raja et al. 1984; Simone et al. 1989; LaMotte et al. 1991; LaMotte 1992; Koltzenburg et al. 1992, 1994b; Treede et al. 1992; Ali et al. 1994; Kilo et al. 1994) (Fig. 2). First is the area of tissue injury—the zone of primary hyperalgesia—in which there is an increased sensitivity for heat and a variety of mechanical and presumably chemical stimuli. Second, in a halo of apparently uninjured tissue—the zone of secondary hyperalgesia—there is hyperalgesia to mechanical stimuli and possibly to cold (Gracely et al. 1993). It is also clear that mechanical hyperalgesia can be further differentiated into at least four subtypes that differ in their temporal and spatial profile and in the relative importance of contributing nociceptive and non-nociceptive primary afferents (Kilo et al. 1994). These subtypes include brush-evoked pain and hyperalgesias to pinprick, blunt pressure or impact stimuli, and can be induced experimentally in humans by mild burn or freeze injury of the skin or application of the algesic chemicals capsaicin or mustard oil (Table I). In neuropathic conditions the distinction between primary and secondary area is less clearly defined, but probably corresponds to the tissue supplied by a damaged nerve and the area outside this territory.

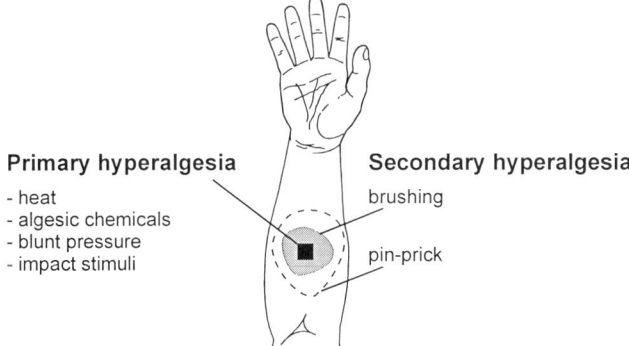

Fig. 2. The spatial pattern of primary and secondary hyperalgesia after an experimental skin injury in normal volunteers. In the primary zone, ■ which has been exposed to a freeze trauma, there is hyperalgesia to heat, pressure, and impact stimuli, and probably also to algesic chemicals. Two types of mechanical hyperalgesia to pinprick (□) and brushing (□ gray shading) stimuli are found in both the secondary and primary zones.

Table I
Mechanisms moderating cutaneous persistent pain and hyperalgesia to heat, cold, algesic chemical, or mechanical stimuli

Stimulus	Location (zone)*	Primary Afferents	Possible Neural Mechanism
None (ongoing pain)	region of injury	Nociceptors (Aδ and C fibers)	*Ongoing activity* of nociceptors
Heat	1° only	Nociceptors (C fibers in hairy skin, Aδ fibers in glabarous skin)	*Peripheral sensitization* of nociceptors
Chemical (including catecholamines)	1° only	Nociceptors (mainly C fibers)	*Peripheral sensitization* of nociceptors
Brush, touch	1° and 2°	Aβ low-threshold mechanoreceptors	*Central plasticity*, induced and sustained by peripheral nociceptor activity
Punctate stimuli (pinprick)	1° and 2°	Nociceptors (Aδ and C fibers)	*Central plasticity*, induced but not dependent on further peripheral nociceptor activity
Blunt pressure	1° only	Nociceptors (mainly C fibers)	*Peripheral recruitment* of nociceptors
Impact stimuli	1° only	Nociceptors (mainly C fibers)	*Peripheral sensitization* of nociceptors
Cold	a. 1° and 2°	a. Sensitive cold receptors	a. *Central plasticity*
	b. 1° only	b. Nociceptors	b. *Central disinhibition*

*1° zone: the area of tissue damage or innervation territory of a lesioned nerve;
2° zone: the area of uninjured tissue surrounding the 1° zone where sensory abnormalities can be detected.

HYPERALGESIA TO HEAT IS MEDIATED BY SENSITIZED NOCICEPTORS

A hallmark of inflammatory pain is the hyperalgesia to heat. Although this symptom occurs only occasionally under neuropathic conditions, the underlying mechanism appears to be similar and is thought to be sensitized nociceptors. As shown by differential nerve blocks, heat hyperalgesia in hairy skin is signaled by unmyelinated, presumably nociceptive afferents (Cline et al. 1989; Culp et al. 1989; LaMotte et al. 1991, 1992; Koltzenburg et al. 1992b, 1994; Treede et al. 1992b; Meyer et al. 1994). In healthy volunteers there is a significant leftward shift of the stimulus-response function that relates the magnitude of pain to the stimulus energy of a heat stimulus following a mild burn injury (LaMotte et al. 1982, 1983, 1984; Thalhammer and LaMotte 1982; Robinson et al. 1983; Torebjörk et al. 1984b), tissue inflammation (Kocher et al. 1987), treatment with algesic chemicals (Beck and Handwerker 1974; Lang et al. 1990; Handwerker et al. 1991), or mechanical tissue damage (Koltzenburg and Handwerker 1994). There is a parallel reduction of the threshold for heat pain and that of mechano-heat-sensitive C fibers (Fig. 3). The hyperalgesic area is strictly confined to the region of tissue injury (primary hyperalgesia), as is the region in which nociceptor sensitization can be observed (Raja et al. 1984; LaMotte et al. 1991; Koltzenburg et al. 1992b; Ali et al. 1994; Kilo et al. 1994). Microneurographic recordings have shown directly that chronic sensitization of nociceptors can occur in patients (Cline et al. 1989; Torebjörk 1990). While heat hyperalgesia is primarily caused by sensitization of primary afferents, there is evidence that additional central sensitization contributes to heat hyperalgesia at temperatures near tolerance level (LaMotte 1984).

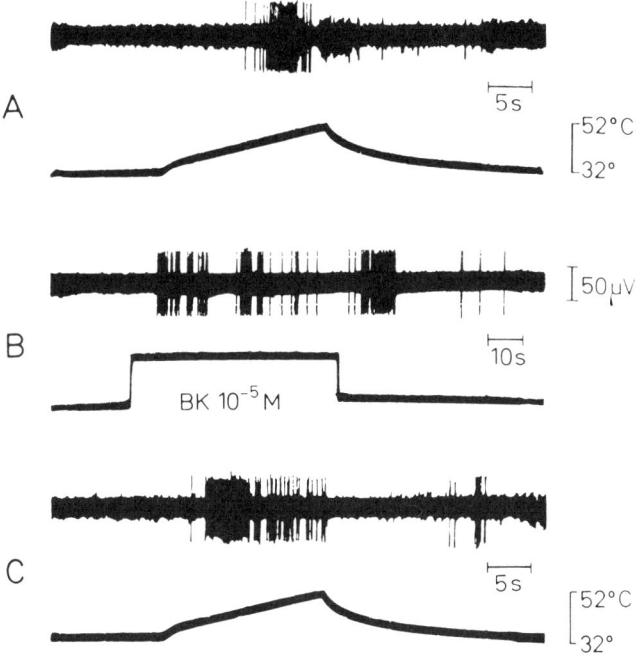

Fig. 3. In vitro record of an unmyelinated nociceptor innervating rat hairy skin. The unit encoded the intensity of noxious radiant heat (**A,** lower trace) and was excited by application of bradykinin to its receptive field (**B**). After exposure to bradykinin there was a drop of the threshold and an increased firing to suprathreshold stimuli (**C**), which indicate sensitization. (Koltzenburg et al. 1992a)

In glabrous skin a different peripheral mechanism signals the hyperalgesia to heat after a mild burn injury. The glabrous skin of primates is supplied by both heat-sensitive unmyelinated nociceptors and heat-insensitive thin myelinated nociceptors (Campbell et al. 1979; Meyer and Campbell 1981; Campbell and Meyer 1983; Torebjörk and Ochoa 1990). In contrast to hairy skin, the unmyelinated nociceptors of the glabarous skin surprisingly do not display an increased responsiveness following burn injury, but desensitize (Campbell and Meyer 1983). Yet, the previously heat-insensitive units start to respond to heat, and it has been concluded that the novel responsiveness of these units signals the magnitude of heat pain in hyperalgesic skin (Meyer and Campbell 1981; Meyer et al. 1994). Little is known about the mechanisms that cause heat hyperalgesia in glabrous skin in neuralgia.

HYPERALGESIA TO ALGESIC CHEMICALS

Few studies have examined the possibility of a hyperalgesia to chemical stimuli. The main information comes from animal studies that suggest the existence of a chemical hyperalgesia in the primary, but not in the secondary zone. For example, while only half the unmyelinated cutaneous nociceptors respond in normal skin to the algesic mediator bradykinin (Beck and Handwerker 1974; Kirchhoff et al. 1990; Lang et al. 1990; Khan et al. 1992; Koltzenburg et al. 1992a), almost all fibers do so in inflamed tissue (Kirchhoff et al. 1990; Handwerker and Reeh 1991). The increased sensitivity to bradykinin can also be acutely mimicked in vitro by addition of a soup of inflammatory mediators containing serotonin, prostaglandins, or protons that are ususally present in exudates of inflamed tissues (Lang et al. 1990; Handwerker and Reeh 1991; Kessler et al. 1992). With persistent tissue inflammation nociceptors may also start to express novel types of bradykinin receptors (Dray and Perkins 1993). Hyperalgesia to inflammatory mediators is probably present in normal volunteers following experimental tissue injury, but it has so far not been systematically examined in neuralgia.

SENSITIZATION OF UNMYELINATED NOCICEPTIVE AFFERENTS TO CATECHOLAMINES CAN BE THE BASIS FOR SYMPATHETICALLY MAINTAINED PAIN

A special case of chemical hyperalgesia may prevail in sympathetically maintained pain states. Animal studies have shown repeatedly that application of catecholamines or activation of sympathetic postganglionic efferents can only minimally modulate the discharge of non-nociceptive afferents or nociceptors under physiological conditions (Jänig and Koltzenburg 1992). It has also been determined beyond doubt that most types of primary afferents, including nociceptors, can develop a sensitivity to catecholamines and are excited by sympathetic stimulation after peripheral nerve injury (Koltzenburg and McMahon 1991; Jänig and Koltzenburg 1992; Devor 1994; Jänig and McLachlan 1994; Perl 1994). Experimental nerve injury in animals has shown that such interaction between sympathetic and sensory systems exists at several points in the peripheral nervous system: (1) the axon tip of regenerating erstwhile nociceptors (Devor and Jänig 1981; Blumberg and Jänig 1984; Häbler et al. 1987) (Fig. 4A); (2) the receptive endings of presumably non-injured nociceptive afferents projecting into the innervation territory of a partially lesioned nerve (Sato and Perl 1991; Selig et al. 1993; Koltzenburg et al. 1994a; Bossut and Perl 1995) (Fig. 4B); and (3) coupling can occur in the dorsal root ganglion that contains axotomized neurons (McLachlan et al. 1993; Devor et al. 1994a).

These unequivocal findings raise the possibility that persisting neuropathic pain in humans may be in part maintained by the sympathetic nervous system. Indeed, the importance of the sympathetic nervous system in the generation of pain has been the focus of a long, if controversial, debate. Two lines of evidence suggest that the persisting pain in some patients is caused or maintained by the sympathetic nervous system. First, sympatholytic therapy can abolish pain and hyperalgesia (Loh and Nathan 1978; Schott 1986; Bonica 1990; Campbell et al. 1992; Treede et al. 1992; Wahren and Torebjörk 1992; Campbell et al. 1994). Second, in patients for whom sympatholytic therapy had provided pain relief, intracutaneous injection of adrenoceptor agonists rekindled pain and hyperalgesia (Wallin et al. 1976; Davis et al. 1991; Torebjörk et al. 1995) (Fig. 5). Furthermore, injections of catecholamines around a stump neuroma can precipitate pain attacks (Chabal et al. 1992).

Given that a pain response can be induced during a differential blockade of myelinated fibers, unmyelinated fibers are sufficient to signal sympathetically maintained pain (Torebjörk et al. 1995). An explanation consistent with these findings is that primary afferents acquire a sensitivity to catecholamines, which extends in some conditions to the receptive terminals innervating a symptomatic skin region (Fig. 4). Importantly, a pain response with a challenging noradrenalin injection is only obtained in patients suffering from sympathetically maintained pains, but not in those with sympathetically independent pain (Torebjörk et al. 1995).

The mechanisms causing this novel and abnormal catecholamine sensitivity are not completely understood. One suggestion is that a general excitability increase of nociceptors may permit preexisting adrenoceptors to become effective (Devor 1994; Devor et al. 1994b). Another explanation supported by animal studies is that injured neurons start to express adrenoceptors (McMahon 1991; Perl 1994). Animal models of inflammatory pain also suggest that catecholamines could act on postganglionic terminals to release mediators that are known to sensitize nociceptors (Koltzenburg and McMahon 1991; Jänig

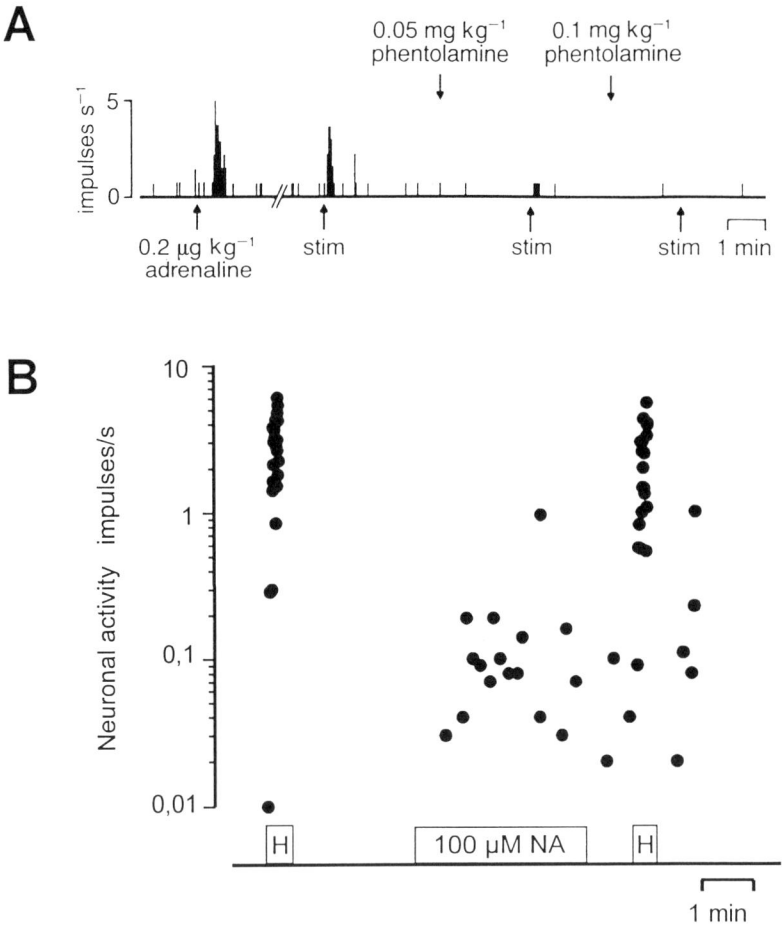

Fig. 4. Excitation of nociceptive C fibers by sympathetic activation after peripheral nerve lesion. **A:** Activation of a single unmyelinated fiber projecting into a neuroma-in-continuity of the cat several months after nerve lesion. The unit had low ongoing activity and responded to intravenous application of adrenaline and electrical stimulation (stim) of postganglionic sympathetic fibers. All responses were blocked and ongoing activity was significantly reduced by the nonselective α-adrenoceptor antagonist phentolamine. From Koltzenburg and McMahon (1991). **B:** Response of a CMH fiber to superfusion of the receptive terminal with noradrenalin recorded from a rat with a chronic constriction injury of the nerve. H, noxious heat stimulus. (Koltzenburg et al. 1994a)

and Koltzenburg 1992; Heller et al. 1994; Levine and Taiwo 1994). However, the pain of neuralgia could be rekindled in patients in whom surgical sympathectomy had produced pain relief, indicating that the pain-provoking action of catecholamines in patients does not involve the presence of post-ganglionic sympathetic fibers (Wallin et al. 1976). In aggregate, several lines of evidence show that sensitization of unmyelinated nociceptive afferents to catecholamines can be the basis for sympathetically maintained pain (Campbell et al. 1992, 1994; Koltzenburg et al. 1994a; Torebjörk et al. 1995). It is theoretically possible that other mechanisms might contribute to sympathetically maintained pain states (Schott 1986; Blumberg and Jänig 1994), although these possibilities have so far not been supported by rigorous experimental studies in humans.

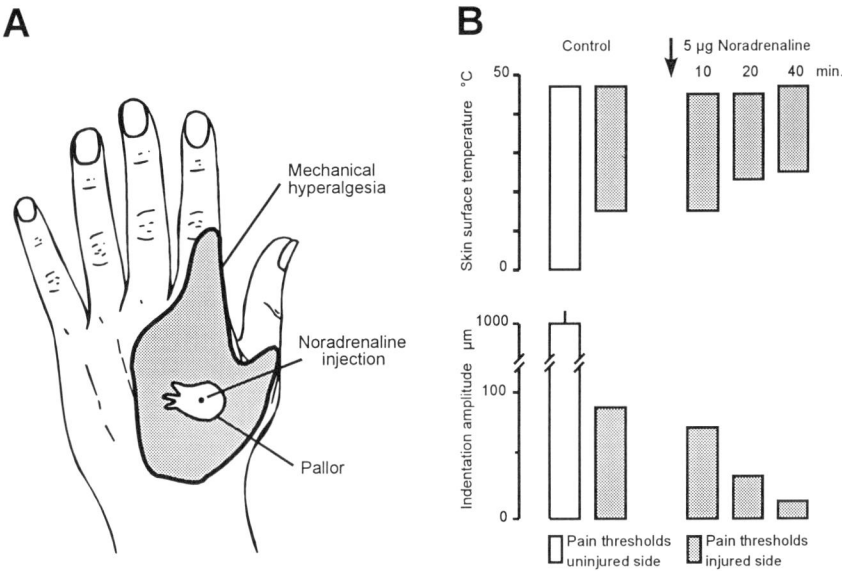

Fig. 5. **A:** Area of pallor and touch-evoked pain 20 minutes after intradermal injection of noradrenalin in a patient with sympathetically maintained pain. The test was performed during a time when the patient was temporarily relieved from pain by a local anesthetic block of the stellate ganglion. **B:** Results of sequential quantitative sensory tests in the same patient (without sympatholytic intervention) in whom injection of 5 μg noradrenalin into the symptomatic skin aggravated stimulus-independent pain and hyperalgesias. Note progressive worsening of hyperalgesia to cold (tested with a Peltier device; upper panel) and to vibratory stimuli (lower panel) starting approximately 20 minutes after injection on the injured side. (Modified from Torebjörk et al. 1995)

TYPES OF MECHANICAL HYPERALGESIA IN HUMANS

Hypersensitivity to mechanical stimuli are extremely diverse and evidence is now forthcoming that at least four distinct types of mechanical hyperalgesia can be identified in humans. While hyperalgesia to heat and algesic chemicals can readily be explained by sensitization of nociceptors, this mechanism is unlikely to play the same important role for mechanical hyperalgesia, as reduction of mechanical thresholds of nociceptors rarely occurs in conditions that produce intense mechanical hyperalgesia. Therefore, other mechanisms are likely to contribute, notably the sensitization of central neurons.

BRUSH-EVOKED PAIN

One of the enigmatic painful symptoms, whose neural basis until recently could hardly be explained, is pain evoked by lightly touching the skin. Several investigations of patients in chronic neuropathic pain have shown some astonishing similarities of the clinical presentation of touch-evoked pain (also known as allodynia) in neuralgia and of experimentally induced pain following application of irritant chemicals (Campbell et al. 1992; Gracely et al. 1992; Koltzenburg et al. 1994b; Koltzenburg and Torebjörk 1995). This observation has led to the conclusion that some of the basic underlying mechanisms in both conditions are similar, if not identical. A string of evidence shows that touch-evoked pain in both conditions is not mediated by nociceptors, but instead is signaled out of the skin by sensitive mechanoreceptors with large myelinated axons that normally encode nonpainful tactile events (Table I). First, differential blockade of large myelinated non-nociceptive afferents abolishes brush-evoked pain (Campbell et al. 1988; Koltzenburg et al. 1992b, 1994b; Torebjörk et al. 1992). Second, transcutaneous (Price et al. 1989, 1992) or intraneural electrical stimulation (Torebjörk 1990; Torebjörk et al. 1992) of these afferents causes painful dysesthesias. Third, reaction time measurements indicate that brush-evoked pain is signaled by fast-conducting myelinated fibers (Fruhstorfer and Lindblom 1984; LaMotte et al. 1991; Lindblom 1994). Finally, light punctate mechanical stimuli that can only activate sensitive mechanoreceptors are often called painful in neuralgia (Price et al. 1989, 1992; Campbell et al. 1992; Lindblom 1994; Torebjörk et al. 1995).

The gist of this reasoning is that the crucial switch from the encoding of tactile sensations to touch-evoked pain has to occur in the CNS, probably to a large extent in the dorsal horn of the spinal cord. However, this qualitative switch of mechanoreceptor function hinges critically on persistent nociceptor input (LaMotte et al. 1991; Gracely et al. 1992; Koltzenburg et al. 1994b). The general principle is a two-step process in which persisting discharge of sensitized nociceptors evokes pain and produces a concomitant sensitization of central pain-signaling neurons to inputs from normal mechanoreceptors (Fig. 6).

Microneurographic recordings and psychophysical studies agree that changes of the ongoing burning pain reflect the different levels of nociceptor firing (Culp et al. 1989; LaMotte et al. 1991, 1992; Koltzenburg et al. 1992b, 1994b) and because of the profound heat sensitization they are strongly affected by skin-surface temperature. Thus, innocuous warming of the skin increases the magnitude of ongoing pain and nociceptor activity, while mild cooling reduces or even abolishes it. Importantly, the severity of touch-evoked pain (reflecting central sensitization) changes strictly in parallel with the magnitude of background pain. The fluctuations can be extremely fast and changes can be induced within seconds in acute experimental inflammation of the skin (Koltzenburg et al. 1994b). Patients in neuropathic pain also report that "spontaneous fluctuation" of persisting pain is usually paralleled by corresponding changes of their hypersensitivity to touch. In those few persons who present with heat hyperalgesia (encoded by sensitized nociceptors) the intentional increase of skin-surface temperature could rapidly aggravate both persisting and touch-evoked pains (Koltzenburg et al. 1994b) (Fig. 7).

Patients without demonstrable heat hyperalgesia do not show this increased pain response following elevation of skin-surface temperature, but frequently complain about parallel fluctuations of both pain measures. An explanation consistent with this finding is that other factors influence the discharge of

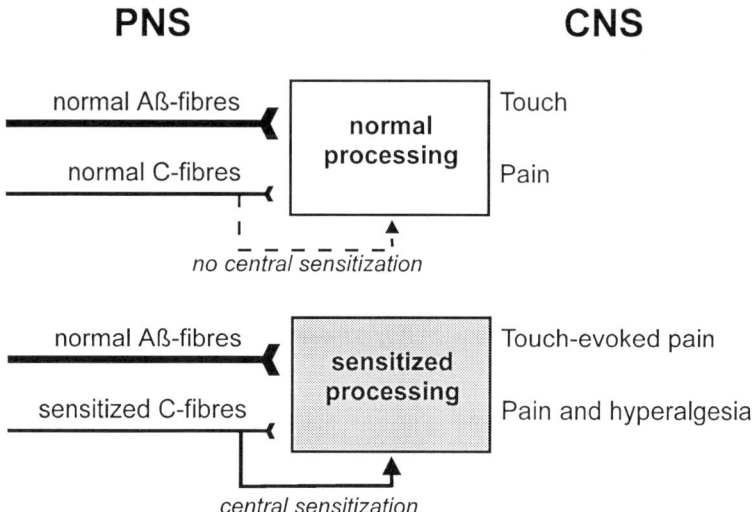

Fig. 6. The mechanism producing pain, hyperalgesia, and touch-evoked pain in neuralgia.

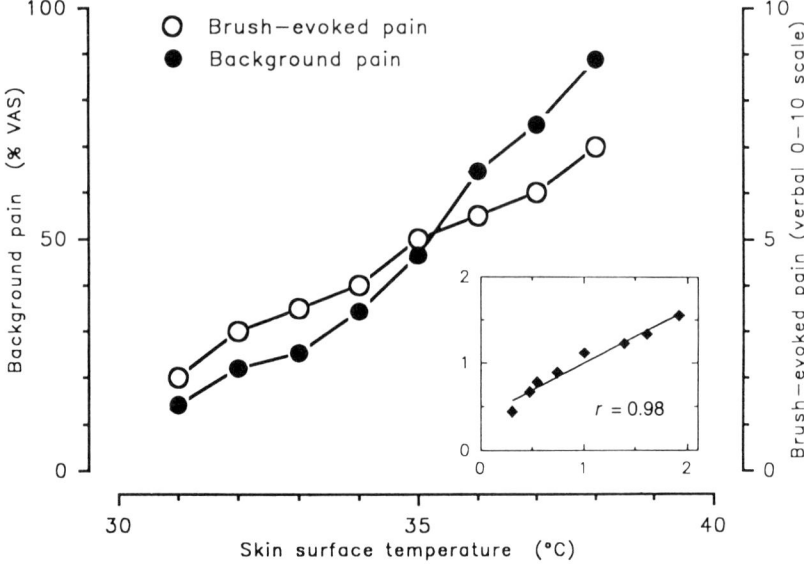

Fig. 7. Parallel increases of background pain (rated on a visual analog scale) and brush-evoked pain (rated on a verbal categorical scale) follow graded increases of skin-surface temperature on the dorsum of the hand in a patient with chronic posttraumatic neuralgia. Inset shows high correlation of normalized ratings. Quantitative sensory tests demonstrated increases of ongoing pain (heat hyperalgesia due to peripheral sensitization), which probably was mediated by unmyelinated nociceptors, while brush-evoked pain (mechanical hyperalgesia due to central sensitization) was signaled by large myelinated mechanoreceptive afferents. (Koltzenberg et al. 1994b)

nociceptors. In patients with sympathetically maintained pain, catecholamines acting on excitatory adrenoceptors expressed on nociceptors may be the culprit (Campbell et al. 1992, 1994; Meyer et al. 1992; Treede et al. 1992; Torebjörk et al. 1995). The kinetic of this process in both chronic neuralgia and acute experimental pains is very fast and requires only few seconds, indicating that the nociceptor-induced CNS processes that allow touch-evoked pain to be expressed are very dynamic. The rapid fluctuations of persisting pains and hyperalgesias provide hope that persistent nociceptor discharge and ensuing central sensitization remain malleable even after years of chronic pain.

PINPRICK HYPERALGESIA

Hyperalgesia to pinprick stimuli can be found in the primary and secondary zone of hyperalgesia after experimental tissue injury and probably in patients suffering from neuralgia. It is distinct from that of brush-evoked pain because of its different spatial and temporal profile. The area of pinprick hyperalgesia is not only larger than that of brush-evoked pain, but its duration is longer after a single application of capsaicin in normal volunteers (Simone et al. 1989; LaMotte et al. 1991; Koltzenburg et al. 1992b; Cervero et al. 1994; Kilo et al. 1994). Moreover, in contrast to brush-evoked pain, hyperalgesia to punctate stimuli appears to be carried out of the skin by nonsensitized nociceptive primary afferents that impinge on a sensitized central nervous system (Kilo et al. 1994). However, we do not yet understand why hyperalgesia is only restricted to mechanical stimuli and cannot be elicited by thermal excitation of nociceptors (Raja et al. 1984; Ali et al. 1994; Kilo et al. 1994). One consistent explanation is that only mechanosensitive nociceptors, but not heat-sensitive fibers, are capable of signaling hyperalgesia to punctate stimuli. Although excitation of unmyelinated afferents is important for the initiation of this type of central sensitization, it is not required for sustaining it (LaMotte et al. 1991; Kilo et al. 1994).

HYPERALGESIA TO BLUNT PRESSURE OR IMPACT STIMULI OCCURS ONLY IN THE PRIMARY ZONE OF INJURY

Two further types of mechanical hyperalgesia can be elicited experimentally in normal humans and are found only in the region of tissue injury (Fig. 8): hyperalgesia to blunt pressure (Culp et al. 1989; Koltzenburg et al. 1992b; Kilo et al. 1994) and hyperalgesia to impact stimuli (Kilo et al. 1994). Both hyperalgesias are mediated by nociceptive, probably unmyelinated, afferents.

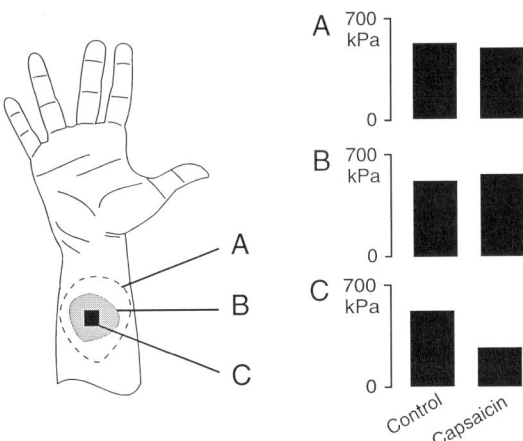

Fig. 8. Reduction of pressure-pain threshold after topical application of capsaicin is only observed in the area of primary hyperalgesia (C), but not in the zone of secondary hyperalgesia as defined by brushing (B) or pinprick (A) stimuli (Kpa = kilo Pascal). (Modified from Koltzenberg et al. 1992b)

Hyperalgesia to pressure that is mediated by unmyelinated nociceptive afferents has also been described in neuralgia patients (Cline et al. 1989; Ochs et al. 1989; Price et al. 1992; Ochoa and Yarnitzky 1993; Koltzenburg et al. 1994b). We do not fully understood how nociceptive afferents can encode these sensations. It seems unlikely that a central sensitization is solely responsible because this hyperalgesia is strictly confined to the region of tissue injury (Culp et al. 1989; Koltzenburg et al. 1992b; Kilo et al. 1994), while humans can localize C-fiber stimuli only with a precision of 10–20 mm (Lewis 1942; Nathan and Rice 1966; Koltzenburg et al. 1993). Yet, following topical application of capsaicin, most mechanosensitive nociceptors do not change their threshold (LaMotte et al. 1992; Schmidt et al. 1995), so other mechanisms are probably involved.

One possibility is that pressure will spread inflammatory mediators further into the tissue, which would cause subsequent excitation of previously nonactive nociceptors (Koltzenburg et al. 1992b; Kilo et al. 1994).

A second explanation is that receptive field size increases and results in a spatial summation at central synapses. In normal skin the receptive fields for mechanical stimuli or heat overlap in individual CMH fibers (Treede et al. 1990). However, following a burn injury (Thalhammer and LaMotte 1982), application of noxious chemicals (Schmelz et al. 1994), or mechanical damage (Reeh et al. 1987), a subpopulation of the cutaneous nociceptors expands their mechanical receptive field (Fig. 9). The expansion is limited to the area of tissue damage and often does not result in a general decrease of the mechanical threshold of the unit. A recent microneurographic investigation using unbiased electrical search procedures indicated that the majority of the unmyelinated afferents had branches that were unresponsive to mechanical stimulation in normal skin. Importantly, about two-thirds of these unresponsive branches became responsive to mechanical stimuli following application of irritant chemicals (Schmelz et al. 1994). The mechanism for this expansion are not completely understood, but it may reflect the sensitization of receptive branches with excessive mechanical thresholds or the removal of a branch-point conduction block. The expansion of receptive fields produces a spatial summation of nociceptive input because more nociceptors will be activated by a given stimulus (Fig. 9).

A third explanation that would also result in a spatial summation is the activation of a novel class of sensory neurons that do not respond to transient noxious mechanical or thermal stimuli but that have a chemical sensitivity that makes them particularly responsive to tissue inflammation (Fig. 10). This type of afferent unit has been given a variety of names such as sleeping nociceptors, silent afferents, or mechanically insensitive afferents (McMahon and Koltzenburg 1990; Meyer et al. 1994; Schmidt et al. 1994). They are ubiquitous and are found in skin and particularly in deep somatic (Schmidt et al. 1994) and visceral tissues (Koltzenburg and McMahon 1995) where up to 50% of the unmyelinated units may fall into this category. Moreover, mechanically insensitive afferents are found in all species examined so far including rat, cat, monkey, and humans, and in structures such as skin (Baumann et al. 1991; Kress et al. 1992; LaMotte et al. 1992; Davis et al. 1993; Lewin and Mendell 1994; Schmidt et al. 1995), joints (Grigg et al. 1986; Schmidt 1985; Schaible and Schmidt 1988; Schaible and Grubb 1993; Schmidt et al. 1994), skeletal muscle (Kniffki et al. 1978), and viscera (Häbler et al. 1988; Häbler et al. 1990; Dmitrieva and McMahon 1994; Wen and Morrison 1994; Koltzenburg and McMahon 1995). In humans these mechanically insensitive afferents may comprise up to 20% of the unmyelinated afferents innervating the hairy skin (Schmidt et al. 1995). They are dormant in healthy tissue, but responded vigorously following application of algesic compounds or during the onset of an inflammation induced by chemical irritants. Importantly, the excitation often requires tens of minutes, which contrasts with the rapid sensitization of nociceptors to heat or the expansion of mechanical receptive

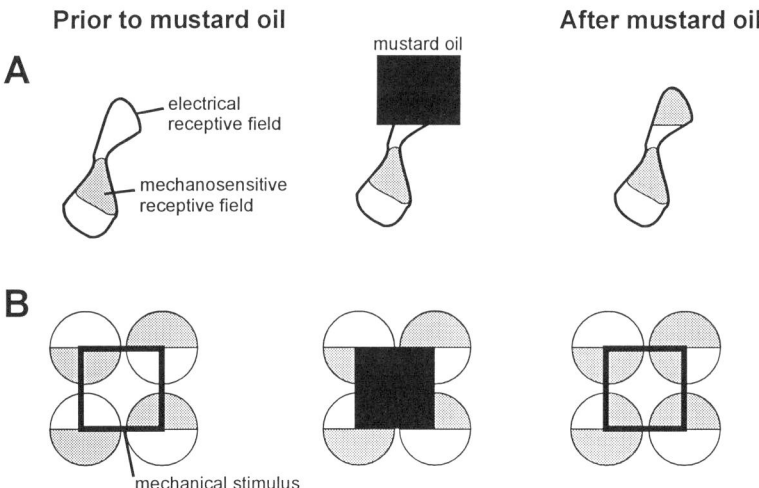

Fig. 9. **A:** Expansion of the mechanosensitive receptive field of a human unmyelinated nociceptor innervating hairy skin. The area of the receptive field of the unit was mapped with transcutaneous electrical or mechanical stimuli. An initially mechanically unresponsive area was treated with the irritant mustard oil and this region strictly confined to the borders of the mustard oil patch and the electrically defined receptive field, became sensitive for mechanical stimuli in the inflamed state. From Schmelz et al. (1994). **B:** Schematic illustration of how the expansion of receptive fields could lead to a spatial summation. In this example, two units fire to a mechanical stimulus prior to mustard oil, while twice as many units would respond thereafter.

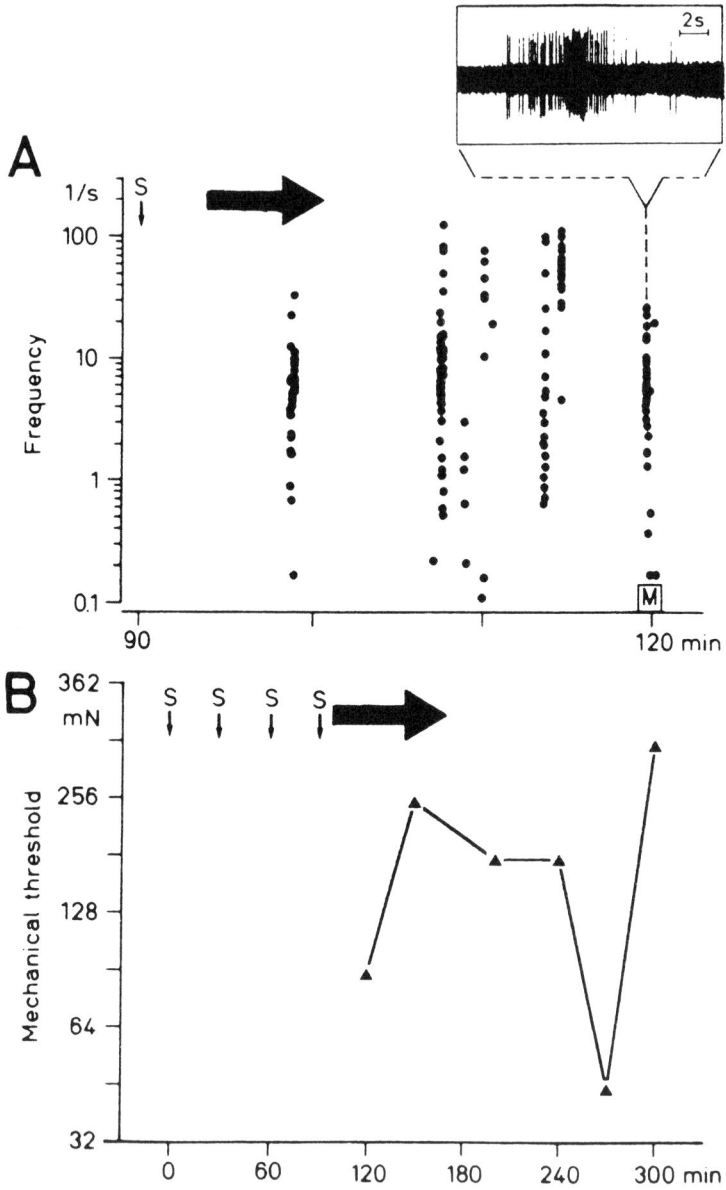

Fig. 10. Recruitment of a previously unresponsive cutaneous C fiber in the rat at the onset of an inflammation (**A**). The receptive field of the unit had been localized with an electrical search procedure. During an initial 90-minute observation interval (**B**), it did not respond to repeated application of noxious mechanical or thermal stimuli (S = mechanical and thermal tests delivered every 30 minutes). After topical application of mustard oil (large horizontal arrows) the unit discharged in bursts (**A**) and started to respond to mechanical stimuli (M). (Kress et al. 1992).

fields. Once excited, the newly responsive afferents remain active for many hours. In some conditions they can quantitatively contribute the majority of the total afferent input signaled at the onset of an acute inflammation to the CNS (Koltzenburg and McMahon 1995).

Although hyperalgesia to pressure stimuli can readily be found following topical capsaicin application, there is no demonstrable hyperalgesia to impact stimuli, indicating that both types of hyperalgesia are distinct and require special conditions (Kilo et al. 1994). *Hyperalgesia to impact stimuli* is a unique sensation that occurs after inflammation of superficial skin layers by UV-irradiation or freeze lesions (Fig. 11). It is commonly experienced by slapping an area of sunburn. Under laboratory conditions quantifiable impact stimuli can be administered by shooting light metal bullets perpendicularly against the skin (Kohllöffel et al. 1991; Koltzenburg and Handwerker 1994). The distinction between these two types of mechanical hyperalgesia is likely to have a clinical correlate. For example, a patient suffering from erythromelalgia had severe, persistent burning pain, an exquisite brush-evoked pain, and hyperalgesia to pinprick and blunt pressure, but not to impact stimuli

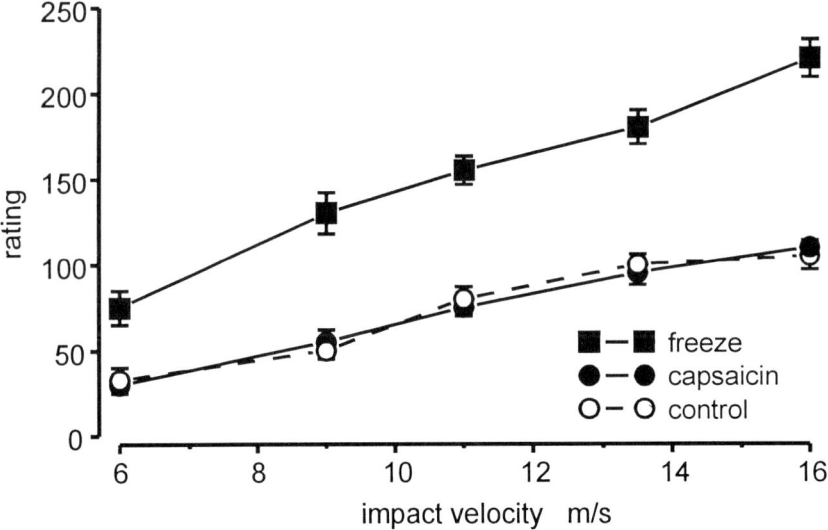

Fig. 11. Hyperalgesia to impact stimuli is present after a freeze lesion, but not after topical capsaicin treatment. Painless or painful graded mechanical impact stimuli were applied by shooting a light metal probe at different impact velocities perpendicularly against the skin. Using magnitude estimation techniques, a group of normal volunteers rated the intensity of the impact stimulus using a value of 100 as pain threshold. A value of 200 is assigned to stimuli that produce pain intensity of twice the threshold intensity. Despite persistent pain and hyperalgesia to heat, pressure, innocuous brushing, and pinprick, capsaicin treatment does not produce hyperalgesia to impact stimuli. (Modified from Kilo et al. 1994).

(Kilo et al. 1994). This constellation exactly matches the sensory abnormalities that are found after topical capsaicin treatment in normal volunteers and indicates that mechanical hyperalgesia in neuralgia is not a nonspecific increase of pain sensitivity.

TWO MECHANISMS MAY CONTRIBUTE TO COLD HYPERALGESIA IN HUMANS

Hyperalgesia to cold is a hallmark of neuropathic pain, and mildly cooling an affected region is often described as burning pain (Frost et al. 1988). Two populations of fine afferent fibers are readily excited by cold, namely sensitive cold receptors, which have myelinated afferents in humans, and nociceptors (LaMotte and Thalhammer 1982; Konietzny 1984; Kress et al. 1992; Simone et al. 1994a). Cold stimuli can also modify the discharge of mechanoreceptive afferents with large myelinated fibers (Konietzny 1984; Jänig and Koltzenburg 1992). Psychophysical studies in normal humans have shown that sensitive cold-specific afferents can inhibit the effect of nociceptor stimulation at a central, probably spinal, level (Bini et al. 1984). Furthermore, studies in healthy volunteers have shown that blockade of sensitive cold receptive afferents would lead to a shift of the cutaneous cold pain threshold to warmer temperatures (Wahren et al. 1989; Yarnitsky and Ochoa 1990), because of a central disinhibition. It is clear that this lack of inhibitory mechanism may be relevant for the hyperalgesia in patients presenting with a preferential loss of myelinated fibers and cold hypoesthesia due to loss of sensitive cold afferents (Ochoa and Yarnitsky 1994).

However, other studies have provided evidence for another mechanism contributing to cold hyperalgesia that may be more important in patients with normal sensitivity to innocuous cold. Reaction time measurements (Fruhstorfer and Lindblom 1984; Lindblom 1994) and differential nerve block experiments (Torebjörk et al. 1995) suggest that thin myelinated cold-sensitive afferents signal pain. Furthermore, cold hyperalgesia, which is probably mediated by myelinated fibers, has also been found in the area of secondary hyperalgesia following the injection of capsaicin (Gracely et al. 1993). The qualitative switch from signaling of innocuous cool sensations to cold pain could be analogous to the mechanisms that mediate brush-evoked pain signaled by large myelinated non-nociceptive fibers.

PAIN AND HYPERALGESIA IN DEEP SOMATIC TISSUES

It is likely that changes of primary afferents innervating deep somatic tissues also play an important role for pain, hyperalgesia, and possibly some motor disturbances (Schott 1986; Bhatia et al. 1993; Marsden 1994; Kaji et al. 1995) after nerve lesion or soft tissue trauma. Systematic studies in normal human volunteers are still rare and are virtually nonexistent in neuralgia patients. It is known that electrical stimulation of thin myelinated or unmyelinated muscle afferents innervating muscle or tendon often causes a dull and cramping pain that frequently is referred to distal locations (Torebjörk et al. 1984; Simone et al. 1994b). Ischemic muscle contraction or injection of chemical irritants into muscle, ligaments, joints, or tendon are painful and produce hyperalgesia to pressure (Lewis et al. 1931; Kellgren 1937; Kellgren 1939; Lewis 1942; Sinclair et al. 1948; Kellgren and Samuel 1950; Simone et al. 1992); both sensations are probably signaled by fine afferents. Researchers conducting animal studies have now analyzed the neural mechanisms in normal and acutely inflamed tissues (Mense 1986; Berberich et al. 1988; Schaible and Grubb 1993; Schmidt et al. 1994), but to date have not systematically investigated the effects of nerve lesions on fine afferents innervating deep somatic tissues.

SUMMARY

Several mechanisms have been identified that mediate persistent pain and hyperalgesia in humans with acute inflammatory lesions or chronic neuralgia. Several studies have shown striking commonalities between both conditions, which suggests that the mechanisms mediating one symptom, such as brush-evoked pain, may be similar, if not identical. The different subtypes of hyperalgesia are mediated by distinct neural mechanisms that reflect adaptive changes of the peripheral and central nervous systems to nerve injury. These changes include the development of ongoing activity, catecholamine sensitivity, or heat sensitization in nociceptors that can persist for months or years. These features are key elements that precede or coincide with powerful changes in central nervous processing of inputs carried by non-nociceptive or nociceptive afferents. These central changes may be instrumental for signaling hyperalgesia to touch, pinprick, or cold. Knowledge about the basis of these peripheral and central excitability increases obviously will be important if their reversal should become the target for causal therapeutic approaches in chronic neuropathic pain states.

ACKNOWLEDGMENT

The author's work is supported by the Deutsche Forschungsgemeinschaft (SFB 353).

REFERENCES

Adriaensen, H., Gybels, J., Handwerker, H.O. and Van Hees, J., Latencies of chemically evoked discharges in human cutaneous nociceptors and of the concurrent subjective sensations, Neurosci. Lett., 20 (1980) 55–59.
Ali, Z., Meyer, R.A., Meleka, S.M. and Campbell, J.N., Capsaicin produces secondary hyperalgesia to mechanical but not heat stimuli, Society for Neuroscience Abstracts, 20 (1994) 1570.
Arnér, S., Lindblom, U., Meyerson, B.A. and Molander, C., Prolonged relief of neuralgia after regional anesthetic blocks: a call for further experimental and systematic clinical studies, Pain, 43 (1990) 287–297.
Baumann, T.K., Simone, D.A., Shain, C. and LaMotte, R.H., Neurogenic hyperalgesia: the search for the primary cutaneous afferent fibers that contribute to capsaicin-induced pain and hyperalgesia, J. Neurophysiol., 66 (1991) 212–227.
Beck, P.W. and Handwerker, H.O., Bradykinin and serotonin effects on various types of cutaneous nerve fibres, Pflügers Arch., 347 (1974) 21–28.
Berberich, P., Hoheisel, U. and Mense, S., Effects of a carrageenan-induced myositis on the discharge properties of group III and IV muscle receptors in the cat, J. Neurophysiol., 59 (1988) 1395–1409.
Bhatia, K.P., Bhatt, M.H. and Marsden, C.D., The causalgia-dystonia syndrome, Brain, 116 (1993) 843–851.
Bini, G., Cruccu, G., Hagbarth, K.-E., Schady, W. and Torebjörk, E., Analgesic effect of vibration and cooling on pain induced by intraneural electrical stimulation, Pain, 18 (1984) 239–248.
Blumberg, H. and Jänig, W., Discharge pattern of afferent fibers from a neuroma, Pain, 20 (1984) 335–353.
Blumberg, H. and Jänig, W., Clinical mainfestations of reflex sympathetic dystrophy and sympathetically maintained pain. In: P.D. Wall and R. Melzack (Eds.), Textbook of Pain, 3rd ed., Churchill Livingstone, Edinburgh, 1994, pp. 685–698.
Bonica, J.J., Causalgia and other sympathetic reflex dystrophies. In: J.J. Bonica (Ed.), The Management of Pain, 2nd ed., Lea & Febiger, Philadelphia, 1990, pp. 220–243.
Bossut, D.F. and Perl, E.R., Effects of nerve injury on sympathetic excitation of Aδ mechanical nociceptors, J. Neurophysiol., 73 (1995) 1721–1723.
Campbell, J.N. and Meyer, R.A., Sensitization of unmyelinated nociceptive afferents in monkey varies with skin type, J. Neurophysiol., 49 (1983) 98–110.
Campbell, J.N., Meyer, R.A. and LaMotte, R.H., Sensitization of myelinated nociceptive afferents that innervate monkey hand, J. Neurophysiol., 42 (1979) 1669–1679.
Campbell, J.N., Raja, S.N., Meyer, R.A. and Mackinnon, S.E., Myelinated afferents signal the hyperalgesia associated with nerve injury, Pain, 32 (1988) 89–94.
Campbell, J.N., Meyer, R.A. and Raja, S.N., Is nociceptor activation by alpha-1 adrenoreceptors the culprit in sympathetically maintained pain, APS Journal, 13 (1992) 344–350.
Campbell, J.N., Raja, S.N., Belzberg, A.J. and Meyer, R.A., Hyperalgesia and the sympathetic nervous system. In: J. Boivie, P. Hansson and U. Lindblom (Eds.), Touch, Temperature, and Pain in Health and Disease: Mechanisms and Assessments, Progress in Pain Research and Management, Vol. 3, IASP Press, Seattle, 1994, pp. 249–265.
Cervero, F., Meyer, R.A. and Campbell, J.N., A psychophysical study of secondary hyperalgesia: evidence for increased pain to input from nociceptors, Pain, 58 (1994) 21–28.

Chabal, C., Jacobson, L., Russell, L.C. and Burchiel, K.J., Pain response to perineuromal injection of normal saline, epinephrine, and lidocaine in humans, Pain, 49 (1992) 9–12.

Cline, M.A., Ochoa, J. and Torebjörk, H.E., Chronic hyperalgesia and skin warming caused by sensitized C nociceptors, Brain, 112 (1989) 621–647.

Culp, W.J., Ochoa, J., Cline, M. and Dotson, R., Heat and mechanical hyperalgesia induced by capsaicin, Brain, 112 (1989) 1317–1331.

Davis, K.D., Treede, R.-D., Raja, S.N., Meyer, R.A. and Campbell, J.N., Topical application of clonidine relieves hyperalgesia in patients with sympathetically maintained pain, Pain, 47 (1991) 309–317.

Davis, K.D., Meyer, R.A. and Campbell, J.N., Chemosensitivity and sensitization of nociceptive afferents that innervate the hairy skin of monkey, J. Neurophysiol., 69 (1993) 1071–1081.

Devor, M., Pathophysiology of injured nerve. In: P.D. Wall and R. Melzack (Eds.), Textbook of Pain, 3rd ed., Churchill Livingstone, Edinburgh, 1994, pp. 79–100.

Devor, M. and Jänig, W., Activation of myelinated afferents ending in a neuroma by stimulation of the sympathetic supply in the rat, Neurosci. Lett., 24 (1981) 43–47.

Devor, M., Jänig, W. and Michaelis, M., Modulation of activity in dorsal root ganglion neurons by sympathetic activation in nerve-injured rats, J. Neurophysiol., 71 (1994a) 38–47.

Devor, M., Lomazov, P. and Matzner, O., Sodium channel accumulation in injured axons as a substrate for neuropathic pain. In: J. Boivie, P. Hansson and U. Lindblom (Eds.), Touch, Temperature, and Pain in Health and Disease: Mechanisms and Assessments, Progress in Pain Research and Management, Vol. 3, IASP Press, Seattle, 1994b, pp. 207–230.

Dmitrieva, N. and McMahon, S.B., NGF acutely sensitises primary sensory neurones, Soc. Neurosci. Abstr., 20 (1994) 238.

Dray, A. and Perkins, M., Bradykinin and inflammatory pain, Trends Neurosci., 16 (1993) 99–104.

Frost, S.A., Raja, S.N., Campbell, J.N., Meyer, R.A. and Khan, A.A., Does hyperalgesia to cooling stimuli characterize patients with sympathetically maintained pain (reflex sympathetic dystrophy). In: R. Dubner, G.F. Gebhart and M.R. Bond (Eds.), Proceedings of the Vth World Congress on Pain, Pain Research and Clinical Management, Vol. 3, Elsevier, Amsterdam, 1988, pp. 151–156.

Fruhstorfer, H. and Lindblom, U., Sensibility abnormalities in neuralgic patients studied by thermal and tactile pulse stimulation. In: U. von Euler, O. Franzén, U. Lindblom and D. Ottoson (Eds.), Somatosensory Mechanisms, Macmillan Press, London, 1984, pp. 353–361.

Gracely, R.H., Lynch, S.A. and Bennett, G.J., Painful neuropathy: altered central processing, maintained dynamically by peripheral input, Pain, 51 (1992) 175–194.

Gracely, R.H., Lynch, S.A. and Bennett, G.J., Evidence for Ab low-threshold mechanoreceptor-mediated mechanoallodynia and cold hyperalgesia following intradermal injection of capsaicin into the foot dorsum. In: Abstracts: 7th World Congress on Pain, IASP Publications, Seattle, 1993, p. 372.

Grigg, P., Schaible, H.-G. and Schmidt, R.F., Mechanical sensitivity of group III and IV afferents from posterior articular nerve in normal and inflamed cat knee, J. Neurophysiol., 55 (1986) 635–643.

Gybels, J., Handwerker, H.O. and Van Hees, J., A comparison between the discharges of human nociceptive nerve fibres and the subject's ratings of his sensations, J. Physiol. (Lond.), 292 (1979) 193–206.

Handwerker, H.O. and Reeh, P.W., Pain and inflammation. In: M.R. Bond, J.E. Charlton and C.J. Woolf (Eds.), Proceedings of the VIth World Congress on Pain, Pain Research and Clinical Management, Vol. 4, Elsevier, Amsterdam, 1991, pp. 59–70.

Handwerker, H.O. and Kobal, G., Psychophysiology of experimentally induced pain, Physiol. Rev., 73 (1993) 639–671.

Handwerker, H.O., Forster, C. and Kirchoff, C., Discharge properties of human C-fibres induced by itching and burning stimuli, J. Neurophysiol., 66 (1991) 307–315.

Hardy, J.D., Wolff, H.G. and Goodell, H., Pain sensations and reactions, Williams & Willkins, Baltimore, 1952.

Häbler, H.-J., Jänig, W. and Koltzenburg, M., Activation of unmyelinated afferents in chronically lesioned nerves by adrenaline and excitation of sympathetic efferents in the cat, Neurosci. Lett., 82 (1987) 35–40.

Häbler, H.-J., Jänig, W. and Koltzenburg, M., A novel type of unmyelinated chemosensitive nociceptor in the acutely inflamed urinary bladder, Agents Actions, 25 (1988) 219–221.

Häbler, H.-J., Jänig, W. and Koltzenburg, M., Activation of unmyelinated afferent fibres by mechanical stimuli and inflammation of the urinary bladder in the cat, J. Physiol. (Lond.), 425 (1990) 545–562.

Heller, P.H., Green, P.G., Tanner, K.D., Miao, F.J.-P. and Levine, J.D., Peripheral neural contributions to inflammation. In: H.L. Fields and J.C. Liebeskind (Eds.), Pharmacological Approaches to the Treatment of Chronic Pain: New Concepts and Critical Issues, Progress in Pain Research and Management, Vol. 1, IASP Press, Seattle, 1994, pp. 31–42.

Jänig, W., Pathophysiology of nerve following mechanical injury. In: R. Dubner, G.F. Gebhart and M.R. Bond (Eds.), Proceedings of the Vth World Congress on Pain, Pain Research and Clinical Management, Vol. 3, Elsevier, Amsterdam, 1988, pp. 89–108.

Jänig, W. and Koltzenburg, M., Possible ways of sympathetic-afferent interactions. In: W. Jänig and R.F. Schmidt (Eds.), Pathophysiological Mechanisms of Reflex Sympathetic Dystrophy, VCH, Weinheim, 1992, pp. 213–243.

Jänig, W. and McLachlan, E.M., The role of modification in noradrenergic peripheral pathways after nerve lesions in the generation of pain. In: H.L. Fields and J.C. Liebeskind (Eds.), Pharmacological Approaches to the Treatment of Chronic Pain: New Concepts and Critical Issues, Progress in Pain Research and Management, Vol. 1, IASP Press, Seattle, 1994, pp. 101–128.

Kaji, R., Rothwell, J.C., Ketayama, M., Ikeda, T., Koburi, T., Kohara, N., Mezaki, T., Shibasaki, H. and Kimura, J., Tonic vibration reflex and afferent block in writer's cramp, Ann. Neurol., 38 (1995) 55–62.

Kellgren, J.H., Observations on referred pain arsing from muscle, Clin. Sci., 3 (1937–1938) 175–190.

Kellgren, J.H., On the distribution of pain arising from deep somatic structures with charts of segmental pain areas, Clin. Sci., 4 (1939–1942) 35–46.

Kellgren, J.H. and Samuel, E.P., The sensitivity and innervation of the articular capsule, J. Bone Joint Surg. Br., 32 (1950) 84–92.

Kessler, W., Kirchhoff, C., Reeh, P.W. and Handwerker, H.O., Excitation of cutaneous afferent nerve endings in vitro by a combination of inflammatory mediators and conditioning effect of substance P, Exp. Brain Res., 91 (1992) 467–476.

Khan, A.A., Raja, S.N., Manning, D.C., Campbell, J.N. and Meyer, R.A., The effects of bradykinin and sequence-related analogs on the response properties of cutaneous nociceptors in monkeys, Somatosens. Mot. Res., 9 (1992) 97–106.

Kibler, R.F. and Nathan, P.W., Relief of pain and paraesthesiae by nerve block distal to a lesion, J. Neurol. Neurosurg. Psychiatry, 23 (1960) 91–98.

Kilo, S., Schmelz, M., Koltzenburg, M. and Handwerker, H.O., Different patterns of hyperalgesia induced by experimental inflammations in human skin, Brain, 117 (1994) 385–396.

Kirchhoff, C., Jung, S., Reeh, P.W. and Handwerker, H.O., Carrageenan inflammation increases bradykinin sensitivity of rat cutaneous nociceptors, Neurosci. Lett., 111 (1990) 206–210.

Kniffki, K.D., Mense, S. and Schmidt, R.F., Responses of group IV afferent units from skeletal muscle to stretch, contraction and chemical stimulation, Exp. Brain Res., 31 (1978) 511–522.

Kocher, L., Anton, F., Reeh, P.W. and Handwerker, H.O., The effect of carrageenan-induced inflammation on the sensitivity of unmyelinated skin nociceptors in the rat, Pain, 29 (1987) 363–373.

Kohllöffel, L.U.E., Koltzenburg, M. and Handwerker, H.O., A novel technique for the evaluation of mechanical pain and hyperalgesia, Pain, 46 (1991) 81–87.

Koltzenburg, M. and McMahon, S.B., The enigmatic role of the sympathetic nervous system in chronic pain, Trends Pharmacol. Sci., 12 (1991) 399–402.

Koltzenburg, M. and Handwerker, H.O., Differential ability of human nociceptors to signal

mechanical pain and to evoke a flare response, J. Neurosci., 14 (1994) 1756–1765.
Koltzenburg, M. and McMahon, S.B., Mechanically insensitive primary afferents innervating the urinary bladder. In: G.F. Gebhart (Ed.), Visceral Pain, Progress in Pain Research and Management, Vol. 5, IASP Press, Seattle, 1995, pp. 163–192.
Koltzenburg, M. and Torebjörk, H.E., Pain and hyperalgesia in acute inflammatory and chronic neuropathic conditions, Lancet, 345 (1995) 1111.
Koltzenburg, M., Kress, M. and Reeh, P.W., The nociceptor sensitization by bradykinin does not depend on sympathetic neurones, Neuroscience, 46 (1992a) 465–473.
Koltzenburg, M., Lundberg, L.E.R. and Torebjörk, H.E., Dynamic and static components of mechanical hyperalgesia in human hairy skin, Pain, 51 (1992b) 207–219.
Koltzenburg, M., Handwerker, H.O. and Torebjörk, H.E., The ability of humans to localise noxious stimuli, Neurosci. Lett., 150 (1993) 219–222.
Koltzenburg, M., Kees, S., Budweiser, S., Ochs, G. and Toyka, K.V., The properties of unmyelinated afferents change in a chronic constriction neuropathy. In: G.F. Gebhart, D.L. Hammond and T.S. Jensen (Eds.), Proceedings of the 7th World Congress on Pain, Progress in Pain Research and Management, Vol. 2, IASP Press, Seattle, 1994a, pp. 511–522.
Koltzenburg, M., Torebjörk, H.E. and Wahren, L.K., Nociceptor modulated central plasticity causes mechanical hyperalgesia in chronic neuropathic and acute chemogenic pain, Brain, 117 (1994b) 579–591.
Konietzny, F., Peripheral neural correlates of temperature sensation in man, Human Neurobiology, 3 (1984) 21–32.
Kress, M., Koltzenburg, M., Reeh, P.W. and Handwerker, H.O., Responsiveness and functional attributes of electrically localized terminals of cutaneous C-fibers in vivo and in vitro, J. Neurophysiol., 68 (1992) 581–595.
LaMotte, R.H., Can the sensitization of nociceptors account for hyperalgesia after skin injury? Human Neurobiology, 3 (1984) 47–52.
LaMotte, R.H., Subpopulations of "nocifensor neurons" contributing to pain and allodynia, itch and alloknesis, APS Journal, 1 (1992) 115–126.
LaMotte, R.H. and Thalhammer, J.G., Response properties of high-threshold cutaneous cold receptors in the primate, Brain Res., 244 (1982) 279–287.
LaMotte, R.H., Thalhammer, J.G., Torebjörk, H.E. and Robinson, C.J., Peripheral neural mechanisms of cutaneous hyperalgesia following mild injury by heat, J. Neurosci., 2 (1982) 765–781.
LaMotte, R.H., Thalhammer, J.G. and Robinson, C.J., Peripheral neural correlates of magnitude of cutaneous pain and hyperalgesia: a comparison of neural events in monkey with sensory judgments in human, J. Neurophysiol., 50 (1983) 1–26.
LaMotte, R.H., Torebjörk, H.E., Robinson, C.J. and Thalhammer, J.G., Time-intensity profiles of cutaneous pain in normal and hyperalgesic skin: a comparison with C-fiber nociceptor activities in monkey and human, J. Neurophysiol., 51 (1984) 1434–1450.
LaMotte, R.H., Shain, C.N., Simone, D.A. and Tsai, E.F., Neurogenic hyperalgesia: psychophysical studies of underlying mechanisms, J. Neurophysiol., 66 (1991) 190–211.
LaMotte, R.H., Lundberg, L.E.R. and Torebjörk, H.E., Pain, hyperalgesia and activity in nociceptive C units in humans after intradermal injection of capsaicin, J. Physiol. (Lond.), 448 (1992) 749–764.
Lang, E., Novak, A., Reeh, P.W. and Handwerker, H.O., Chemosensitivity of fine afferents from rat skin in vitro, J. Neurophysiol., 63 (1990) 887–901.
Levine, J. and Taiwo, Y., Inflammatory pain. In: P.D. Wall and R. Melzack (Eds.), Textbook of Pain, 3rd ed., Churchill Livingstone, Edinburgh, 1994, pp. 45–56.
Lewin, G.R. and Mendell, L.M., Regulation of cutaneous C-fiber heat nociceptors by nerve growth factor in the developing rat, J. Neurophysiol., 71 (1994) 941–949.
Lewis, T., Pain, Macmillan, New York, 1942.
Lewis, T., Pickering, G.W. and Rothschild, P., Observations upon muscular pain in intermittent claudication, Heart, 15 (1931) 359–383.
Lindblom, U., Analysis of abnormal touch, pain, and temperature sensation in patients. In: J.

Boivie, P. Hansson and U. Lindblom (Eds.), Touch, Temperature, and Pain in Health and Disease: Mechanisms and Assessments, Progress in Pain Research and Management, Vol. 3, IASP Press, Seattle, 1994, pp. 63–84.

Loh, L. and Nathan, P.W., Painful peripheral states and sympathetic blocks, J. Neurol. Neurosurg. Psychiatry, 41 (1978) 664–671.

Marsden, C.D., Peripheral movement disorders. In: C.D. Marsden and S. Fahn (Eds.), Movement Disorders 3, Butterworth-Heinemann, Oxford, 1994, pp. 406–417.

McLachlan, E.M., Jänig, W., Devor, M. and Michaelis, M., Peripheral nerve injury triggers noradrenergic sprouting within dorsal root ganglia, Nature, 363 (1993) 543–546.

McMahon, S.B., Mechanisms of Sympathetic Pain, Br. Med. Bull., 47 (1991) 584–600.

McMahon, S.B. and Koltzenburg, M., Novel classes of nociceptors: beyond Sherrington, Trends Neurosci., 13 (1990) 199–201.

Mense, S., Slowly conducting afferent fibres from deep tissues: neurobiological properties and central nervous actions, Progress in Sensory Physiology, 6 (1986) 139–219.

Meyer, R.A. and Campbell, J.N., Myelinated nociceptive afferents account for the hyperalgesia that follows a burn to the hand, Science, 213 (1981) 1527–1529.

Meyer, R.A., Raja, S.N., Treede, R.-D., Davis, K.D. and Campbell, J.N., Neural mechanisms of sympathetically maintained pain. In: W. Jänig and R.F. Schmidt (Eds.), Pathophysiological Mechanisms of Reflex Sympathetic Dystrophy, VCH, Weinheim, 1992, pp. 57–66.

Meyer, R.A., Campbell, J.N. and Raja, S.N., Peripheral neural mechanisms of nociception. In: P.D. Wall, R. Melzack (Eds.), Textbook of Pain, 3rd ed., Churchill Livingstone, Edinburgh, 1994, pp. 13–44.

Nathan, P.W. and Rice, R.C., The localization of warm stimuli, Neurology, 16 (1966) 533–540.

Nurmikko, T., Wells, C. and Bowsher, D., Pain and allodynia in postherpetic neuralgia: role of somatic and sympathetic nervous systems, Acta Neurol. Scand., 84 (1991) 146–152.

Ochoa, J.L. and Yarnitzky, D., Mechanical hyperalgesias in neuropathic pain patients: dynamic and static subtypes, Ann. Neurol., 33 (1993) 465–472.

Ochoa, J.L. and Yarnitsky, D., The triple cold syndrome: cold hyperalgesia, cold hypoaesthesia and cold skin in peripheral nerve disease, Brain, 117 (1994) 185–197.

Ochs, G., Schenk, M. and Struppler, A., Painful dysaesthesias following peripheral nerve injury: a clinical and electrophysiological study, Brain Res., 496 (1989) 228–240.

Perl, E.R., Causalgia and reflex sympathetic dystrophy revisited. In: J. Boivie, P. Hansson and U. Lindblom (Eds.), Touch, Temperature, and Pain in Health and Disease: Mechanisms and Assessments, Progress in Pain Research and Management, Vol. 3, IASP Press, Seattle, 1994, pp. 231–248.

Price, D.D., Bennett, G.J. and Rafii, A., Psychophysical observations on patients with neuropathic pain relieved by a sympathetic block, Pain, 36 (1989) 273–288.

Price, D.D., Long, S. and Huitt, C., Sensory testing of pathophysiological mechanisms of pain in patients with reflex sympathetic dystrophy, Pain, 49 (1992) 163–173.

Raja, S.N., Campbell, J.N. and Meyer, R.A., Evidence for different mechanisms of primary and secondary hyperalgesia following heat injury to the glabrous skin, Brain, 107 (1984) 1179–1188.

Reeh, P.W., Bayer, J., Kocher, L. and Handwerker, H.O., Sensitization of nociceptive cutaneous nerve fibers from the rat's tail by noxious mechanical stimulation, Exp. Brain Res., 65 (1987) 505–512.

Robinson, C.J., Torebjörk, H.E. and LaMotte, R.H., Psychophysical detection and pain ratings of incremental thermal stimuli: a comparison with nociceptor responses in humans, Brain Res., 274 (1983) 87–106.

Rowbotham, M.C. and Fields, H.L., Topical lidocaine reduces pain in post-herpetic neuralgia, Pain, 38 (1989) 297–301.

Rowbotham, M.C., Davies, P.S. and Fields, H.L., Topical lidocaine gel relieves postherpetic neuralgia, Ann. Neurol., 37 (1995) 246–253.

Sato, J. and Perl, E.R., Adrenergic excitation of cutaneous pain receptors induced by peripheral

nerve injury, Science, 251 (1991) 1608–1610.
Schaible, H.-G. and Grubb, B.D., Afferent and spinal mechanisms of joint pain, Pain, 55 (1993) 5–54.
Schaible, H.-G. and Schmidt, R.F., Effects of an experimental arthritis on the sensory properties of fine articular afferent units, J. Neurophysiol., 54 (1985) 1109–1122.
Schaible, H.-G. and Schmidt, R.F., Time course of mechanosensitivity changes in articular afferents during a developing experimental arthritis, J. Neurophysiol., 60 (1988) 2180–2195.
Schmelz, M., Schmidt, R., Ringkamp, M., Handwerker, H.O. and Torebjörk, H.E., Sensitization of insensitive branches of nociceptors in human skin, J. Physiol., 480 (1994) 389–394.
Schmidt, R.F., Schaible, H.-G., Messlinger, K., Heppelmann, B., Hanesch, U. and Pawlak, M., Silent and active nociceptors: structure, functions and clinical implications. In: G.F. Gebhart, D.L. Hammond and T.L. Jensen (Eds.), Proceedings of the 7th World Congress on Pain, Progress in Pain Research and Management, Vol. 2, IASP Press, Seattle, 1994, pp. 213–250.
Schmidt, R.F., Schmelz, M., Forster, C., Ringkamp, M., Torebjörk, H.E. and Handwerker, H.O., Novel classes of responsive and unresponsive C nociceptors in human skin, J. Neurosci., 15 (1995) 333–341.
Schott, G.D., Mechanisms of causalgia and related clinical conditions: the role of the central and of the sympathetic nervous system, Brain, 109 (1986) 717–738.
Selig, D.K., Meyer, R.A. and Campbell, J.N., Noradrenaline excitation of cutaneous nociceptors two weeks after ligation of spinal nerve L7 in monkey, Society for Neuroscience Abstracts, 19 (1993) 326.
Simone, D.A., Baumann, T.K. and LaMotte, R.H., Dose-dependent pain and mechanical hyperalgesia in humans after intradermal injection of capsaicin, Pain, 38 (1989) 99–107.
Simone, D.A., Caputi, G., Marchettini, P. and Ochoa, J.L., Cramping pain and deep hyperalgesia following intramuscular injection of capsaicin, Society for Neuroscience Abstracts, 18 (1992) 134.
Simone, D.A., Gilchrist, H.D. and Kajander, K.C., Responses of primate cutaneous nociceptors evoked by noxious cold, Society for Neuroscience Abstracts, 20 (1994a) 1379.
Simone, D.A., Marchettini, P., Caputi, G. and Ochoa, J.L., Identification of muscle afferents subserving sensation of deep pain in humans, J. Neurophysiol., 72 (1994b) 883–889.
Sinclair, D.C., Weddell, G. and Feindel, W.H., Referred pain and associated phenomena, Brain, 714 (1948) 184–211.
Thalhammer, J.G. and LaMotte, R.H., Spatial properties of nociceptor sensitization following heat injury of the skin, Brain Res., 231 (1982) 257–265.
Torebjörk, H.E., Clinical and neurophysiological observations relating to pathophysiological mechanisms in reflex sympathetic dystrophy. In: M. Stanton-Hicks, W. Jänig and R.A. Boas (Eds.), Reflex Sympathetic Dystrophy, Kluwer Academic Publishers, Boston, 1990, pp. 71–80.
Torebjörk, H.E. and Ochoa, J.L., New method to identify nociceptor units innervating glabrous skin of the human hand, Exp. Brain Res., 81 (1990) 509–514.
Torebjörk, H.E., Ochoa, J.L. and Schady, W., Referred pain from intraneural stimulation of muscle fascicles in the median nerve, Pain, 18 (1984a) 145–156.
Torebjörk, H.E., LaMotte, R.H. and Robinson, C.J., Peripheral neural correlates of magnitude of cutaneous pain and hyperalgesia: simultaneous recordings in humans of sensory judgments of pain and evoked responses in nociceptors with C-fibers, J. Neurophysiol., 51 (1984b) 325–339.
Torebjörk, H.E., Lundberg, L.E. and LaMotte, R.H., Central changes in processing of mechanoreceptive input in capsaicin-induced secondary hyperalgesia in humans, J. Physiol. (Lond.), 448 (1992) 765–780.
Torebjörk, H.E., Wahren, L.K., Wallin, B.G., Hallin, R.G. and Koltzenburg, M., Noradrenaline-evoked pain in neuralgia, Pain, 63 (1995) 11–20 .
Treede, R.-D., Meyer, R.A. and Campbell, J.N., Comparison of heat and mechanical receptive fields of cutaneous C-fiber nociceptors in monkey, J. Neurophysiol., 64 (1990) 1502–1513.
Treede, R.-D., Davis, K.D., Campbell, J.N. and Raja, S.N., The plasticity of cutaneous hyperalgesia during sympathetic ganglion blockade in patients with neuropathic pain, Brain, 115 (1992a) 607–621.

Treede, R.-D., Meyer, R.A., Raja, S.N. and Campbell, J.N., Peripheral and central mechanisms of cutaneous hyperalgesia, Prog. Neurobiol., 38 (1992b) 397–421.

Van Hees, J. and Gybels, J., C nociceptor activity in human nerve during painful and nonpainful skin stimulation, J. Neurol. Neurosurg. Psychiatry, 44 (1981) 600–607.

Wahren, L.K. and Torebjörk, E., Quantitative sensory tests in patients with neuralgia 11 to 25 years after injury, Pain, 48 (1992) 237–244.

Wahren, L.K., Torebjörk, E. and Jorum, E., Central suppression of cold-induced C fibre pain by myelinated fibre input, Pain, 38 (1989) 313–319.

Wallin, B.G., Torebjörk, H.E. and Hallin, R.G., Preliminary observations on the pathophysiology of hyperalgesia in the causaligic pain syndrome. In: Y. Zotterman (Ed.), Sensory Functions of the Skin in Primates, Pergamon Press, Oxford, 1976, pp. 489–499.

Wen, J. and Morrison, J.F.B., The effects of changing urinary composition on silent afferents in the rat urinary bladder, J. Physiol. (Lond.), 476 (1994) 50P–51P.

Yarnitsky, D. and Ochoa, J.L., Release of cold-induced burning pain by block of cold-specific afferent input, Brain, 113 (1990) 893–902.

Correspondence to: Martin Koltzenburg, Dr med, Department of Neurology, University of Würzburg, Josef-Schneider-Str. 11, D-97080 Würzburg, Germany. Tel: 49-931-201-2621; Fax: 49-931-201-2697; E-mail: Neuk115@rzbox.uni-wuerzburg.de.

Reflex Sympathetic Dystrophy: A Reappraisal,
Progress in Pain Research and Management,
Vol. 6, edited by W. Jänig and M. Stanton-Hicks,
IASP Press, Seattle, © 1996.

9

Quantitative Sensory Testing in Patients with Complex Regional Pain Syndrome (CRPS) I and II

Richard H. Gracely,[a] Donald D. Price,[b] William J. Roberts,[c] and Gary J. Bennett[a]

[a]Neuropathic Pain and Pain Measurement Section, Neurobiology and Anesthesiology Branch, National Institute of Dental Research, National Institutes of Health, Bethesda, Maryland, [b]Pain Management Center, Department of Anesthesiology, Medical College of Virginia, Richmond, Virginia, [c]R.S. Dow Neurological Sciences Institute, Portland, Oregon, USA

Patients described in this volume present with a heterogeneous mix of symptoms including autonomic, somatic sensory, and motor abnormalities. This chapter will focus on the evaluation of the sensory abnormalities in this diverse population. It will describe specialized laboratory techniques and also easily performed clinical tests that are often completely adequate for the assessment of specific abnormalities.

THE PURPOSES OF SENSORY TESTING

Patients with complex regional pain syndrome (CRPS) I and II almost invariably have symptoms of sensory abnormalities within pathological zones of skin or other body tissue. The incidence, type, and extent of these abnormalities vary considerably across these patients, so that no single type of abnormality nor its extent can be used as an exclusionary criterion to diagnose CRPS I or II. Nevertheless, the presence of one or more sensory abnormalities can be helpful in further confirming the presence of these diseases. For example, of the 31 patients studied by Price et al. (1992), all had cutaneous mechanical allodynia; 34.5% (10 of 29 tested) had temporal summation of mechanical allodynia, and 54.8% (17 of 31 tested) had thermal hyperalgesia. Cutaneous mechanical allodynia/hyperalgesia is relatively easy to establish with simple tests, so testing CRPS I and II patients for this specific sensory abnormality would seem helpful in confirming the presence of CRPS I and II. Thus, one major reason for sensory testing of these patients is that it serves as an important adjunctive aid in confirming the diagnosis of these diseases.

A second and related reason for sensory testing is that it could be helpful in characterizing pathophysiological pain mechanisms and hence in matching such mechanisms to appropriate therapies. To give a hypothetical example, temporal summation of Aβ-mediated mechanical allodynia may be mediated by N-methyl-D-aspartate (NMDA) receptor activity. If this is so and if temporal summation of Aβ-mediated mechanical allodynia is present in one-third of CRPS I patients, then a clinical trial of a NMDA receptor blocker would detect a clinical benefit only if patients had been carefully examined for the presence of this particular sensory abnormality. In another example, evoked pains that radiate (i.e., shooting pain) may be particularly responsive to treatment with anticonvulsants.

A very important point is that the kinds of sensory testing described here can, if done in an aggressive manner, cause the patient considerable distress that may last for days. We have found that the examiner must exercise great patience. Sufficient time, often 10 minutes or more, must be taken to permit test-evoked pain, and the lingering "soreness" that follows, to dissipate before commencing the next test. Patients must, of course, be specifically instructed that they have the right to terminate testing at any time and that such a decision will not prejudice their treatment. The amount of sensory testing to be performed should be appropriate to the context. The bedside and "clinical" tests presented in this chapter are, in our view, appropriate to a careful and thorough pain examination in a situation centered on patient care. Additional testing might be best considered in an experimental context, requiring the patient's informed consent. Before addressing this diverse array of symptoms in CRPS I and II and methods of evaluation, we will define important distinctions and a common nomenclature.

DEFINITIONS AND NOMENCLATURE

SPONTANEOUS AND EVOKED PAIN

This chapter refers to the pain experienced by the patient in the absence of stimulation or movement as "spontaneous" pain; it also can be termed "ongoing" or "background" pain. A distinguishing feature of these syndromes is that usually nonpainful stimulation such as room-temperature metal or contact with clothing produces pain sensations that sometimes can be quite intense. The pain produced by any form of stimulation or by movement is termed "evoked" pain.

THRESHOLD VERSUS SUPRATHRESHOLD STIMULATION AND SENSATION

Threshold stimulation is defined as the minimal amount of stimulation required to produce a predetermined subjective state. The predetermined state is usually either the detection of the presence of any sensation regardless of quality (detection threshold), or the presence of pain (pain threshold). It is also useful to classify stimulation near these levels such as "detection-level" stimulation or stimulation at "pain threshold levels." In contrast, "suprathreshold stimulation" implies stimulation at levels well above the specified threshold, although technically it refers to any stimulation that the subject perceives at the detection threshold, or that is painful at the pain threshold.

These terms are not limited to the common cases of detection threshold or pain threshold. Other examples include thresholds for specific sensory qualities such as burning or spreading, or for discomfort.

NOCICEPTION

Nociception refers to the serial neural events extending from activation of receptors specialized to detect tissue damage or stimuli that would result in tissue damage if maintained over time (i.e., nociceptors) to central neural events closely associated with the conscious perception of pain. Nociception is the normal operation of the pain sensory system in the absence of any injury or disease to the nervous system.

NOCICEPTIVE VERSUS NEUROPATHIC PAIN

The adjective "nociceptive" may be used to refer to a specific class of peripheral sensory nerves, specifically the $A\delta$ and C-fiber primary afferents (see below). It is also useful to apply this adjective to the experience of pain because it serves as a counterpoint to the adjective "neuropathic." Nociceptive pain is pain arising from nociception, from the normal operation of the pain sensory system. In contrast, neuropathic pain results from abnormal operation of the system after it has been damaged. It is defined formally by the International Association for the Study of Pain (IASP) as, "pain initiated or caused by a primary lesion or *dysfunction* in the nervous system" (Merskey and Bogduk 1994, emphasis added). If nociceptive pain accurately reflects real or threatened tissue damage, neuropathic pain is like a ghost image. It does not arise from stimulus-evoked activation of transducers, but from nerve activity originating from nerve injury or other pathophysiological processes. It can result in a sensation of pain referred to a region that has not been injured, or to a region that appears to have long since healed. If nociception can be compared to activation of a burglar alarm by opening a window, neuropathic pain is activation of the alarm by a "short circuit" in the wires leading to the window.

ALLODYNIA AND HYPERALGESIA

Allodynia is defined as, "pain due to a stimulus which does not normally provoke pain," while hyperalgesia is defined as "an increased response to a stimulus which is normally painful" (Merskey and Bogduk 1994). These terms are not used consistently, especially in the older literature. Many follow the tradition of Hardy et al. (1952) and use the term hyperalgesia to refer to both increases in pain sensitivity and to pain evoked by light tactile stimuli. We follow the IASP position and define allodynia as pain evoked by innocuous stimulation that would not evoke pain under normal conditions. For example, light brushing by a cotton wisp usually would not evoke pain, no matter how rapidly applied. The term allodynia is useful because it delineates this striking feature. The reader should be aware that many writers will describe allodynia as hyperalgesia, or perhaps dynamic hyperalgesia.

The problem of nomenclature arises when the stimulus modality can evoke both painful and nonpainful sensations. For example, thermal stimuli produce pain at temperatures of about 45°C and above. Increased pain to 46°C would indicate hyperalgesia, but how is a pain threshold lowered to 43°C described? While this lowered threshold can be termed hyperalgesia (and is by many), what if the threshold is lowered much further to stimulus temperatures that only produce warmth under normal conditions or produce no thermal sensation? Can this condition be termed heat allodynia? The answer is controversial, depending on several theoretical issues such as the distribution of firing thresholds in the nociceptive primary afferents. Here we accept the position that a pain threshold in the pathological area that is lower than the threshold in normal skin (e.g., contralateral homologous area) is defined as allodynia.

Dynamic and static allodynia/hyperalgesia

Pain evoked by innocuous touch stimuli can be divided into two classes. Dynamic mechanical allodynia (referred to also as dynamic hyperalgesia) is characterized by pain to lightly stroking the skin. In contrast, firm pressure without movement can result in pain at innocuous intensities and enhanced pain at noxious intensities. These conditions are properly referred to as static allodynia and static hyperalgesia, respectively, although the term "static hyperalgesia" as been used in the literature to describe both conditions.

Stimulus-defined versus mechanistic-defined abnormalities

The literature on sensory abnormalities contains both stimulus-defined descriptions, e.g., allodynia, brush-evoked pain, and mechanistic descriptions such as $A\beta$-mechanical-allodynia. One does not imply the other. For example, allodynia can result from at least two mechanisms: sensitized nociceptors, or central interpretation of activity in low-threshold touch afferents as pain instead of touch.

This specialized nomenclature is supplemented by medical terms used to describe altered sensation. Commonly used terms and the IASP definitions (Merskey and Bogduk 1994) are listed in Table I with parenthetical comments.

Table I
IASP definitions of medical terms commonly
used to describe altered sensations

Hyperalgesia
  Increased sensitivity to stimulation, excluding the special senses (includes both allodynia and hyperalgesia)

Hypoesthesia
  Decreased sensitivity to stimulation, excluding the special senses

Hypoalgesia
  Diminished pain in response to a normally painful stimulus

Dysesthesia
  An unpleasant abnormal sensation, whether spontaneous or evoked (that is not described as painful)

Paresthesia
  An abnormal sensation, whether spontaneous or evoked

Hyperpathia
  A painful syndrome characterized by an abnormally painful reaction to a stimulus, especially a repetitive stimulus, as well as an increased threshold (the pain usually radiates and persists after the stimulus, often with an abnormal delay between stimulus onset and sensation onset)

MECHANICAL STIMULATION: SENSE OF TOUCH

DYNAMIC MECHANICAL ALLODYNIA

Both the presence and area of allodynia can be quantified easily in the clinic. The presence of mechanical allodynia is determined by two stimulus characteristics: light pressure and movement. Thus, dragging any light stimulus, for example a cotton applicator, gauze pad, camel-hair brush, or piece of clothing, is painful. Often, blowing on the skin or brushing body hair without touching the skin evokes pain. A cotton wisp or a brush are commonly applied to determine the area of allodynia. Starting outside the area and moving inwards along radial spokes, the clinician strokes the skin until the patient reports a change in sensation from "touch" to "distinct pain." The point at which the evoked sensation changes to pain is marked on the skin and the area is traced onto transparencies. From these tracings the area can be computed by using available computerized tracing tablets, or acceptable accuracy can be obtained by the classic method of tracing the area onto quality paper, cutting out this template, and weighing it on a laboratory scale.

The patient's description of allodynia is extremely important. The clinician must be sure that the patient is reporting a pain sensation and not just an unpleasant dysesthetic sensation. It is useful to take some time to explain the difference between pain and dysesthesia, giving examples and analogies. Often the point will be moot, because the patient may flinch or show other reflexive behavior indicative of pain. However, an accurate report of pain is more critical than the choice of mechanical stimulus or method of stimulation. This distinction is also an issue in interpreting the literature, because some investigators have defined allodynia as the point at which the sensation changes, without specifying that it be painful.

In addition, the clinician should note the quality of the evoked sensations and all unusual characteristics. Distinctions such as radiating pain, prolonged pain, or temporal pain summation may identify patients selectively responsive to a specific therapy. The magnitude of dynamic mechanical allodynia has been quantified with the use of mechanical stimuli by two different methods.

The first method involves obtaining a pain rating to a standard stimulus applied to the allodynic area. The simplest method is the application of punctate pressure by von Frey hairs. Originally, horse hairs of varying stiffness were mounted in handles; the modern equivalent is a series of nylon monofilaments of varying diameter mounted in plastic handles. The hairs are applied perpendicular to the skin surface with enough force to slightly bend the filament, which produces a constant pressure. While quantitative, the static, punctate pressure produced by this method is not the ideal stimulus for allodynic skin, which responds much more vigorously to a moving stimulus (i.e., dynamic allodynia). Although a von Frey hair can be dragged across the skin at a constant rate, the laboratory standard has been a cotton applicator attached to a piece of flexible saw blade (LaMotte et al. 1991). The applicator is dragged across the skin with the blade just noticeably bent. Parameters such as the length of the blade and stroking speed (3–5 cm/s) are standardized. In a laboratory adaptation of this method, Anderson et al. (1995) mounted 4-cm-long nylon filaments perpendicular to a nylon shaft. The shaft was rotated by a controllable motor and the tips of the filaments were allowed to contact the skin. The number and diameter (stiffness) of the filaments and the rotational speed could be varied. Essick and Edin (1995) earlier developed a device that rotated various brushes through varying sized apertures at varying speeds, and recently developed a multiple-pin, tactile contactor surface controlled by a computer. This method has not yet been applied to the evaluation of allodynia.

The second method uses a controlled mechanical stimulus intensity to obtain a presumably lowered pain threshold in the allodynic area. The easiest clinical application is the use of calibrated monofilaments (von Frey hairs) described above. A typical procedure uses the Method of Constant Stimuli. A range of filaments that spans the threshold interval is used, i.e., the lowest is not painful and the highest is always painful. Each filament is applied 10 times and the patient, who does not observe the application, rates the each stimulus as not painful or painful. No response indicates no detection. The pain threshold can be defined by varying criteria, such as the filament that produces pain 50% of the time, or the smallest filament to produce pain 100% of the time.

Because dynamic mechanical allodynia is most sensitive to a moving stimulus, the pain threshold might be best evaluated by the methods discussed above that move a filament or brush against the skin. These methods have not yet been used for this evaluation. A vibrating tuning fork can be used to characterize a symptomatic extremity by placing the vibrating base on a finger or toe nail, or by placing the vibrating tips or counterweights lightly against the skin.

The methods used to assess thresholds can vary from simple to complex; the need for complexity will depend on the resolution required. Diagnosis of the salient features of dynamic mechanical allodynia can be demonstrated by simple procedures, while the time course of the magnitude of this allodynia or the effect of a therapeutic intervention may require more sensitive (and time-consuming) methods. In the above example in which varying nylon filaments are administered 10 times each, the simplest procedure would apply each filament 10 times, and then proceed to the next filament in either descending or ascending order. If greater sensitivity and resistance to biases are required, the order of the filaments can be randomized for each presentation. Additional controls would include the inclusion of blank stimuli, a trial in which the skin is not touched by the filament. Methods that employ blank stimuli provide a measure of sensitivity that is independent of response bias (e.g., two-alternative forced choice, Sensory Decision Theory [SDT]), and may also provide an estimate of such bias (SDT) if it is needed.

MECHANICAL HYPERALGESIA

Dynamic mechanical hyperalgesia is assessed by response to a sharp stimulus such as the neurologist's standard safety pin or the wooden handle of a cotton swab cut at a diagonal. The skin is pricked, but not pierced. With practice, the operator can administer a reasonably constant stimulus. A calibrated stimulus can also be used; a simple, sterile stimulator can be constructed by cutting the sharp arm of a sterile safety pin and crimping this "straight pin" into the bore of a large (16-gauge, 1.5-in) blunt irrigating needle. This assembly is passed down the bore of a 3-cc syringe, which serves as a handle and a guide for adjustable weights that are placed in the barrel.

Regardless of method, these punctate stimulators determine the presence of mechanical hyperalgesia by evoking a pain sensation that is distinctly different (i.e., noticeably more painful) from the sensation evoked from a control area of skin. The area of mechanical hyperalgesia can be mapped using the same strategy described above for mapping the area of mechanical allodynia.

STATIC MECHANICAL ALLODYNIA AND HYPERALGESIA

Firm pressure applied to the affected extremity can produce pain at pressure levels that do not result in pain on the unaffected extremity (Atkins and Kanis 1989; Bryan et al. 1991; Ochoa and Yarnitsky 1993). Lowered pain thresholds to pressure also have been observed in experimental models that administer topical capsaicin or mustard oil (Koltzenburg et al. 1992). The area of this sensitivity can be mapped on the skin, although the nature of the stimulus does not allow the determination of precise borders. As with the assessment of dynamic mechanical-allodynia, pain ratings can be made to a constant stimulus, or pain thresholds can be determined with a controllable stimulus. Several commercial pressure stimulators are available; the best allow the application of pressures at a constant increasing rate, an important feature because the threshold is influenced by rate (Jensen et al. 1986). The composition of the stimulated region, e.g., skin over muscle, or skin and muscle over bone, may influence the result. In addition, animal studies have shown that the response of spinal neurons with deep somatic fields is dependent also on both the area of the stimulating surface and on the duration of the pressure (W.J. Roberts, personal communication).

MECHANISMS: DYNAMIC MECHANICAL ALLODYNIA

The demonstration of pain to light touch does not specify the mechanism of dynamic mechanical allodynia. This pain could be due to high-threshold nociceptors that are sensitized to the point that they respond to gentle mechanical stimulation. Alternatively, activation of the primary afferents that usually respond to light touch, the Aβ low-threshold-mechanoreceptors (Aβ-LTMs), could under pathological conditions result in the perception of pain. While there is evidence of the former mechanism of sensitized nociceptors (Cline et al. 1989), there is now considerable evidence that dynamic mechanical allodynia is mediated by Aβ-LTM afferents. This conclusion is based on five lines of evidence shown in Table II. The methods shown in this table make extensive use of electrical skin stimulation. In addition to precise control, electrical stimuli possess two related properties useful for sensory assessment. First, these stimuli bypass receptors and directly stimulate the axons of primary afferents. Thus, the results of electrical stimulation are independent of alterations in receptor functioning, such as sensitization or suppression. Second, the sensitivity of primary afferents to electrical stimulation is based on axon diameter. The large-diameter myelinated Aβ axons are the most sensitive, the smaller-diameter thinly myelinated Aδ axons are less sensitive, and the smallest, unmyelinated C fibers are the least sensitive.

1. *The sensations produced by electrical stimulation at the threshold for detection are painful.*

Electrical stimuli of increasing intensity first activate Aβ fibers, so we can assume that these fibers are selectively activated at the threshold for detection. Under normal conditions, the sensations evoked at threshold and

Table II
Aβ-mediated mechanical allodynia: five lines of evidence

1. The sensations produced by electrical stimulation at the threshold for detection are painful.
2. Reaction time latencies to painful detection-level electrical or mechanical stimuli are consistent with Aβ conduction velocities.
3. Differential cuff or nerve compression block
4. Differential local anesthetic block
5. Microneurography

stimulus intensities near threshold are described as a light tactile, tapping sensation when the stimulus rate is low (e.g., 1 Hz) and as a "buzzing," vibratory sensation when short trains of high frequency are used (e.g., one second at 100 Hz). Sensations evoked by stimulation applied to the allodynic area in patients with neuropathic pain have been described as both tactile and pain sensations, strongly suggesting that the Aβ-LTMs mediate dynamic mechanical allodynia (Price et al. 1989; Gracely et al. 1992; Price and Harkins 1992).

Electrical stimuli used for threshold assessment have included single, brief, one-millisecond constant-current pulses (Gracely et al. 1992), or one-second trains of pulses (60 μsec, 110 Hz, Price et al. 1989; one millisecond, 100 Hz, Gracely et al. 1992). Constant-current stimulators allow the measurement of stimulus intensities at threshold (Gracely et al. 1992). However, a simple transcutaneous electrical nerve stimulation (TENS) stimulator can provide an adequate assessment in a clinical situation because the important finding is pain at detection threshold, regardless of the stimulus intensity needed to evoke the sensation. In addition, equal TENS stimulation can be applied to a contralateral "control" area, and the evoked sensations compared. Electrical stimuli also may be applied transcutaneously to the nerve innervating the pathological territory, and to a contralateral control nerve and territory (Price et al. 1989). Such stimulation produces sensation localized to both the stimulation site and the innervated area. Care must be taken to selectively evaluate the sensations evoked in the innervated area, and to delay stimulation until the sensations produced by previous stimuli have waned. In the authors' experience, short trains of high-frequency stimulation are the most effective for either skin or nerve stimulation.

2. *Reaction-time latencies to painful detection-level electrical or mechanical stimuli are consistent with Aβ conduction velocities.*

The Aβ-LTM afferents conduct impulses quite rapidly (> 30 m/s) while the small-diameter C fibers are very slow (1 m/s). (If you stub your toe, the messages from the C fibers will arrive at the spinal cord about a second after the messages from the Aβ fibers). The conduction velocity of the thinly-myelinated Aδ fibers is in between, ranging from six to 30 m/s. The conduction velocity can be estimated by measuring the reaction time latency to applied electrical or mechanical stimuli (Lindblom and Verrillo 1979; Fruhstorfer and Lindblom 1984; Campbell et al. 1988; Gracely et al. 1992). The time of conduction in the primary afferent is determined by subtracting a constant time that represents spinal and supraspinal processing and the motor response. This primary afferent traverse time is divided by an estimate of the length of the primary afferent from the stimulation site to the appropriate spinal cord segment. The result is an estimated conduction velocity for the primary afferent mediating the sensation.

Several issues surround the use of reaction time methods. First, these methods assume that the quality of the evoked sensation, when it is first felt, is painful. Thus, the reaction time represents the reaction to painful sensation, and not to a sensation that becomes painful slowly. Second, there is an overlap in the conduction velocities between Aβ and Aδ fibers. Thus, reaction times may readily distinguish between A and C fibers, but not necessarily between subclasses of A fibers (Aβ, Aδ, etc.). Third, the same stimulus intensity may produce different sensations in the test and control areas. The sensations in the control area will be painful, and may be both more intense and of different quality. Reaction times may depend on the subjective intensity of the stimulation-evoked sensations, so the stimulus intensity may need to be adjusted to produce sensations of equal overall intensity in the test and control areas.

The influence of these factors may be controlled to some extent by experimental designs. For example, the component due to central processing and motor response may be estimated by measuring the reaction time to an auditory stimulus, or to a somatosensory stimulus applied to an area with a short primary afferent distance to the spinal cord. One modification of this approach is the Helmholtz technique in which the reaction times to stimuli applied to both proximal and distal portions of the affected extremity are subtracted to give a measure of conduction time over the distance between the stimulation sites. Alternatively, comparison to a control stimulation of Aβ fibers in an unaffected area may be adequate. For example, Gracely et al. (1993) showed that the reaction times to detection-level electrical stimuli were faster when the same site was located in an area of dynamic mechanical allodynia following an intradermal injection of the irritant capsaicin. These stimuli evoked a light tactile sensation before the injection and a pain sensation after the injection, which suggested that the painful allodynic sensations were mediated by the same fast afferents mediating touch in normal skin.

3. *Differential cuff or nerve compression block*

Direct nerve compression or occlusion of blood flow by application of a tourniquet such as a blood pressure cuff (termed a cuff block because it may also include a component of nerve compression) results in a progressive loss of sensation. The order in which sensations are lost is related to the diameter of the primary afferents mediating the specific sensations, with the largest diameter fibers being blocked first and the smallest diameter fibers being blocked last. Thus, touch sensations mediated by the large-diameter Aβ fibers are lost first. The sensation of cold and the sensation of first, pricking pain are both mediated by populations of the thinly myelinated Aδ afferents, and these fibers are lost next. The sensations of warmth and of second, burning pain, mediated by the unmyelinated C fibers, are lost last.

This method has been used to investigate the primary afferents mediating Aβ mechanical allodynia in both patients (Campbell et al. 1988; Gracely et al. 1992) and normal volunteers (Gracely et al. 1993) receiving intradermal injections of capsaicin. As the block progresses, both the sensation of touch and the mechanical allodynia are lost when the sensations of cold and warmth are present. This result suggests that the mechanical allodynia is mediated by the Aβ fibers that also mediate touch sensation, and not by Aδ or C fibers, which also mediate cool and warm sensation.

4. *Differential local anesthetic block*

Local anesthetics block primary afferents, but in the opposite order than compression or ischemia; the small, unmyelinated C fibers are blocked first, followed by the Aδ fibers and then the Aβ fibers. Although the onset of local anesthesia is usually too rapid for any differential assessment, a differential evaluation can be made as the block wanes. Aβ fibers recover first, followed by Aδ and then C fibers. This method has been used to infer Aβ-evoked pain (Wallin et al. 1976; Ochoa 1982; Campbell et al. 1988; Gracely et al. 1992) by the observation that these symptoms returned after the recovery of Aβ function but at a time when both Aδ- and C-fiber activity were still blocked. With this test it is important to control for the systemic effects of the anesthetic by giving an equivalent dose either systemically or locally in a region distant from the symptomatic region.

5. *Microneurography*

The activity in specific afferents can be evaluated directly in human subjects by recording and stimulating through microelectrodes. The logic of these studies follows that of electrical skin stimulation. For example, electrical intraneural stimuli that produce only touch sensations produce painful sensations after an intradermal injection of capsaicin in adjacent skin. The pain detection threshold approaches the detection threshold, indicating that the Aβ afferents mediating touch are now mediating a pain sensation (Torebjörk et al. 1992).

In addition to these five methods, at least two clinical findings suggest the presence of Aβ mechanical allodynia. In many cases, pain can be evoked by moving hair without touching the skin. This finding is strong evidence for Aβ allodynia because hair movement is known to activate Aβ afferents. In addition, pain is often evoked when pressure from a nylon filament is quickly removed. Such pain is likely mediated by Aβ afferents because only these afferents are capable of responding to this dynamic stimulus (W.J. Roberts, personal communication).

TEMPORAL SUMMATION OF MECHANICAL ALLODYNIA

Repetitive mechanical stimulation can be used to test for the presence of slow temporal summation of mechanical allodynia. Summation to mechanical stimulation can be assessed easily with simple tools. A brush, cotton applicator, von Frey hair, gauze, or similar item is used to touch or brush the symptomatic area with sufficient force or velocity to cause pain. The stimulus is repeated at least three to four times with an interstimulus interval of about two to three seconds (not greater than four seconds) and a stimulus duration of about one second (Price et al. 1977, 1992; Dubner et al. 1987). Care must be taken to not increase stimulus intensity with each successive stimulus.

The magnitude of the summation can be evaluated by several methods, including simply asking subjects if the intensity increased over the course of the multiple stimulations. Our experience indicates that at least four trials are necessary to confirm temporal summation.

In the clinic, summation also can be evaluated by electrical stimulation, as both detection-level electrical stimulation and mechanical stimulation activate Aβ-LTM afferents. The stimulation parameters obviously can be achieved most easily with electrical as opposed to mechanical stimuli, particularly if electrical stimulators with controllable timing circuits (e.g., Grass stimulators) are available. With these methods, a stimulus intensity is selected that is just above the threshold of pain. Thus, the stimulus-evoked sensation, not the physical stimulus intensity, is equated across patients. The stimulus parameters are the same as those used for mechanical stimulation; three to four stimuli are delivered every two to three seconds, and the trial is repeated four times. Stimulus duration of electrical stimuli, however, can be much shorter—in the range of one to two milliseconds. The summation can be evaluated by the same method as at bedside, by asking if the sensations increased during the successive stimulations. Other methods appropriate for the clinic include asking subjects to quantify this increase on a ratio scale (Andersen et al., personal communication), or rating each stimulus-evoked sensation by methods such as cross-modality matching to handgrip force (Dubner et al. 1987) or by a visual analog scale (VAS) rating (Price et al. 1992).

THERMAL STIMULATION: THE SENSE OF WARMTH AND COLD

CLINICAL TESTS FOR ABNORMAL HEAT-EVOKED PAIN

Testing for heat hypoalgesia, hyperalgesia, and allodynia requires a controlled source of noxious heat stimulation. Simple clinical methods include the use of test tubes filled with heated water or objects such as brass rods kept in controlled-temperature water baths. More complicated methods include radiant-heat stimulation (Hardy-Wolff-Goodell dolorimeter) and a variety of controlled-contact thermodes including those using Peltier devices and electrically heated thermodes that also can be cooled by circulating water. These stimulators must be able to deliver brief (a few seconds) stimuli from neutral temperatures (30°C) up to those in the nociceptive range (45–51°C). The simplest approach (Fruhstorfer et al. 1976; Yarnitsky et al. 1995) uses a slowly increasing (e.g., 1°C/s) stimulus temperature to assess whether heat-induced sensations are altered within pathological cutaneous zones as compared to contralateral control zones within the same patient. Increased pain thresholds indicate heat hypoalgesia, and decreased pain thresholds indicate heat allodynia. Multiple determination of thresholds (N = 3–6) within each of these regions would be sufficient to determine whether an altered threshold exists within the pathological zone. This method is sufficient to detect the dramatic threshold changes often observed in patients with neuropathic pain, but may not be sufficient to detect subtle changes in the pain threshold. A further limitation is that only the presence of heat allodynia (often termed heat hyperalgesia) can be established by this method.

The determination of heat hyperalgesia and hyperpathia requires testing with noxious temperatures. The slow ramps used to establish pain thresholds with a Peltier stimulator described above could conceivably be continued past the pain threshold into the suprathreshold pain range. However, such continuous stimulation would transfer a great deal of heat energy, likely resulting in tissue damage or at the least considerable discomfort for the patient. This continuous stimulation is avoided in methods that present a broad range of brief stimuli in random sequence and collect the patient's judgments of pain intensity with a rating scale. For example, Fig. 1 shows a patient's ratings of five-second duration heat stimuli delivered by a 1-cm diameter contact thermode. The baseline temperature was set to 35°C, which was not painful when applied to the pathological area. This baseline temperature and the use of a contact thermode normalizes the small baseline skin temperature differences between the pathological and contralateral control areas. In this example, stimulus intensities were restricted to 43, 45, 47, and 49°C because such temperatures are sufficient to establish the presence or absence of heat allodynia and hyperalgesia and because many patients with heat hyperalgesia find it difficult to tolerate higher temperatures or extensive stimulation. These temperatures were presented three times each in random sequence to both the pathological site and the contralateral control site. Stimulus presentations were separated by at least a minute; and care was taken to delay stimulation until the pain evoked by the previous stimulus had subsided completely. As can easily be discerned from Fig. 1, heat allodynia and hyperalgesia were clearly established in this patient. Responses to both the innocuous temperature of

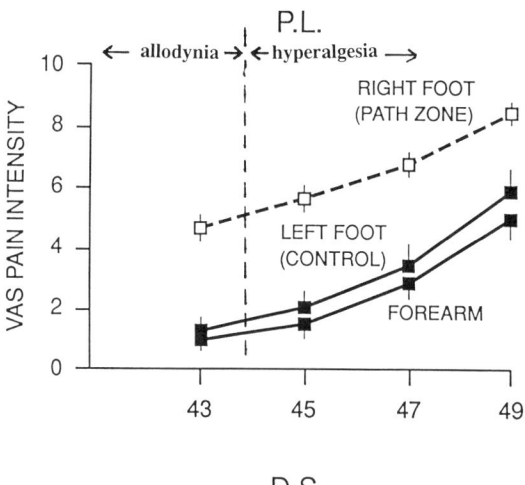
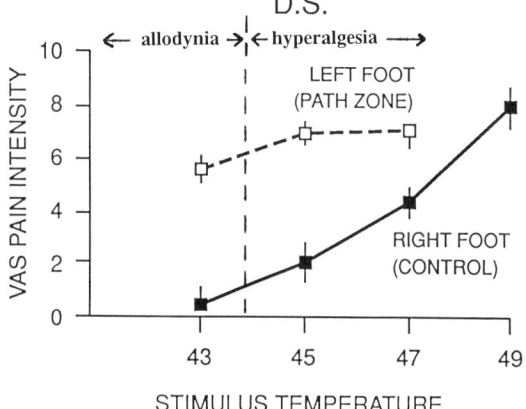

Fig. 1. Visual analog scale (VAS) ratings of pain intensity in two patients (P.L. and D.S.) who had both heat-induced allodynia and hyperalgesia. The vertical dotted line represents a theoretical pain threshold in normal skin. Ratings of thermal pain intensity evoked by stimulation of normal skin should be zero or near zero for stimulation to the left of this line and increase for stimulation to the right of the line. Ratings of sensations evoked from the pathological zone indicate allodynia if they are elevated to the left of this line (innocuous stimulus intensities evoke pain), and hyperalgesia if they are elevated to the right of this line (painful stimulus intensities evoke greater pain).

43°C and the noxious temperatures of 45, 47, and 49°C were distinctly greater on the pathological side.

Ratings of randomized discrete stimulation can also demonstrate hyperpathia; the resulting psychophysical function would show an increased threshold and an enhanced response above this threshold. However, this method may present an extremely painful stimulus early in the series, and present such stimuli more than once. If hyperpathia is suspected, a better alternative is to administer an ascending series of discrete stimuli, terminating the series once a hyperpathic response has been observed.

Evaluation of thermal pain sensation duration

The majority of pain measurement methods evaluate only the sensory intensity of the pain sensation. Recognition is increasing of the need to assess also the discomfort or unpleasantness of this pain sensation (Gracely 1992; Price and Harkins 1992) and its sensory qualities (e.g., burning, shooting, squeezing). In addition, pain sensations produced by external stimulation can also be characterized by their latency and by the variation of intensity over both time (e.g., hyperpathia) and space (e.g., spreading or radiating pains).

The temporal characteristics of an evoked pain sensation can be evaluated by methods in which subjects continuously rate the magnitude of the evoked sensation. For example, Fig. 2 shows the response to thermal stimuli applied to the pathological arm in a patient with peripheral neuropathic pain. The patient used a track ball to adjust the height of a vertical analog scale calibrated with 13 verbal descriptors of pain intensity, seven of which are shown in the figure. In this example, the patient received an ascending series of three-second thermal stimuli delivered by an 8-mm diameter contact thermode with a baseline temperature of 37°C. Stimulation of the symptomatic arm by a normally nonpainful 43°C stimulus (contralateral pain threshold was 45°C)

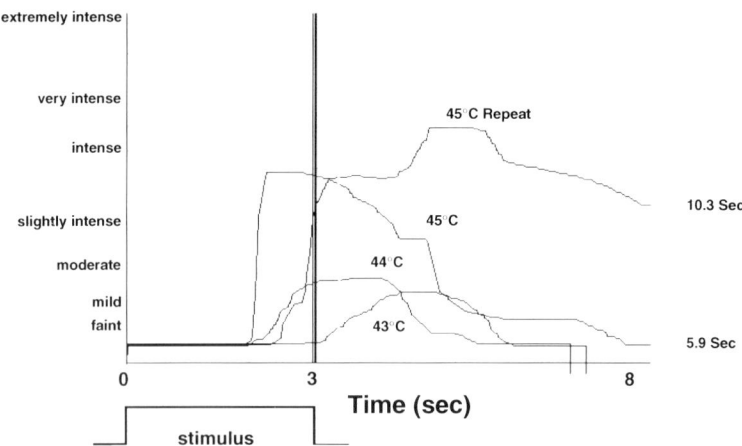

Fig. 2. Response of patient with peripheral neuropathic pain to thermal stimuli applied to the affected arm. Stimuli applied to the affected arm show a graded but hyperalgesic response to thermal stimulation. In comparison to a normal 45°C threshold on the control side, 43°C was rated as mildly painful (duration 2.9 seconds), 44°C was rated as moderately painful (duration 3.5 seconds), and 45°C as intense pain. Pain duration also increased with temperature. Repeating the 45°C stimulus produced a slight increase in pain magnitude and an increase in pain duration from 5.9 to 10.3 seconds. (Modified from Gracely 1991)

produced a pain sensation characterized as "mild;" increasing stimuli of 44°C and 45°C evoked more intense pain sensations, and the duration of the sensation to 45°C (5.9 seconds) was almost twice the duration observed on the contralateral limb or in normal subjects. Repeating the 45°C stimulus resulted in a slightly increased and delayed peak pain sensation, and a prolonged duration of 10.3 seconds. Thus, this figure demonstrates thermal allodynia, hyperalgesia, summation, and prolonged thermal sensations. Conventional rating methods would not have revealed this pronounced effect of repeating the 45°C stimulus.

Use of standard probe temperatures if a heat stimulator is not available

In the most basic clinical situation, the presence of heat allodynia and hyperalgesia can be evaluated by noting the response to the administration of constant-temperature stimuli. The stimuli can be metal probes immersed in water baths and calibrated informally by contact with the examiner's skin or with the skin of the patient in an unaffected area. A thermometer can add a degree of quantification, either by noting the temperature of the bath or by calibrating a warming procedure (for example one cup of water in a microwave for X seconds will provide a warm stimulus, and for Y seconds will provide a weak pain stimulus). Verbal responses such as "neutral, warm and not painful, hot and not painful, faint pain, mild pain, moderate pain, intense pain, extremely intense pain" (Gracely et al. 1988) would be sufficient to classify responses to determine heat allodynia and heat hyperalgesia.

Inferring functional status of C-fiber nociceptors

Both burning pain sensations and the sense of warmth are mediated by specific populations of C fibers. Therefore, the functional status of C-fiber nociceptors can be inferred by assessing warmth perception. Considerable spatial summation is required for the perception of warmth, so the surface area stimulated must be larger than that needed for thermal pain stimulation. Peltier probes of approximately 16 cm^2 are ideal for this application, while many of the 0.5–1.0 cm^2 contact probes are too small and yield irregular results. The need for a large surface area causes difficulty in the evaluation of small pathological areas.

CLINICAL TESTS FOR ABNORMAL COLD-EVOKED PAIN

Sensitivity to cold is a striking feature of many patients with CRPS I and II. Even contact with metal objects at room temperature often is quite painful. The assessment of cold hypoalgesia, hyperalgesia, and allodynia mirrors the evaluation of heat abnormalities. The description of altered responses can be confusing because the direction of a threshold change may be the opposite of a temperature change. For example, a decreased cold pain threshold indicates that cold pain was evoked by a higher temperature.

Quantified testing of cool/cold sensation must use thermal stimulators that can approach 0°C. As with heat stimulation, the simplest approach (Fruhstorfer, 1976; Yarnitsky et al. 1995) uses a slowly decreasing (e.g., 1°C/s) stimulus temperature from a neutral baseline (e.g., 30°C) to assess whether cold-induced sensations are altered within pathological cutaneous zones as compared to contralateral control zones within the same patient. Increased cold-detection thresholds and increased cold-pain thresholds indicate heat hypoalgesia, and decreased cold-pain thresholds indicate cold allodynia. Multiple determination of thresholds (N = 3–6) within each of these regions would be sufficient to determine whether an altered threshold exists within the pathological zone. The caveats associated with heat testing also apply. This method may not be sufficient to detect subtle changes in the pain threshold, and only the presence of cold allodynia (often termed cold hyperalgesia) can be established by this method.

Similar to the use of heat, the determination of true cold hyperalgesia requires testing with noxious temperatures that are painful when applied to normal skin. The possible damage of continuous heat stimulation with Peltier probes is not a critical issue when delivering cold stimuli. However, the use of slow ramps to evaluate cold hyperalgesia is limited by the discomfort that must be endured by the patient.

The use of thermodes perfused with cold water can achieve very fast cooling rates and thus minimize overall cooling by delivering discrete thermal stimuli of varying cool and cold temperatures. This capability has not been studied extensively in patients with CRPS. Evidence described below indicates that cold pain sensations may be sensitive to the rate of cooling, a dependence that could be fruitfully addressed with such devices.

Use of standard probe temperatures if a cold stimulator is not available

As noted above, one of the striking findings in patients with CRPS is that contact with room-temperature metal (23°C) is often quite painful. Such sensitivity can be easily assessed with simple tools in the clinical situation. F.A. Lenz (personal communication) has described a simple procedure in which one of the weights in a neurological tuning fork is warmed for a few minutes in the hand of the examiner. This weight is first applied to the pathological zone, followed by the identical, room-temperature weight that was not warmed. Patients often describe a nonpainful mechanical sensation when the warmed weight is applied, and a distinct, intense pain sensation when the room-temperature weight is applied, accompanied by flinching and a withdrawal reaction.

Variability in response requires a variety of probes. Standard temperatures colder than room temperature can be applied by the use of cold tap water, or objects placed in a refrigerator. Colder temperatures can be achieved by the use evaporative liquids such as alcohol, acetone, or a clinical vapo-coolant spray such as fluoromethane. These probes can be applied in order of increasing coldness and the trial stopped when pain is reached. For example, if room-temperature metal is not painful, refrigerated metal, metal from an ice bath, and a vapo-coolant spray can be applied in turn. If a thermal probe is available, ramps of decreasing temperature can be applied. If these do not evoke pain at abnormally high temperatures, fixed cold temperatures can be applied in a series of increasing coldness. We have observed many cases in which precooled probes were painful while decreasing thermal ramps were not, and in which only vapo-coolant sprays produced a pain response (Gracely et al. 1992, 1993). In all cases, responses in the pathological area are compared to responses in normal skin.

SUMMARY

Table III categorizes the methods discussed in this chapter into those that can be presented at bedside and in the clinic. At bedside, the use of minimal tools (a cotton applicator with the handle-end sharpened, a tuning fork, metal objects at room temperature [warmed in the hand or in a water bath] and cooled in a refrigerator, and vapo-coolants) can be used to determine mechanical allodynia, mechanical hyperalgesia, heat allodynia, heat hyperalgesia, cold allodynia, and temporal summation to mechanical stimulation.

More extensive testing in the clinic could use these tools and: (1) von Frey hairs to quantify detection and pain thresholds, temporal summation, and reaction to quick removal of a von Frey stimulus; (2) a pressure algometer to assess pressure-pain thresholds and determine the presence of static allodynia or hyperalgesia; (3) an electrical stimulator to assess $A\beta$-LTM-mediated mechanical allodynia and temporal summation; (4) a thermal stimulator to perform quantified thermal testing; and (5) a standard blood pressure cuff to perform differential cuff blocks.

Further tests in a laboratory setting could include continuous rating of evoked pain sensations to assess abnormal characteristics such as prolonged duration, reaction time equipment to infer conduction velocities, and other laboratory techniques such as physiological measures of nociceptive reflexes (Andersen et al. 1995).

Table III
Simple sensory testing in CRPS I and II

Bedside	Compare Symptomatic Area with Control Area
Dynamic mechanical allodynia	Stroking with a brush, gauze, or cotton applicator Hair movement Vibration by a tuning fork
Static mechanical allodynia	Manual light pressure
Mechanical hyperalgesia	Manual pinprick by safety pin, sharpened wood stick, or a calibrated stimulator
Mechanical summation	Apply dynamic stimuli every 2–3 seconds, 3–6 times.
Heat allodynia	Contact with objects kept immersed in 40–42°C water, or objects that feel warm to clinician, and to patient when applied to control area. Also compare to contact with identical object warmed to skin temperature (to control for contact-evoked pain).
Heat hyperalgesia	Contact with objects kept immersed in 45–47°C water, or objects that feel weekly painful to clinician, and to patient when applied to control area
Cold allodynia	Contact with room-temperature metal object
	Also compare to contact with identical object warmed to skin temperature (to control for contact-evoked pain)
	Contact with refrigerated object (metal or nonmetal)
	Contact with coolants (ice water, alcohol, acetone, flurometholone)
Clinic	**Additional Tests**
Touch sensitivity	von Frey hairs
Dynamic mechanical allodynia	Electrical stimulation Release of von Frey hair Differential cuff block (all above to determine Aβ involvement)
Mechanical summation	Deliver electrical stimuli every 2–3 seconds, 3–6 times.
Static mechanical allodynia	Pressure algometer
Heat allodynia	Quantitative thermal stimulator
Heat hyperalgesia	Quantitative thermal stimulator
Cold allodynia	Quantitative thermal stimulator
Cold hyperalgesia	Quantitative thermal stimulator

REFERENCES

Andersen, O.K., Gracely, R.H., Bjerring, P. and Arendt-Nielsen, L., Facilitation of the human nociceptive reflex by stimulation of Aβ-fibres in a secondary hyperalgesic area sustained by nociceptive input from the primary hyperalgesic area, Acta Physiol. Scand., 155 (1995) 87–97.

Atkins, R.M. and Kanis, J.A., The use of dolorimetry in the assessment of posttraumatic algodystrophy, Br. J. Rheumatol., 28 (1989) 404–409.

Bryan, A.S., Klenerman, L. and Bowsher, D., The diagnosis of reflex sympathetic dystrophy using an algometer, J. Bone Joint Surg. Br., 73 (1991) 644–646.

Campbell, J.N., Raja, S.N., Meyer, R.A. and MacKinnon, S.E., Myelinated afferents signal the hyperalgesia associated with nerve injury, Pain, 32 (1988) 89–94.

Cline, M.A., Ochoa, J. and Torebjörk, H.E., Chronic hyperalgesia and skin warming caused by sensitized C nociceptors, Brain, 112 (1989) 621–647.

Dubner, R., Sharav, Y., Gracely, R.H. and Price, D.D., Idiopathic trigeminal neuralgia: sensory features and pain mechanisms, Pain, 31 (1987) 23–33.

Essick, G.K. and Edin, B.B., Receptor encoding of moving tactile stimuli in humans, II. The mean response of individual low-threshold mechanoreceptors to motion across the receptive field, J. Neurosci., 15 (1995) 848–864.

Fruhstorfer, H. and Lindblom, U., Sensibility abnormalities in neuralgic patients studied by thermal and tactile pulse stimulation. In: C. von Euler, O. Franzen, U. Lindblom and D. Ottoson (Eds.), Somatosensory Mechanisms, Wenner-Gren International Symposium, Vol. 41, Macmillan, London, 1984, pp. 353–361.

Fruhstorfer, H., Lindblom, U. and Schmidt, W.G., Method for quantitative estimation of thermal thresholds in patients, J. Neurol. Neurosurg. Psychiatry, 39 (1976) 1071–1075.

Gracely, R.H., Theoretical and practical issues in pain assessment in central pain syndromes. In: K.L. Casey (Ed.), Pain and Central Nervous System Disease, Raven Press, New York, 1991, pp. 85–101.

Gracely, R.H., Affective dimensions of pain: how many and how measured? APS Journal, 1 (1992) 243–247.

Gracely, R.H., Lota, L., Walther, D.J. and Dubner, R., A multiple random staircase method of psychophysical pain assessment, Pain, 32 (1988) 55–63.

Gracely, R.H., Lynch, S.A. and Bennett, G.J., Painful neuropathy: altered central processing maintained dynamically by peripheral input, Pain, 51 (1992) 175–194.

Gracely, R.H., Barcellos, S.A., Saltzman, S.J., Byas-Smith, M.G., Max, M.B. and Bennett, G.J., Aβ mechano-allodynia and cold hyperalgesia following large doses of intradermal capsaicin, Society for Neuroscience Abstracts, 1993, p. 1073.

Hardy, J.D, Wolff, H.G. and Goodell, H., Pain Sensation and Reactions, Williams & Wilkins, Baltimore, 1952.

Jensen, K., Andersen, H., Oleson, J. and Lindblom, U., Pressure-pain threshold in human temporal region: evaluation of a new pressure algometer, Pain, 25 (1986) 313–323.

Koltzenburg, M., Lundberg, L.E.R. and Torebjörk, H.E., Dynamic and static components of mechanical hyperalgesia in human hairy skin, Pain, 51 (1992) 207–219.

LaMotte, R.H., Shain, C.N., Simone, D.A. and Tsai, E.-F.P., Neurogenic hyperalgesia: psychophysical studies of underlying mechanisms, J. Neurophysiol., 66 (1991) 190–211.

Lindblom, U. and Verrillo, R.T., Sensory functions in chronic neuralgia, J. Neurol. Neurosurg. Psychiatry, 42 (1979) 422–424.

Merskey, H. and Bogduk, N. (Eds.), Classification of Chronic Pain, 2nd ed., IASP Press, Seattle, 1994.

Ochoa, J.L., Pain in local nerve lesions. In: W.J. Culp and J. Ochoa (Eds.), Abnormal Nerves and Muscles as Impulse Generators, Oxford University Press, Oxford, 1982, pp. 568–587.

Ochoa, J.L. and Yarnitsky, D., Mechanical hyperalgesias in neuropathic pain patients: dynamic and static subtypes, Ann. Neurol., 33 (1993) 465–472.

Price, D.D. and Harkins, S.W., The affective motivational dimension of pain: a two-stage model, APS Journal, 1 (1992) 229–239.
Price, D.D., Bennett, G.J. and Rafii, A., Pyschophysical observations on patients with neuropathic pain relieved by a sympathetic block, Pain, 36 (1989) 237–288.
Price, D.D., Hu, J.W., Dubner, R. and Gracely, R.H., Peripheral suppression of first pain and central summation of second pain evoked by noxious heat pulses, Pain, 3 (1977) 57–68.
Price, D.D., Long, S. and Huit, C., Sensory testing of pathophysiological mechanisms of pain in patients with reflex sympathetic dystrophy, Pain, 49 (1992) 163–173.
Torebjörk, H.E., Lundberg, L.E.R. and LaMotte, R.H., Central changes in processing of mechanoreceptive input in capsaicin-induced secondary hyperalgesia in humans, J. Physiol., 448 (1992) 765–780.
Wallin, B.G., Torebjörk, E. and Hallin, R.G., Preliminary observations on the pathophysiology of hyperalgesia in the causalgic pain syndrome. In: Y. Zotterman (Ed.), Sensory Functions of the Skin of Primates with Special Reference to Man, Pergamon Press, Oxford, 1976, pp. 489–499.
Yarnitsky, D., Sprecher, E., Zaslansky, R. and Hemli, J.A., Heat pain thresholds: normative data and repeatability, Pain, 60 (1995) 329–332.

Correspondence to: Richard H. Gracely, PhD, Building 10, Room 1N-103, National Institutes of Health, Bethesda, MD 20892, USA. Tel: 301-496-5238; Fax: 301-496-2443; E-mail: Gracely@yoda.nidr.nih.gov.

10

The Challenge and the Problem of Placebo in Assessment of Sympathetically Maintained Pain

Donald D. Price,[a] Richard H. Gracely,[b] and Gary J. Bennett[b]

[a]*Anesthesiology Department, Medical College of Virginia, Richmond, Virginia, and* [b]*Neurobiology and Anesthesiology Branch, National Institute of Dental Research, National Institutes of Health, Bethesda, Maryland, USA*

The role of the sympathetic efferent system in complex regional pain syndrome (CRPS) I and II has been extremely controversial for two major reasons. First, several technical problems are associated with diagnostic tests of sympathetic efferent involvement in these pain states. Second, the testing situation fosters a placebo response that is particularly difficult to evaluate when diagnosing sympathetically maintained pain (SMP). Part of this latter problem relates to a widespread misunderstanding of what is required to establish the presence of a placebo effect and to rule it out in the assessment of an active treatment.

This chapter will explain the basis on which placebo effects, in general, are established, and explain these problems as they specifically relate to the challenge of assessing the role of the sympathetic efferent system in CRPS I and II. The basis for establishing a placebo effect requires an understanding of the nature of placebo analgesia and the factors that contribute to its presence and magnitude.

FACTORS THAT POTENTIALLY CONTRIBUTE TO PLACEBO ANALGESIA

A strong need to be relieved of pain, expectations that pain relief will occur as a result of a treatment, and a treatment situation that reproduces in some way a previously effective treatment may promote a placebo analgesic response. A better understanding of how placebo manipulations (e.g., saline injections) can reduce pain requires explicit attention to determine which dimensions of pain are most affected by such manipulations and the most important psychological factors that contribute to the placebo effect. Considerations in analysis of placebo analgesia include environmental or situational factors, learning, and cognitive factors such as perceived need of pain relief and expectancy. The following discussion will deal briefly with each type of factor.

ENVIRONMENTAL AND SITUATIONAL FACTORS

Evidence is strong that the magnitude of placebo analgesia is influenced by the degree of threat that is present in the context of placebo treatments. Based on comparisons of placebo analgesic effects across studies of different types of pain, both Beecher (1955, 1959) and Jospe (1978) asserted that the magnitudes of analgesic response to an explicit placebo manipulation are, in general, much greater in studies of clinical pain than in studies of experimental pain. Although both authors base this assertion on numerous studies, a serious limitation in this comparison is that the clinical studies rarely consider the natural history of the patients' or subjects' pain. However, among studies using experimental pain, which more often include assessments of the natural history and or baseline reliability, placebo analgesic effects are larger for those forms of experimental pain that are of longer duration or are more stressful (Jospe 1978). These types of experimental pain are more likely to simulate the psychological conditions of most acute clinical pains. Thus, while placebo treatment produces large reductions in experimental limb ischemic pain, which continuously increases in intensity over several minutes (Grevert et al. 1983; Grevert and Goldstein 1985), placebo has no effect on brief pains produced by five-second heat stimuli applied to the skin (Price et al. 1985, 1986) or one-second electrical stimuli applied to the tooth pulp (Gracely 1979).

Situational factors that influence perceived threat are likely to vary considerably according to the external circumstances of the patient and the specific meanings the patient gives to these circumstances. These factors are likely to contribute to the large variability in mean magnitude of the placebo effect across studies (Jospe 1978; White et al. 1985). Systematic differences in natural history across different types of pain also may have contributed to this variability.

THE CONTRIBUTION OF COGNITIVE FACTORS

The study of cognitive factors has the potential for increasing understanding of how learning influences the placebo effect and how factors not directly related to classical conditioning influence placebo responses. First, conditioning stimuli (e.g., syringes, doctors in white coats) and conditioned responses (e.g., pain relief) may well have concomitant cognitive dimensions. For example, conditioning stimuli occurring during the visit to the doctor and during the prescription and ingestion of medication (via pills and syringes) become associated with active pharmacological agents (unconditioned stimuli) and with the reduction in pain (unconditioned responses). Conditioned stimuli can indicate that the period of pain, uncertainty, fear, and depression is over or that relief and healing are imminent.

While the consideration of cognitive factors extends and supports the role of learning and even classical conditioning in placebo analgesia, cognitive factors also help to resolve some of the limitations and inconsistencies of classical conditioning as an explanation for placebo analgesia. Although evidence is ample that prior exposure to an effective treatment enhances placebo effects, such prior exposure is not necessary for a placebo response. Because of the important roles that meanings, attributions, imagery, and information have in mediating beliefs, desires, and expectations, it is plausible that the placebo response is more directly controlled by these cognitive factors than by the immediate and direct association of a specific treatment with pain reduction as required for classical conditioning (i.e., conditioned stimuli or CS and unconditioned stimuli or UCS).

Indeed, consideration of the nature of suggestions inherent in placebo manipulations strongly indicate that cognitive factors operate to influence and even determine the nature and magnitude of the placebo response. The suggestion in placebo analgesia is that pain relief is being provided from an outside authoritative source (e.g., pain medicine prescribed by a knowledgeable professional). The placebo literature contains evidence that greater placebo effects are achieved by more believable and more technically convincing agents. Thus, Traut and Passarelli (1957) claimed that placebo injections are more effective than placebo pills and placebo morphine is more effective than placebo aspirin. Implicit in the overall suggestion inherent to a placebo analgesic manipulation is the idea that in the absence of this outside authoritative agent, pain would not be relieved.

THE CONTRIBUTION OF LEARNING AND EXPECTATION

It is common clinical experience that patients learn to expect therapeutic effects from various treatments. Several psychologists have independently proposed that the placebo response can be at least partly explained by classical conditioning, thereby providing a formal, testable scientific model for the role of learning in the placebo response (Watkins and Mayer 1982; Wickramasekera 1985). Human studies clearly show that prior experience with an effective analgesic drug enhances the analgesic effectiveness of a subsequent placebo. To take one of the more salient examples from the literature, Laska and Sunshine (1973) designed a clinical trial in which a second medication, always placebo, followed graded doses of propoxyphene HCL (three dose levels), propoxyphene napsylate (three doses), or placebo. There were seven groups with 14 to 20 patients in each group. Their results showed convincing evidence of a dose-response relationship between the dose of the first medication and the analgesic response to the subsequent placebo, though the magnitudes of placebo effects were lower than were their corresponding doses of the active drug. Placebo given as a second treatment acted as an effective analgesic when it followed an effective analgesic, whereas placebo following a placebo continued to have the same slight analgesic effect as did the first placebo. We can easily interpret their results as supportive of learning, even classical conditioning.

This possible role of *expectation* in placebo responses is supported both by new alternative models of learning (Reiss 1980) and by some evidence that expectation plays a critical role in the placebo response. Recognizing that classical conditioning itself may reflect a cognitive process, Reiss argues that what is learned in Pavlovian conditioning is an expectation regarding the occurrence or nonoccurrence of an unconditioned stimulus onset or a change in its magnitude or duration. However, although classical conditioning is one way to change expectation, other types of learning can contribute. For example, expectation can reflect knowledge about the therapeutic agent, the circumstances under which it is administered, and the condition to be treated. Classical conditioning could result in increased knowledge about the efficacy of the therapeutic agent by producing a memory of past effects. A person could also read a book about the agent's therapeutic efficacy. In either case, increased information indicating an agent's effectiveness could increase expectation of relief. What this implies for placebo analgesia is that *expectation* for relief may cause a placebo response in a subject who has no prior exposure to a therapeutic agent, though such exposure certainly will increase expectation (Laska and Sunshine 1973). Evidence exists that the expectation of the clinician administering the placebo can influence the placebo response (Gracely et al.

1985). Belief in the efficacy of the treatment may lead to subtle behaviors that increase the "authority" of the placebo administrator. Indeed, it may be useful to consider the placebo response not from the view of only the patient or only the clinician, but as a social interaction between the two.

THE ROLE OF DESIRE FOR RELIEF OR MOTIVATION

Although expectation may be a salient factor that influences the magnitude of the placebo response, it does not appear to operate alone. Placebo effects are commonly observed in circumstances wherein it is likely that subjects not only expect therapeutic effects but also strongly want them to occur. Although desire for relief, or motivation, which is not quite the same thing, has been directly or indirectly implicated in the placebo response, less explicit recognition has been given to this factor than to that of expectation. In one exceptional study of placebo manipulations suggesting possible sedative or stimulant effects, Jensen and Karoly (1991) assessed the separate contributions of *motivation* and *expectancy* to placebo responses. They manipulated both these factors by separate instructions and then later checked (by subject self-ratings) to determine whether either or both factors had been influenced. Thus, the study was a 2 × 2 factorial design that contained four groups (high motivation–high expectancy, etc.). They found that motivation accounted for a significant amount of variance in the placebo responses that included both perceived sedation or stimulant effect, but they obtained equivocal results from expectation. Nevertheless, they maintained that both factors are likely to contribute to placebo responses.

Desire for a specific treatment or agent to produce relief may account for the increase in placebo response with increasing severity of clinical pain and for the generally greater placebo effect for clinical pain as compared to experimental pain (Beecher 1959; Jospe 1978). Thus, the greater and more open-ended is the threat related to the pain, the greater the need for relief and the greater the placebo response.

DESIRE FOR RELIEF AND EXPECTATION

The combined factors of desire and expectation may account for the association between the placebo response and anxiety. Anxiety represents a combination of desire to avoid negative consequences coupled with an uncertain expectation of avoiding those consequences (Price et al. 1980, 1985). These two dimensions comprise the anxiety that is associated with acute clinical pain. To the extent that patients increase their expectation that a given treatment or agent will reduce their pain, their anxiety decreases when they receive the treatment. This reduction in anxiety would be expected to reduce the unpleasantness associated with pain (Price 1988).

Repeated treatments that are efficacious in reducing pain lead to increased expectations for relief. However, while repetition of the treatments and hence conditioning may be sufficient for such an effect, it may not be necessary. Cognitive influences that have a direct, immediate, and unique impact on a person's desire for relief and expectation might occur without prior exposure to the treatment under question. Thus, the combination of these two factors accounts for the several studies that directly or indirectly indicate that *expectation* is a salient determinant of placebo analgesia (Laska and Sunshine 1973; White et al. 1985) and for the general association between severity of pain or extent of threat and magnitude of placebo analgesia.

EFFECTS OF COGNITIVE FACTORS ON MULTIPLE DIMENSIONS OF PAIN

Just as multiple psychological dimensions or factors contribute to placebo responses, the placebo responses themselves are likely to be comprised of multiple dimensions. Pain has both a sensory-discriminative and an affective-motivational dimension. A research strategy for characterizing the critical psychological factors that mediate placebo analgesia could be integrated with one that assesses how these factors influence the different dimensions of pain. The potential strength of this strategy requires use of accurate, sensitive, and valid methods of pain measurement. This may be accomplished by using methods that fulfill criteria for ideal pain measurement (Gracely and Dubner 1981; Price 1988). Direct magnitude scaling of sensory and affective dimensions of pain would seem essential, especially if placebo effects differentially influence the two dimensions of pain. Tursky has recommended the use of more sophisticated scaling methods and has pointed out the deficiencies of category and other assessment methods as they relate to the assessment of placebo effects.

Under some circumstances, placebo effects in pain patients may involve only a reduction in anxiety and therefore a selective reduction in the affective dimension of pain. Such a selective antianxiety effect could occur if the patient was led to expect that the therapeutic agent would make the pain less threatening, bothersome, or distressing, but not necessarily less intense (e.g., "I am going to give you something to make it easier to tolerate the pain."). The patient's expectation that the agent will have such an effect might in itself reduce anxiety both before and after a painful procedure, thereby reducing both the anxiety of anticipating pain and the unpleasantness of the pain. Thus far, only one study has shown a selective effect of a placebo on the affective dimension of pain. Gracely (1979) found that saline placebo reduced affective but not sensory ratings of experimental pain, and that this effect was greater toward the low end of the nociceptive stimulus range. This pattern of effect is similar to that produced by diazepam, an anxiety-reducing agent (Gracely et al. 1978), and by cognitive manipulations that are likely to reduce anxiety (Price et al. 1988).

It is unlikely that all placebo manipulations selectively influence the affective dimension of pain by reducing anxiety. In fact, such a possibility is inconsistent with the observation that placebo effects are larger for severe pain as compared to mild pain, a pattern at variance with Gracely et al.'s (1979) finding that an antianxiety agent reduced the unpleasantness of mild but not more intense pain. It is also inconsistent with other studies showing placebo effects on sensory intensive aspects of pain and the reversal of these effects by naloxone (Grevert and Goldstein 1985). We must consider the possibility of multiple placebo analgesic effects. Clearly, different desires and expectations could be induced in patients and subjects by the way placebo suggestions are framed, and even the same placebo instructions could lead some persons to expect reductions in unpleasantness and others to expect reductions in both pain sensation intensity and unpleasantness. These possibilities are indirectly supported by studies of hypnotic analgesia wherein different subjects show vastly different reductions in pain-affect and pain-sensation intensity (Price and Barber 1987; Kiernan et al. 1995).

Both the situational context and level of pain converge to influence a person's desire for relief and expectation that a given therapeutic agent will result in relief. These cognitive factors, in turn, are likely to strongly influence the magnitude of pain relief produced by a placebo treatment. The consequent magnitudes of reduction in pain sensation and pain unpleasantness are likely to vary considerably across subjects and clinical contexts. Nevertheless, it is possible to measure both the factors that are most directly responsible for producing placebo analgesia and the pain dimensions that are affected, and thereby provide a potential scientific analysis of placebo analgesia.

RATIONALE FOR ASSESSMENT OF PLACEBO EFFECTS IN CLINICAL ANALGESIA STUDIES

CONSIDERATION OF NATURAL HISTORY

Unlike experimental pain, whose intensity can be controlled by controlling stimulus factors, investigators must rely on the natural history of pain intensity in clinical studies, that is, the temporal profile of pain intensity that occurs without any treatment whatsoever. Natural histories of pain vary according to type of clinical pain and circumstances. For example, the natural history of most postoperative pains is that of a slow increase in intensity over time, whereas that of migraine headaches is often that of a gradual rise in pain intensity to a severe level followed by a decline to no pain at all. Natural histories of pain also vary considerably across patients. Thus, any treatment may be followed by a reduction in pain level as a result of the natural history rather than the treatment itself. To attribute a reduction in pain to any antecedent treatment, including placebo, is an inference. Without a natural history control condition, this attribution is not valid because we do not know the change in pain intensity that would have occurred without the treatment. For this reason, the assessment of the mean magnitude of a placebo analgesic effect in a group of patients can only be carried out by comparing a no-treatment condition with that of the placebo treatment condition. Since few studies of placebo analgesia have included an untreated comparison group or condition (in crossover studies), little knowledge exists with regard to the magnitude, time course, or frequency of occurrence of placebo effects. Indeed, in the absence of a no-treatment group, it is difficult to know whether a placebo treatment has produced any effect at all.

THE PROBLEMS OF OBSERVING INDIVIDUAL PLACEBO RESPONSES

Lack of consideration of these issues has resulted in the frequently unwarranted conclusion that a placebo response has occurred if a patient's pain is observed to decrease following placebo treatment. Without a natural history control comparison, we can neither exclude the possibility that a placebo effect is absent nor confirm that it has occurred. The two types of pain mentioned above can serve as examples. Giving a placebo treatment at the peak of a migraine headache would likely be followed by a reduction in pain, regardless of whether the placebo had any effect. The reduction, however, does not establish the presence of a placebo response. Likewise, a postoperative pain that steadily increased in intensity may continue to increase in intensity despite any small reduction in pain produced by the placebo treatment. The absence of an overall reduction in pain does not mean that a placebo response did not occur. In both examples, the placebo effect is the measured difference between the level of pain with and without the presence of the placebo treatment. In a situation where there is a strong placebo response, it may be difficult or impossible to determine anything about the effects of the test agent.

Given the variability in individual natural histories and different types of clinical pain, group comparisons are usually the only reliable way to assess the magnitudes and time course of placebo analgesia. It is possible to establish an individual's placebo response, but this would require extensive analysis and procedures. An individual occurrence of placebo analgesic effect could possibly be determined by comparing the patient's postplacebo pain level at any given time with a group-derived mean. If this patient's response was significantly below the group mean, we could infer (at a defined level of confidence) that a response to placebo had occurred. Alternatively, a clinician could administer multiple placebo treatments to a patient and compare the mean analgesic response to these treatments with that for multiple untreated occurrences of the same pain condition in the same patient. This latter approach has practical, theoretical, and ethical problems. It requires extensive experimentation on the same patient, which may be costly, time consuming, and greatly discomforting and stressful. It could even produce long-term increases in pain, particularly in neuropathic pain patients.

Given this difficulty in identifying an individual placebo response, the assumption that an individual placebo responder can be identified seems unwarranted, as is the idea that the fraction of placebo responders can be identified within a given study. Although the figure of 33% is commonly quoted in papers and textbooks, it is extremely misleading because the "fraction" varies enormously (from close to 0 to 100%) depending on the exact circumstances of the study and probably on numerous subject-related factors (Wall 1994, for review). Closely allied with the fixed fraction myth is the notion that the tendency toward responding to a placebo represents a stable personality trait. Based on a review of 36 studies by Turner et al. (1980) and those described in White et al. (1985), most papers report no significant correlation between placebo response and personality, and the remainder are contradictory.

SPECIFIC METHODS OF CONTROLLING FOR PLACEBO EFFECTS IN CLINICAL STUDIES

There are presently two accepted methods for controlling for placebo response: (1) double-blind comparison of active treatment versus placebo control, and (2) hidden infusion wherein the active drug is infused at a time unbeknownst to the patient (or subject). A combination of both approaches is possible. An important point is that nearly all studies that include a placebo condition do not directly assess a placebo effect. Such an assessment can only be carried out by comparing the results of a placebo condition with that of a natural history control condition. Nevertheless, when effects of an active drug or treatment condition are compared with a placebo condition, the latter includes both the natural history and the placebo.

The first method is a subtractive method wherein the placebo influence is present in both conditions, but the active treatment is present only in one. The difference in analgesic effects between the two conditions is believed to represent the unique contribution of the treatment or active ingredient to analgesia. The validity of this comparison requires the psychological factors that contribute to the placebo effect to be the same for both conditions. This may be accomplished if neither the patient nor the person who administers the treatment knows whether the active ingredient is contained in the treatment and if the procedures for administrating the treatment are the same across the two conditions. If the patient can somehow detect the presence of the active ingredient, then the double-blind is rendered invalid. Clinicians and researchers sometimes attempt to solve this problem by including an active agent in the placebo control condition, for example, by administering a barbiturate or tranquilizer in comparison to morphine, the "active" ingredient. The problems with this approach are that the active placebo controls are by no means neutral with regard to their effects on pain, and no agent other than morphine produces the exact subjective effects of morphine. This is not a trivial concern if the subjective effects of morphine provide the strongest signal that pain relief is imminent and increase the patient's expectation for such relief.

A second method is to reduce the contribution of psychological factors that influence the placebo response during administration of both the active ingredient and the saline (or vehicle) control substance. This reduction may be accomplished by the technique of hidden infusion wherein the injection is carried out behind a screen (Gracely et al. 1983). If a stable baseline of pain intensity occurs prior to the infusion and if the patient cannot detect the time of infusion, then the reduction in pain intensity that occurs after the infusion can be attributed to the influence of the active ingredient. Unlike the first method described, psychological factors that are likely to contribute to placebo effects are greatly reduced under both experimental conditions. There are no doctors with white coats and no large syringes. However, the psychological factors that may contribute to the placebo response are not totally eliminated because the mere context of the procedure may produce some degree of placebo response. That is why a stable baseline over time is necessary, not only to control for the infusion of the vehicle (e.g., saline), but also to control for possible placebo effects related to the general context as well as the immediate natural history of the pain intensity.

Similar to the first method, that of hidden infusion requires that the patient not be able to detect the possible subjective effects of the active agent. Thus, although it may be possible to assess the relative contribution of active ingredients of an analgesic drug, it is often difficult, and several conditions need to be established to control for placebo effects. Clearly, this method is limited to injections and could not likely be used for many types of pain treatments, such as somatosensory stimulation therapies, or even with pills. The potential validity of both methods also requires that accurate, sensitive, and valid methods of pain measurement be used.

ASSESSMENT OF PLACEBO EFFECTS IN IDENTIFYING THE ROLE OF THE SYMPATHETIC EFFERENT SYSTEM IN CRPS I AND II

What constitutes the placebo effect and how to assess its influence have emerged as controversial issues in diagnostic tests of sympathetically maintained pain. Indeed, these problems seem to be magnified within this particular clinical circumstance. Factors known or suspected to strongly influence placebo, such as anxiety, desire for relief, or expectancy, appear to be maximized under conventional diagnostic anesthetic sympathetic blocks. The patients usually have constant and often severe pain, and the block procedure is somewhat invasive, so patients are often anxious prior to and during the procedure and relieved after it is over. Their desire for relief is likely to be strong and the expectations for pain reduction may be optimized by the elaborateness and invasiveness of the procedure itself, thereby maximizing the placebo effect. In addition, because their pain may be sympathetically maintained, their sympathetic efferent outflow may be high prior to block and reduced after a placebo saline block. Thus, an irony of distinguishing placebo from active sympathetic blocks is that all the psychological factors that may enhance placebo responses appear to be present during conventional sympathetic block, including the possibility that anxiety may enhance sympathetic efferent outflow. Thus, the issues discussed above with regard to assessment of the contribution of placebo effects in research studies are especially applicable to the assessment of the role of SMP in CRPS I and II.

ASSESSMENT OF SMP BY ANESTHETIC BLOCK OF SYMPATHETIC GANGLIA

Given the considerable problems of rigorously controlling for placebo responses in clinical research settings in general, and in clinical diagnosis of sympathetically maintained pain, what can the clinician do in ordinary clinical settings to assess the placebo response, albeit using imperfect methods? Specific guidelines have been recommended to help increase the certainty of the diagnostic value of anesthetic blockade of the relevant sympathetic ganglia, and consideration of possible placebo effects has figured prominently in these guidelines. Thus, Bonica (1990) has recommended repeating the block at least three times with local anesthetics with different durations of action, and Lindblom and Nemeth (1992) have recommended a direct comparison between local anesthetic and placebo injections. Unfortunately, none of these guidelines control for placebo effects.

Unless the clinician can know the magnitude of the placebo effect that should occur under the specific circumstances of a sympathetic block, it is difficult to rely on a comparison between placebo and the active anesthetic agent. Similarly, setting a criterion for percent pain relief produced by the local anesthetic would be arbitrary, particularly in view of the strong possibility that placebo effects may be maximized during procedures of sympathetic blockade. The comparison of local anesthetics with saline is difficult to interpret because saline has some local anesthetic properties (Urban and McKain 1978). Finally, the reliability of the blocking effect does not in itself serve to eliminate the possibility of a placebo effect, particularly without a comparison to repeated placebo blocks and with repeated observations of natural history. For these reasons and for the general considerations discussed earlier, it is difficult to determine whether a placebo response has occurred in a given patient. Placebo effect magnitudes are best assessed in studies of group responses and even they present considerable difficulty.

To further illustrate the complexity of assessing a placebo response in an individual patient, let us consider the data presented in Figs. 1 and 2 for a patient with CRPS I who had previous successful sympathetic anesthetic blocks. This patient went through a double-blind test with an active local anesthetic block (lidocaine) and a saline block. As shown in Fig. 1, both saline injection and local anesthetic injection of the stellate ganglion had virtually equal and powerful effects on this patient's pain. Based on the lack of differential effects between the local anesthetic and saline, we may be tempted to conclude that the effect of the local anesthetic injection was that of a powerful placebo, although direct effects of saline on the stellate ganglion cannot be ruled out. However, close monitoring of the patient's pain for hours and days after each injection clearly showed that the pain-reducing effect of the saline injection subsided within the first few hours, whereas that of the local anesthetic injection persisted for several days (Fig. 2). These effects, in turn, can be compared to those produced by a natural history control condition of having the patient lay quietly on the hospital bed for one and a half hours. This latter condition produced no reduction in pain intensity. Thus, local anesthetic block of the stellate ganglion produced an analgesic effect that long outlasted the durations of many influences that are considered to produce placebo effects. The critical difference between effects of active sympathetic blockade and alternative control

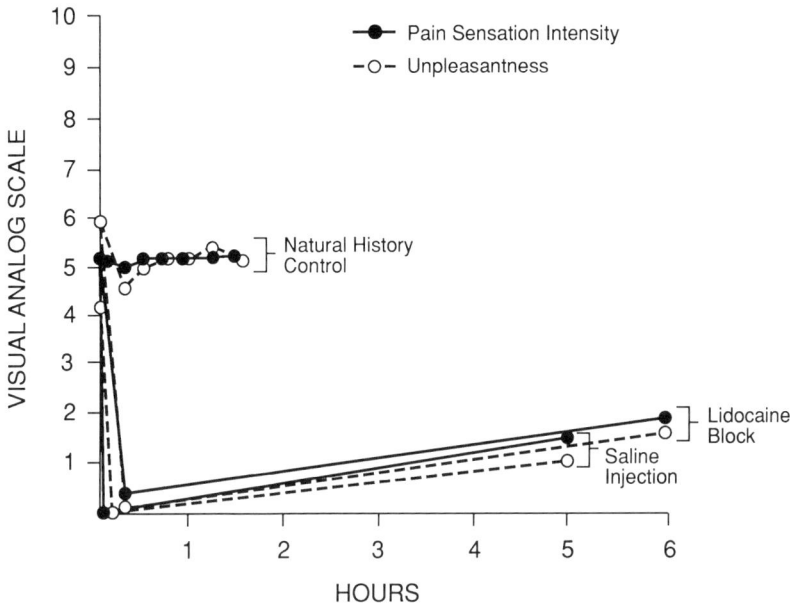

Fig. 1. A patient's visual analog scale ratings of pain sensation and unpleasantness for six hours after receiving a saline injection or local anesthetic injection of the stellate ganglion. Both injections had virtually equal and powerful effects.

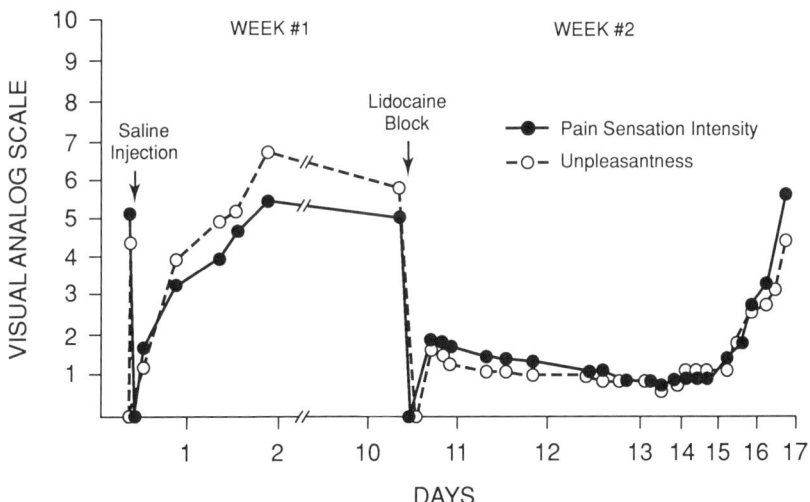

Fig 2. Close monitoring of the patient's pain for 17 days after each injection showed that the pain-reducing effect of the saline injection subsided within a few hours, whereas that of the local anesthetic lasted for several days.

conditions may not occur in the first few hours after treatment but in the several hours and days that follow treatment. The robust differential duration of analgesic action between a strong (i.e., lidocaine) and weak (i.e., saline) local anesthetic might be interpreted as evidence against the former as being simply the result of a placebo effect.

Other technical and interpretational problems can potentially confound diagnostic tests of sympathetic block by local anesthetics. The first relates to potential effects of local anesthetics independent of their effects on sympathetic ganglia. Systemic uptake of local anesthetics occurs within minutes of injection, particularly within the highly vascularized region near the stellate ganglion (Dellemijn et al. 1994). The consequent elevation in blood levels of local anesthetic reach well into the therapeutic range for local anesthetic antiarrhythmic effects, and such effects are now known to reduce abnormal generators of nerve impulses that occur in neuropathic pain conditions. Furthermore, depending on the volume of injected solution and individual factors, local anesthetic can spread to nearby nerve roots or proximal brachial plexus (in the case of stellate block) and can even spread across the midline. A second interpretational problem is that a response to either saline or local anesthetic will be highly problematic if the patient has a pain that is only partly sympathetically dependent (as is interpretation of a response to phentolamine). Thus, partial relief may be obtained as a result of several potential phenomena: placebo response, psychological effects on sympathetic outflow, partial sensory block, and systemic effects of local anesthetic on abnormal neural generators of nociceptive afferent activity. The extent to which these problems actually confound diagnostic tests of anesthetic sympathetic block has yet to be empirically determined. Thus, while local anesthetic blocks of sympathetic ganglia can be useful as screening for their potential therapeutic value, they are not likely to be specific tests of SMP and their results can be easily misinterpreted.

THE USE OF THE PHENTOLAMINE TEST IN ASSESSING SMP

Raja and colleagues have attempted to solve many of the problems related to the placebo effect by using a hidden infusion method to inject systemic phentolamine, an alpha adrenergic antagonist (Raja et al. 1991). The test is probably more specific than that of anesthetic sympathetic block in that the infusion procedure permits the time of changes in pain intensities to be correlated with the time of phentolamine infusion and thereby helps to differentiate drug-related effects from placebo effects. Moreover, a strong correlation between pain reduction during phentolamine infusion and pain reduction during sympathetic ganglia block has been found in 18 patients even after excluding those who had prominent reductions in pain intensity during the placebo phase of the phentolamine test (Raja et al. 1991). However, the phentolamine dose that may be effective in reversing sympathetically maintained pain is not yet determined, and there exists the possibility that the effective dose is detectable in patients who receive a hidden infusion. A more practical problem is that this approach is somewhat elaborate and requires considerable technician time and expense. It is becoming apparent that no single type of test for SMP is without considerable problems of interpretation.

CONCLUSIONS ABOUT THE PROBLEM OF PLACEBO IN ESTABLISHING SMP

Multiple lines of evidence demonstrate a sympathetic efferent involvement in various types of neuropathic pain diseases (Chapters 2, 5–10, 12, this volume). Studies of SMP in rat models provide evidence that SMP and sympathetically independent pain (SIP) coexist for different types of pain diseases and even that SMP and SIP may exist in combination in the same body region (Chapter 7, this volume). Thus, the role of the sympathetic efferent system in various types of neuropathic pain diseases has become increasingly clear in recent years. Although it quite evident that SMP exists and is an integral though variable manifestation of various pathophysiological pain syndromes, the presence or absence of SMP in individual patients is always questionable because of the problems elaborated above, particularly the problem of placebo effect. Placebo effects are measured in groups and in well-controlled studies, not in individual patients. It would be of great importance to conduct well-controlled studies to determine the relative extent of SMP in groups of patients with fully characterized pain diseases because such studies could elucidate the mechanisms of these diseases and the general extent to which treatments using sympathetic efferent blocking agents may be effective. It also may be of great potential therapeutic value to provide each patient with a series of multiple sympathetic blocks separated by brief intervals (e.g., a few days), simply to determine whether such blocks are effective treatments, *regardless of their exact neural mechanisms*. Indeed, such an approach has long been known to have significant practical value (Bonica 1990). Nevertheless, using multiple blocks and multiple control treatments, including natural history and placebo conditions to determine the exact extent to which a given patient's pain is SMP does not appear feasible given the considerations discussed in this chapter.

Finally, it is important to emphasize that assessments of placebo effects in clinical studies of multiple patient groups (or at least multiple conditions across a group of patients) are necessary to determine both the efficacy and the mechanisms of sympatholytic agents for pain. Placebo responses in individual patients are extremely difficult to establish. Many patients who have a documented organic basis for their pain may experience a temporary reduction in pain intensity when given a placebo (which doesn't necessarily mean that they have a placebo response). Such a reduction cannot and should not be used to provide information about the veracity, severity, or "psychogenicity" of a patient's pain. Many psychological factors, such as placebo, hypnotic suggestions, and even naturally occuring psychological contexts can, under the right conditions appropriate to each individual, powerfully alter the experience of many types of pain, including experimental pain. There is no reason to believe that because such psychological influences can exert a potent influence in a given person, the pain experienced by that person is unrelated to an organic cause or unrelated to nociceptive information in ascending afferent pathways.

ACKNOWLEDGMENTS

The authors wish to acknowledge the conceptual contribution from Dr. Howard L. Fields concerning the necessity of considering natural history in evaluating placebo effects. We also wish to thank the staff of the pain management center at the Medical College of Virginia and a pain patient (N.G.) for providing the data shown in Fig. 1.

REFERENCES

Barber, J. and Adrian, C., Psychological Approaches to the Management of Pain, Brunner/Mazel, New York, 1982.

Beecher, H.K., The powerful placebo, JAMA, 159 (1955) 1602–1606.

Beecher, H.K., Measurement of Subjective Responses: Quantitative Effects of Drugs, Oxford University Press, New York, 1959.

Bonica, J.J., Causalgia and other reflex sympathetic dystrophies. In: J.J. Bonica (Ed.), The Management of Pain, Lea & Febiger, Philadelphia, 1990, pp. 220–256.

Bootzin, R.R., The role of expectancy in behavior change. In: L. White, B. Tursky and G.E. Schwartz (Eds.), Placebo: Theory, Research, and Mechanisms, Guilford Press, New York, 1985.

Campbell, J.N., Raja, S.N., Belzberg, A.J. and Meyer, R.A., Hyperalgesia and the sympathetic nervous system. In: J. Boivie, P. Hansson and U. Lindblom (Eds.), Touch, Temperature, and Pain in Health and Disease: Mechanisms and Assessments, Progress in Pain Research and Management, Vol. 3, IASP Press, Seattle, 1994.

Dellemijn, P.L., Fields, H.L., Allen, R.R. and Rowbotham, M.C., The interpretation of pain relief and sensory changes following sympathetic blockade, Brain Res., 117 (1994) 1475–1487.

Evans, F.J., Expectancy, therapeutic instructions, and the placebo response. In: L. White, B. Tursky and G.E. Scwhartz (Eds.), Placebo: Theory, Research, and Mechanisms, Guilford Press, New York, 1985.

Fields, H.L. and Basbaum, A.I., Endogenous pain control mechanisms. In: P.D. Wall and R. Melzack (Eds.), Textbook of Pain, 3rd ed., Churchill Livingstone, Edinburgh, 1994.
Fields, H.L. and Price, D.D., Toward a Neurobiology of Placebo Analgesia, Harvard University Press, Cambridge, MA, in press.
Gracely, R.H., Psychophysical assessment of human pain. In: J.J. Bonica, J.C. Liebeskind and D.G. Albe-Fessard (Eds.), Proceedings of the Second World Congress on Pain, Advances in Pain Research and Therapy, Vol. 3, Raven Press, New York, 1979.
Gracely, R.H. and Dubner, R., Pain assessment in humans: a reply to Hall, Pain, 11 (1981) 109–120.
Gracely, R.H., McGrath, P. and Dubner, R., Validity and sensitivity of ratio scales of sensory and affective verbal pain descriptors: manipulation of affect by diazepam, Pain, 2 (1978) 19–29.
Gracely, R.H., Dubner, R. and McGrath, P.A., Narcotic analgesia: fentanyl reduces the intensity but not the unpleasantness of painful tooth pulp sensations, Science, 203 (1979) 1261–1263.
Gracely, R.H., Dubner, R., Deeter, W.R. and Wolskee, P.J., Naloxone and placebo alter postsurgical pain by separate mechanisms, Nature, 306 (1983) 264–265.
Gracely, R.H., Dubner, R., Deeter, W.R. and Wolskee, P.J., Clinician's expectations influence placebo analgesia, Lancet, 1, 8419 (1985) 43.
Grevert, P. and Goldstein, A., Placebo analgesia, naloxone, and the role of endogenous opioids. In: L. White, B. Tursky and G.E. Schwartz (Eds.), Placebo: Theory, Research, and Mechanisms, Guilford Press, New York, 1985.
Grevert, P., Albert, L.H. and Goldstein, A., Partial antagonism of placebo analgesia by naloxone, Pain, 16 (1983) 129–143.
Jensen, M.P. and Karoly, P., Motivation and expectancy factors in symptom perception: a laboratory study of the placebo effect, Psychosom. Med., 53 (1991) 144–152.
Jospe, M., The Placebo Effect in Healing, Lexington Books, Lexington, MA, 1978.
Kiernan, B.D., Dane, J.R., Phillips, L. and Price, D.D., Hypnotic analgesia reduces R-111 nociceptive reflex: further evidence concerning the multifactorial nature of hypnotic analgesia, Pain, 60 (1995) 39–47.
Kirsch, I., Changing Expectations: A Key to Effective Psychotherapy, Brooks/Cole, Pacific Grove, CA, 1990.
Lasagna, L., Laties, V.G. and Dohan, J.L., Further studies on the "pharmacology" of a placebo administration, J. Clin. Invest., 37 (1958) 533–537.
Laska, E. and Sunshine, A., Anticipation of analgesia a placebo effect, Headache, 13 (1973) 1–11.
Levine, J.D., Gordon, N.C., Bornstein, J.C. and Fields, H.L., Role of pain in placebo analgesia, Proc. Natl. Acad. Sci. USA, 76 (1979) 3528–3531.
Lindblom, U. and Nemeth, G., Types of pain with neglected differenital diagnosis, Lakartidningen, 89 (1992) 1392–1393.
Mowrer, O.H., Learning Theory and Behavior, Wiley, New York, 1962.
Price, D.D., Psychological and Neural Mechanisms of Pain, Raven Press, New York, 1988.
Price, D.D. and Barber, J., An analysis of factors that contribute to the efficiency of hypnotic analgesia, J. Abnorm. Psychol., 96 (1987) 46–51.
Price, D.D. and Fields, H.L., The Contribution of Desire and Expectation to Placebo Analgesia: Implications for New Research Strategies, Harvard University Press, Cambridge, MA, in press.
Price, D.D., von der Gruen, A., Miller, J., Rafii, A. and Price, C., A psychophysical analysis of morphine analgesia, Pain, 22 (1985) 320–330.
Price, D.D., Harkins, S.W., Rafii, A. and Price, C., A simultaneous comparison of fentanyl's analgesic effects on experimental and clinical pain, Pain, 24 (1986) 197–203.
Raja, S.N., Treede, R.-D., Davis, K.D. and Campbell, J.N., Systemic alpha-adrenergic blockade with phentolamine: a diagnostic test for sympathetically maintained pain, Anesthesia, 74 (1991) 691–698.
Reiss, S., Pavlovian conditioning and human fear: an expectancy model, Behav. Ther., 11 (1980) 380–396.

Rowbotham, M.C., Topical analgesic agents. In: H.L. Fields and J.C. Liebeskind (Eds.), Pharmacological Approaches to the Treatment of Chronic Pain: New Concepts and Critical Issues, Progress in Pain Research and Management, Vol. 1, IASP Press, Seattle, 1994.

Traut, E.F. and Passarelli, E.W., Placebos in the treatment of rheumatoid arthritis and other rheumatic conditions, Ann. Rheum. Dis., 16 (1957) 18–22.

Turner, J.L., Gallimore, R. and Fox-Henning, C., An annotated bibliography of placebo research, Journal of the Supplemental Abstract Service of the American Psychological Association, 10(2) (1980) 22.

Tursky, B., The 55% analgesic affect: real or artifact? In: L. White, B. Tursky, and G.E. Schwartz (Eds.) Placebo: Research, Theory, and Mechanisms, Guilford Press, New York, 1985.

Urban, B.J. and McKain, C.W., Local anesthetic effect of intrathecal normal saline, Pain, 5 (1978) 43–52.

Wall, P.D., The placebo and the placebo response. In: P D. Wall and R. Melzack (Eds.), Textbook of Pain, Churchill Livingstone, Edinburgh, 1994.

Watkins, L.R. and Mayer, D.J., Organization of endogenous opiate and nonopiate pain control systems, Science, 216 (1982) 1185–1192.

White, L., Tursky, B. and Schwartz, G.E. (Eds.), Placebo: Theory, Research, and Mechanisms, Guilford Press, New York, 1985.

Wickramasekera, I., A conditioned response model of the placebo effect: predictions from the model. In: L. White, B. Tursky and G.E. Schwartz (Eds.), Placebo: Theory, Research, and Mechanisms, Guilford Press, New York, 1985.

Correspondence to: Donald D. Price, PhD, Anesthesiology, MCV Station Box 516, Medical College of Virginia, Richmond, VA 23298-0516, USA. Tel: 804-828-1984; Fax: 804-828-8300.

11

Psychological Issues in Reflex Sympathetic Dystrophy

Edward C. Covington

Chronic Pain Rehabilitation Program, The Cleveland Clinic Foundation, Cleveland, Ohio, USA

We have come to our current understanding of reflex sympathetic dystrophy (RSD), recently renamed as complex regional pain syndrome (CRPS) (Merskey et al. 1994; Stanton-Hicks et al. 1995), via a convoluted route that began with the description of causalgia (Mitchell et al. 1864). The boundaries of the condition have changed through the years, and nomenclature has been a Tower of Babel. Rizzi et al. (1984) located 21 terms thought to describe the illness. At this publishing, diagnostic criteria remain phenomenological and without a foundation in well-defined pathophysiology. We hope the adoption of generally accepted terminology and diagnostic criteria, which was the goal of the consensus development conference, will facilitate research into the etiology and treatment of this condition. The ultimate criteria, of course, await neurophysiological explanations.

The question of psychological components in the syndrome further complicates matters. RSD is not unique in this regard, as the physiology remains enigmatic in many other conditions that are similarly complicated by questions of the role of the psyche in pathogenesis. Fibromyalgia, irritable bowel syndrome, and chronic fatigue syndrome are current examples. A review of the literature on psychological factors in pain in general reveals that conceptual and methodological flaws substantially limit conclusions (Gamsa 1994a,b).

This chapter will summarize information regarding psychological factors in RSD. At times it will draw upon information concerning chronic nonmalignant pains in general to fill in gaps in knowledge regarding the specific condition under discussion. Some techniques for diagnostic discrimination are described, and the therapeutic strategies that result from the conclusions are presented. It is important to recognize that the mind plays a role in all forms of suffering and dysfunction, and it is the mind that copes and adapts or fails to do so. It is self-evident that among intractable cases, failures of coping and adaptation will be disproportionately represented. While the language of the chapter may suggest linear hypotheses, multicausality and feedback loops probably are more important (e.g., pain causes autonomic arousal that increases pain).

The subject of this chapter has been discussed in five recent reviews (Haddox 1990b; Bruehl and Carlson 1992; Lynch 1992a; Van Houdenhove et al. 1992; Weiss 1994). All have required implicit or explicit decisions as to the boundaries of the concept. For example, most assumed that studies of causalgia were pertinent to RSD and that RSD in children was similar to that in adults. Such choices may modify conclusions, because the likelihood of psychological causation may be less in causalgia, following clear nerve trauma, than in RSD, and the precipitation and course of RSD in children may differ from that in adults (Chapter 4, this volume).

RSD has several postulated psychological components: the obvious one is the expected emotional reaction to pain and dysfunction. It is theorized as well that personality traits or psychiatric illnesses could cause the illness or could create a diathesis toward it, perhaps through biochemical alterations. Additionally, RSD could represent a conversion reaction/psychogenic pain phenomenon. Behaviors, volitional or unconscious, could modify the course and symptoms of the illness. Psychological issues known to be important in other chronic pain syndromes could be operative in RSD as well. These issues include operant conditioning, cognitive issues, coping skills, and such psychiatric illnesses as chemical dependency (primary or secondary to the condition) and mood disorders.

Lynch (1992b) has summarized the serious limitations in the adult and pediatric literature on this subject. These limitations include inconsistent diagnostic criteria, poorly defined/quantified behavioral criteria, lack of objective measurements of psychological constructs, incorrect use of psychiatric terminology (usually in studies whose primary aim was to assess nonpsychiatric questions), lack of blinding and controls, and perpetuation of misinformation through uncritical citations. Bruehl and Carlson (1992) reviewed 20 articles against seven criteria for quality of research design and concluded that most studies were scientifically inadequate.

Unfortunately, unsubstantiated statements in the literature purport to describe the personalities of RSD patients, often in pejorative terms, e.g., ". . . often described by psychiatrists as 'fearful, suspicious, emotionally labile, inadequate, chronic complainer, dependent, insecure, and unstable.' I almost never discover a . . . patient with RSD who is . . . stoic or Spartan" (Lankford 1978); or "It has long been recognized clinically, but seldom discussed in the literature, that only a certain type patient develops RSD" (Lankford 1982). Lynch concludes, along with Haddox (1990b), that "Unsupported statements by established authorities have occurred more frequently than studies designed to address these issues."

PSYCHIATRIC SEQUELAE OF RSD

Perhaps the *least* controversial issue in the psychology of RSD is that severe pain engenders emotional suffering and promotes behavioral changes that are subject to misinterpretation. This observation seems best established with causalgia, and numerous dramatic historical reports describe the extraordinary suffering seen in soldiers following nerve injury and the remarkable efforts they made to diminish it (e.g., Mayfield and Devine 1945). Their responses to pain included maintaining an affected extremity wrapped at all times in damp cloths, withdrawal to darkness and solitude in an effort to minimize stimulation, and anguish to the point that suicide was feared (Miller and De Takats 1942). The augmentation of RSD pain by adrenergic stimulation, together with the likelihood that these soldiers experienced a near autonomic storm, creates a strong likelihood of a circular relationship in which emotional anguish exacerbated the pain that was its source.

What may be more surprising than the anxiety and depression so typical of causalgia is the *absence* of these reactions in some cases. Wilson (1981) compared injured patients with and without RSD symptoms and reported that "None of the patients with pain demonstrated any pathologic deviations by the standard interpretations of Minnesota Multiphasic Personality Inventory (MMPI) results." This incidence of abnormalities is remarkably low, perhaps lower than would be expected from chance alone. Grunert et al. (1990) reported "1 and 3 profiles" (elevated scales 1 and 3 only) on the MMPIs of 18 of 20 RSD patients who were treatment failures. This profile is characterized by a relative *lack* of depression and reflects somatic preoccupation and tendencies toward denial, repression, and somatization. Subbarao and Stillwell (1981) studied 125 patients, of whom 45 had completed MMPIs. Of these, 42% had abnormal scales 1 and 3 only, while 40% had an elevated depression scale as well; 20% were normal. Bernstein et al. (1978) reported that in 23 children without known trauma, of 12 assessed for illness concerns, 100% were *indifferent* to their illness. Thus, we encounter the puzzling situation of one group of patients thought to have psychogenic pain because they display excessive suffering, while another group is similarly suspect for suffering too little.

PSYCHOLOGICAL CAUSATION IN RSD

It is not surprising that a condition in which symptoms are disproportionate to injury, with ill-defined pathogenesis and diagnostic criteria, would be considered to be of psychological origin; however, it remains unclear whether and how psychological factors might cause, trigger, or exacerbate the condition. The fact that some persons with trivial injuries are affected, while others more severely injured are not, spurs speculation about underlying psychological factors (though genetic factors may play a role; Mailis and Wade 1994). The sometimes bizarre behaviors of those with causalgia/RSD have contributed to the suspicion. The fallacy of such reasoning lies in its unsubstantiated attribution of the idiopathic to the psychogenic, much as earlier societies attributed solar eclipses to supernatural causes.

PSYCHOPHYSIOLOGIC FACTORS

Often a psychological stressor, such as witnessing an auto accident, will produce a demonstrable physiologic response, such as emesis. Psychophysiologic processes may constitute a significant component of RSD. Significantly, Van Houdenhove (1986) reported that 31 of 32 RSD patients referred for psychiatric evaluation had experienced a major life stressor, usually a loss, coincident with onset of RSD. Egle and Hoffman (1990) found that eight of eight patients were experiencing "an extraordinarily difficult period in their lives" coincident with the trauma or surgery that precipitated RSD.

It has long been known that sympathetic stimulation increases pain in causalgia, as can strong emotions, noises, bright light, or the excitement of cinema (Doupe et al. 1944; Drucker et al. 1959; Bonica 1979). Autonomic arousal, a major component of anxiety disorders and stress reactions, is associated with catecholamine release. Ecker (1989) described the interaction of this arousal with the pain of RSD and proposed a mechanism for exacerbation of RSD through a feedback loop. Bruehl and Carlson (1992) expanded on this idea. Adrenergic discharge and anxiety can be severe in those with alcoholism and other chemical dependencies, especially as trough levels of anxiolytics, sedatives, or opioids are approached. Bruehl and Carlson felt the studies they reviewed were at least compatible with a model in which depression, anxiety, or stress could influence RSD through α-adrenergic mechanisms.

Chronic states of hyperarousal could also predispose to the development of RSD. Haddox (1990b) cites several authors who held to this position, but without benefit of data. Lankford (1982), for example, thought many of these patients were "sympathetic hyperreactors" with cold extremities, hyperhidrosis, "sick headaches," Raynaud's phenomenon, etc. In the only study providing data, Shumacker and Abramson (1949) found that 25 of 142 patients described premorbid cold extremities and the same number had excessive sweating. Additionally, those with "type A personality," (driven, competitive, angry, impatient) may have elevated sympathetic activity, which increases their susceptibility to RSD (Contrada and Drants 1988). Finer and Graf (1968) demonstrated the potential for psychological modulation of the physiology of RSD with their finding that under hypnotically induced hyperalgesia, causalgic extremities showed marked changes in blood flow, with reductions in the distal extremities and increase in the proximal, large muscle areas.

BEHAVIORAL FACTORS

Behavioral responses to RSD range from fully preserved function to complete invalidism; however, this variability has no particular etiologic significance, as the same can be said for most chronic pain conditions. We cannot compare nociception among individuals, so we are unable to ascertain the extent to which a person's behavior reflects the experience of pain itself versus the role of extrinsic factors, although indirect evidence may be provided by the consequences of alterations in extrinsic factors. Pilowsky (1960, 1984) notes that "illness behaviors" may be adaptive or maladaptive, and coined the term "abnormal illness behavior," which in essence indicates that the person solicits more perquisites of the "sick role" than authorities, such as physicians, consider warranted.

Behavioral responses may be especially important in RSD because disuse, overprotection, and immobilization may lead to exacerbations, and may themselves produce or exacerbate demineralization (Steinert et al. 1990), vasomotor changes (Ochoa 1995a), and edema (Cooke and Ward 1990). Drucker (1959) cited disputes as to whether the bony changes of reflex sympathetic dystrophy could be distinguished from those of disuse, while Moberg (1960) went so far as to attribute the entire syndrome to immobilization and disuse. Holden (1948) noted that many mild cases of RSD recover spontaneously or with physical therapy. These factors, together with reports of reversal of RSD in response to normal activity, strongly suggest that inactivity may contribute to the pathology. White and Sweet (1969) agreed that many of the trophic sequelae are due to prolonged disuse occasioned by pain, and that the physiological changes and cutaneous dysesthesia develop in persons "who are poorly motivated to get well and unwilling to make the effort needed to overcome the discomfort and stiffness that follows immobilization after trauma." Shumacker and Abramson (1949), in 142 cases, indicated that active exercise, which is the best treatment, caused reversal of edema, trophic changes, and vasomotor signs.

In a demonstration of ways that psychological stress could interact with behavior in RSD, Lidz and Payne (1945) described a wounded soldier who developed causalgic symptoms following what he believed to be unjust accusations. After emotional ventilation facilitated by amobarbital, his emotional distress resolved, he began working on rehabilitation, and his trophic/vasomotor changes abated, permitting return to duty. Thus, we can be sure that the behaviors of the patient can and do influence the severity and outcome of RSD, but we lack information as to how often behavioral responses are a liability and how often an asset to the recovery process.

MAJOR PSYCHIATRIC ILLNESS

Psychiatric illnesses could both exacerbate RSD and reduce ability to cope with it. The incidence of severe psychiatric illness in RSD is unknown, as most studies have not used standard diagnostic criteria, have tended to lump different illnesses into such categories as "unstable," and have studied highly selected samples. The most frequent psychiatric illnesses in pain center patients are probably anxiety disorders, depression, and substance abuse (Katon et al. 1985; Fishbain et al. 1986, 1988; Poulsen et al. 1987). Kramlinger et al. (1983) cite estimates of depression in chronic pain patients that range from 10–83%. We can question to what extent depression represents a consequence of the pain itself, as Rudy et al. (1988) found that it is associated more with helplessness/loss of control and interference by pain in life activities (social, work, recreation, family) than with pain *per se*. The hopelessness experienced in major depression may play an important role in delaying recovery—those without hope exert less effort in their own behalf (Haddox 1990a).

Chemical dependence, including alcoholism, is a common correlate of chronic pain *syndrome*, though its incidence is not well established. Fishbain et al. (1992) reviewed the literature and reported that the prevalence of drug abuse/dependence/addiction ranged from 3.2–18.9% in chronic pain patients. The national alcoholism prevalence is probably 14–18%, so we might expect that these figures are underestimates. Our experience is that a large minority of referrals have a true addictive disorder (as opposed to simple physiologic tolerance and dependence).

We are reduced to speculation on the question of the impact of psychiatric illness until the actual studies are done. We can safely assume that depression occurs in RSD as in other chronic pain syndromes, and that it exacerbates overall suffering. We can also assume that anxiety disorders, perhaps especially panic disorder and posttraumatic stress disorder, would produce exacerbations of RSD through episodic catecholamine release. Addictive disorders can be expected to increase anxiety and depression, while impairing coping. Finally, we can predict that the prevalence of these psychiatric illnesses will be highest in the most refractory cases, i.e., those referred to pain centers, thus causing a bias in the samples most likely to be studied.

PERSONALITY

Perhaps the most controversial question concerning the psychology of RSD is whether these patients are in some way different from other persons/ patients and, if so, what is the nature of their difference. The answer may vary depending on whether causalgia is included in the conditions under study, as several authors report that these patients show less constitutional predisposition, anxiety, and hypochondriasis than do those with RSD (Holden 1948; Drucker et al. 1959). There is not total agreement on this issue, however, as Tamoush (1981) was unable to psychologically distinguish a group of patients with a causalgia-like syndrome from a second group with symptoms suggesting RSD. (His study is quite weak because he evaluated only eight subjects, tested only with the McGill Pain Questionnaire, and some patients diagnosed with RSD had neurological damage.)

It is difficult to think that personality alone could cause a disease process; however, such theorizing has a long history. Asthma, migraine, irritable bowel syndrome, and Crohn's disease are among several conditions once thought to be associated with specific personality types; however, these theories were abandoned for lack of support. Cassileth et al. (1984) argued that conceptions of disease-specific psychiatric traits were invalid, and cited earlier notions of "diabetic personalities" and "arthritic personalities." Merskey (1986) reviewed evidence that ideas of a "migraine personality" actually reflected a characteristic "clinic personality," and that the more nearly the study group approached a general sample, the weaker the evidence for migraine personality.

Haddox (1990b) has thoroughly summarized and reviewed older concepts of a specific personality type associated with RSD and demonstrates that they do not hold up to scrutiny. Thus, there is no "RSD personality." Selection bias surely explains some of the appearance of personality abnormalities in RSD. Even when not selected for psychopathology, pain clinic patients represent a biased sample: those who come to chronic pain clinics report more intense pain and report it to be more constant and associated with greater functional impairment. They also had higher likelihood of depression, withdrawal, and substance abuse, and half the improvement rate of family practice patients (Crook and Tunks 1985). It is a challenge for investigators of the psychology of RSD to avoid such biased samples.

Bonica (1979) and later Lynch (1992a) cited several reports that abnormalities in personality and behavior in causalgia disappeared after relief of pain, which strongly suggests that the abnormalities were sequelae of RSD and not predisposing factors. Sternbach et al. (1975) also found normalization of MMPI after pain-relieving surgery (and psychological treatment and rehabilitation).

Perhaps the greatest difficulty in determining the role of personality in RSD is the absence of prospective studies. Cross-sectional studies of psychiatric symptoms and personality traits in those with RSD reveal little about causality. Nevertheless, if we define personality as a bias toward certain ways of feeling and behaving, it becomes clear that it must affect the strategies used for coping with pain, and their efficacy. Personality also affects stress tolerance and would be expected to have autonomic concomitants. In addition, people vary in the degree to which they find the sick role aversive versus a welcome respite from demands, stress, and responsibility, so that personality modifies incentives for recovery.

Haddox (1990b) critically reviewed the use of standardized tests in this population and reports that, not only were these tests performed *after* the development of RSD, but that the most commonly used instrument, the MMPI, was not standardized on those with pain and may exaggerate their psychopathology. This is true of other instruments for measuring psychopathology, and they perhaps are not as useful for comparing scores of pain patients with "normal scores" as for contrasting scores of patients with various pain syndromes.

Conclusions are further limited because many studies addressed populations preselected for psychiatric referral or failure to respond to treatment, so that even issues of correlation, much less the inappropriate inference of causality, are confounded. In effect, authors have drawn conclusions about this particular form of chronic pain based on studies of those with so-called chronic pain *syndrome* (U.S. Commission on the Evaluation of Pain, 1987), which is a largely psychiatric condition characterized by abnormal illness behavior. Although such studies can contribute to a qualitative understanding of salient psychological issues, using them to determine prevalence figures is tautologous.

Prospective studies are needed to circumvent this problem; however, Van Houdenhove et al. (1992) could find only two such studies of personality in RSD. In the first, Zachariae (1964) reported that preoperative psychiatric assessment predicted which patients with Dupuytren's contracture would develop postoperative dystrophy. Of 47 patients, 32 were predicted to do well and did so (despite 17 "unstable," six "demented," and two with "real mental diseases.") Ten patients seem to have had an ambiguous prediction. Of these, eight had edema, fibrosis, and stiffness for three months (no cases of dystrophy) and two did well. Five cases were predicted to be at serious risk due to "sthenic characters" (the opposite of "asthenic") and other traits. It appears that one developed dystrophy, two did quite well, and two developed prolonged stiffness and swelling, one of whom had edema as well. Van Houdenhove reported that the second study (Van Spaendonck 1992) was unable to distinguish those patients with radius fracture who developed RSD, but the number of patients was small.

Strategies devised to circumvent the difficulty of obtaining prospective data have included retrospective evaluations of premorbid traits of RSD patients, comparisons of RSD patients with other pain or nonpain patients, and efforts to distinguish, from among those with RSD, those with good and poor outcomes.

Retrospective personality assessment

Several efforts have been made to retrospectively determine premorbid characteristics of those with RSD. Hemler (1988) reported that 12 of 19 active-duty servicemen with RSD had records showing conflict with authorities, nonjudicial punishment, slow promotion rates, and repeated sick calls for non-specific symptoms. He does not indicate the prevalence of these characteristics in randomly selected evaluated servicemen or in military personnel with other illnesses. He concludes that the concept of personality diathesis has been overemphasized and argued that psychotherapy, while useful, should not delay "medical intervention into the reflex and inflammatory mechanisms of the disease." He favored a multidisciplinary approach and noted that the patients tend to be "poorly compliant, creating an atmosphere of both dependence and frustration between therapist and patient." In another study, Pak (1970) reported that 37% of 140 RSD patients had premorbid psychiatric problems or emotional disturbance. (Those seen by psychiatrists *during* the episode were thought to suffer primarily from anxiety, depression, or conversion disorders.) In yet another study, Horowitz (1984) reported that of 11 patients who developed RSD as a procedural complication, six were diagnosed with premorbid dependent personality disorder.

In reviewing the literature on RSD in children, Lynch (1992a) found only 48 cases with any psychological assessment. One study of 17 cases (Bernstein et al. 1978) described premorbid characteristics. Parental conflict had been present in 10 of 12, marked hyperresponsibility in 11 of 13, and nonassertiveness in 9 of 10.

Comparisons of RSD with other pain syndromes

Haddox et al. (1988) used the Dartmouth Pain Questionnaire and the State Trait Anxiety Inventory to compare RSD patients with those having radiculopathy. They found no differences, even though outcome was better in the radiculopathy patients. Additionally, DeLeo and Magni (1983), using Eysenck's Personality Inventory, found Sudek's atrophy patients to be no more neurotic (albeit somewhat more introverted) than a comparison group of patients with fractures and no Sudek's. Waylett-Rendell (1978) studied patients with industrial injuries in a hand rehabilitation center and compared those with definite, probable, or non-RSD. The Buhler-Coleman Life Goals Inventory was used, in addition to unstructured observation sheets prepared by four observers. In the definite RSD group, only 50% were able and willing (five of 12 refused) to complete the test, and none of the completed tests were in the normal range. This finding compared with 16 of 17 normal profiles in the non-RSD group. Observations indicated that patients in the RSD group were more somatically focused in conversation, less able to achieve independent exercise performance, more inconsistent in symptom presentation, and less able to retain instructions. (This study is obviously compromised by the refusal rate among the "definite RSD" group.) DeGood et al. (1993) compared RSD patients with headache and low back pain patients (all in a pain center). Even though they had the most reported pain, vocational impairment, and financial compensation, the RSD patients showed less emotional distress on the SCL-90R than did the comparison groups.

The reasonable conclusions seem to be that, despite the well-publicized emotional distress of causalgia patients, there is no consistent evidence that RSD patients have more distress than do other pain patients, and indeed, some seem to have less. The notion of an RSD personality has been thoroughly and repeatedly debunked, but questions remain as to whether personality traits are significant predisposing or exacerbating factors in RSD.

Psychiatric correlations with Outcome

In 125 patients, Subbarao and Stillwell (1981) had follow-up information on 77 and MMPI results on 45. The MMPI showed no association with outcome, nor did outcome correlate with litigation status or psychiatric care. Parenthetically, one of the few items that correlated with outcome was narcotic status. Of 12 patients continuing to use narcotics at follow-up, only one was functioning as a worker, homemaker, or student. (Again, the study is compromised by biased sampling: not all patients were administered the MMPI, not all completed the test, and not all completed the follow-up questionnaire.)

Sherry and Weisman (1988) found that all of 21 affected children had a "significant underlying psychological component," and reported that "all were completely normal in a matter of weeks." On the Child Behavior Checklist, 20 of 21 subjects were in the normal range; they were also normal on the Brief Symptom Inventory. (The contrast between clinical impressions of psychopathology and normal responses to psychometrics impedes conclusions.) Bernstein et al. (1978) studied 23 children, of whom 17 had psychological consultation. Follow-up data on 20 of 23 revealed all to be functioning normally.

These studies do not support the idea that psychopathology necessarily is associated with adverse outcomes. In children, such an association might be masked by a favorable prognosis or because the studies appropriately addressed psychological needs.

PSYCHOLOGICAL FACTORS NOT SPECIFIC TO RSD

Several psychological factors play a role in the perception of and response to pain. These are summarized below.

PERSONALITY

While there is no personality disorder specific to RSD, traits that facilitate or impede coping with other chronic pains may be expected to play a role in RSD as well. Fishbain et al. (1986), for example, found that of 283 consecutive pain center admissions, 58% fulfilled rigorous criteria for personality disorders, primarily dependent, passive-aggressive, and histrionic.

LOCUS OF CONTROL

One important trait has been referred to as "perceived locus of control." This trait reflects a person's tendency to attribute important events to personal behavior (internal locus of control) or to such external forces as fate or powerful others. Internal locus of control correlates strongly with active coping responses, while the converse is associated with passivity and depression. This trait is a major determinant of coping with chronic pain (Harkapaa et al. 1991). Chronic pain patients with a "chance external" locus of control reported depression and anxiety, felt helpless to deal with their pain, and relied on maladaptive coping strategies (Crisson and Keefe 1988). Beliefs in personal helplessness also are important in those disabled with pain (Ciccone and Grzesiak 1984).

COGNITION

The role of cognition in psychiatric conditions has won increasing recognition during the last 15 years (Turk et al. 1983), and cognitive factors have an important impact on pain (Jensen et al. 1991; Affleck et al. 1992). Appreciation of pain is modified by the person's understanding of the significance of the pain and its implications for health and future function. Additionally, efficacy in coping with pain is diminished by such cognitive errors as tendencies to catastrophize (i.e., interpret minor mishaps as catastrophic), negative overgeneralizations, selective negative abstraction (noticing and responding preferentially to negative aspects of a situation that contains positive or neutral characteristics as well).

OPERANT CONDITIONING

Operant conditioning refers to the increase in the frequency of behaviors (often without the subject's awareness) when they are rewarded. Behavior modification addresses this important influence on responses to illness. Rewards (reinforcements) for "illness behavior" include solicitous responses from others, escape from responsibility and stressful/dangerous work environments, and entitlements to narcotics, nurture, and financial compensation. They play a major role in determining the extent of pain behaviors and disability (Fordyce et al. 1973; Fordyce 1976). For example, numerous studies suggest that pain-related disability is more a function of job satisfaction and status than of illness severity (Osterweis et al. 1987; Bigos et al. 1991).

Several studies of children with CRPS suggest that reinforcements for illness behaviors are relevant, in that they provide relief from parental demands without the confrontation that rebellion would elicit (Bernstein et al. 1978, Sherry and Weisman 1988). Sherry and Weisman felt the illness provided the children with access to the nurturing they were denied due to family pathology.

FEAR

Fear of injury promotes inordinate inactivity and thereby impedes coping with other conditions, and it likely plays a role with RSD as well. Kori et al. (1990) referred to chronic pain syndrome as "kinisophobia"—a fear of movement—to reflect the important role of fear in causing inactivity that leads to invalidism. Doupe et al. (1944) point out how easily RSD could lead to conditioned fear responses: any stimulus previously associated with pain would cause apprehension and sympathetic discharge on reexposure, thereby producing a recurrence of the pain through the sympathetic mediation.

PSEUDO-RSD: PSYCHOGENIC PAIN AND MALINGERING

Despite controversy regarding the existence of psychogenic pain, several signs lead to its consideration. Psychogenic pain is often suspected when there is a large discrepancy between complaints and observable pathology, which can be minimal in RSD and especially in sympathetically maintained pain (Schwartzman and McLellan 1987). The reported response of RSD symptoms to amobarbital (Roe et al. 1994a,b) and benzodiazepines, known to interrupt such conditions as psychogenic paralysis and mutism, further raises questions of psychogenicity. Dystonic features, as yet unexplained neurologically, may have the appearance of conversion or volitional symptoms (Bhatia et al. 1993).

Our poor understanding of these cases and the absence of good diagnostic criteria invite misdiagnosis. Livingston (1943) notes that "to classify certain types of pain as 'psychic' pain is purely arbitrary, because all pain is a psychic perception." Nevertheless, the term is useful for cases in which dysfunction seems to be at the level of information processing (a "software" function) as opposed to tissue stimulation or neurological dysfunction (hardware).

Psychogenic pain, malingering, and factitious illness may be misdiagnosed as RSD. This error creates the impression that RSD patients are characterized by marked psychopathology. De Takats (1965) held that ". . . particularly in traumatic and the compensation cases, . . . a certain amount of malingering, neurosis, and hysteria have to be ruled out," and distinguished these states from anxiety, which affects autonomic reflexes. De Takats and Miller (1943) thought that the "state of mind" generally played a role in the symptoms. Thus, importantly, the *modulation* of symptoms by psychic factors was distinguished conceptually from the *simulation* of symptoms by psychic factors.

The issues are of considerable practical importance. The misdiagnosis of a psychiatric condition as organic exposes the patient to futile, expensive, and potentially hazardous interventions, while the misdiagnosis of organic conditions as psychogenic exposes the patient to futile interventions, stigma, and potential loss of entitlements. Both errors deprive the patient of optimal treatment.

Unfortunately, "political correctness" has entered the discussion, and erroneous diagnoses of psychiatric illness are decried, while erroneous diagnoses of organic illness are accepted in our zeal to take the patient at his or her word. Either error is potentially harmful.

PSYCHOGENIC PAIN

Psychogenic pain is a conceptual conundrum. We can diagnose conversion blindness, in which there is preserved opticokinetic reflex, and psychogenic seizures, in which EEGs remain normal. In conversion paralysis, normal muscle function can be demonstrated in sleep or with distraction. Psychogenic pain is a different matter, because there is no objective confirmation of pain or its absence.

To minimize covert bias in this chapter, I share my understanding, based on unsystematic observation of numerous cases, which surely affects my perspective. We see patients diagnosed with psychogenic pain who seem to experience extreme suffering and demonstrate impaired sleep, anorexia, or suicidal tendencies. Others similarly diagnosed seem cheerful, often appear quite comfortable when unobserved, sleep well, and have depression inventory scores in the low range of normal. They may not show physiologic hyperarousal on biofeedback assessment. It is difficult to believe that these cases have similar pathology, despite the same diagnosis. Rather, it seems that in some persons pain represents an appreciation of psychological suffering in physical terms. The suffering is real, but its source is disguised or "unconscious." In other cases, the illness seems more a solution than a problem, and what seems to be "unconscious" (dissociated?) is the exaggeration or perhaps even fabrication of complaints. In the latter group, malingering could be considered as a possibility, except that antisocial character traits are absent and these patients welcome rather than resist diagnostic investigations.

Miller (1988) has described the difficulty in diagnosing even classical (as opposed to pain-related) conversion. An essential requirement is that the patient be unaware of the psychogenic nature of the symptoms, and must experience them as "real," e.g., a hysterically paralyzed patient must truly believe himself to be incapable of movement, else the diagnosis would be malingering. Yet, no examiner can know the contents of a patient's awareness. Miller cited three studies showing that patients with hysterical blindness, deafness, and dissociative disorder could not be distinguished on objective tests from subjects asked to fake these syndromes. He concluded that it was impossible to prove that a patient with hysterical illness was feigning, and equally impossible to prove that he was not. Therefore, he suggested remaining "agnostic," focusing on reasons for symptom maintenance, and addressing those, without speculating about consciousness awareness.

It is common to see patients diagnosed with RSD whose allodynic legs are shaven, allodynic hands are manicured or calloused, and who have inexplicable persistence of symptoms despite regional anesthesia. Others with chronically immobilized shoulders may show normal range of motion under sedation (when capsulitis or contractures might be expected). Some have hypersensitivity that ablates with distraction. It is likely that such patients will be overrepresented in pain centers because they tend to confound primary care physicians. Their prevalence is unknown.

Diagnostic criteria for somatoform pain disorder in DSM-III-R and for pain disorder, psychological type, in DSM-IV (American Psychiatric Association 1987, 1994) provide little help, because they refer mainly to pain in excess of or without organic cause and pain thought to have psychological causation. The way to establish this conclusion is left obscure, as is the methodology for determining whether pain complaints are appropriate for a given condition. Diagnostic difficulties are highlighted by back-to-back articles entitled "Regional pain is usually hysterical" (Weintraub 1988) and "Regional pain is rarely hysterical" (Merskey 1988). It may be that diagnosis is more accurate if based on nonphysiologic findings and responses to intervention, rather than on the detection of overt psychological issues, which are likely to be obscured on initial interviews.

Nevertheless, this problem is significant, and Purtel et al. (1951) report that in patients with multiple psychogenic physical and emotional symptoms (Briquet's syndrome or hysteria; Guze 1975), one of the most common symptoms was pain. In 50 "hysterics," headache, abdominal, back, and extremity pain, as well as dysmenorrhea and dyspareunia, were many times more common than in controls. Interestingly, the authors found that pain was a more frequent feature than the more classical and expected neurological symptoms, such as paralysis, blindness, and amnesia.

Ochoa has written extensively on the subject of RSD, which he considers a group of physiologically diverse conditions (as do others, e.g., Schott 1995), many or most of them psychogenic (Ochoa 1992; Ochoa et al. 1994). Many of these patients are misdiagnosed, he believes, because they are not examined neurologically and because placebo responses confound diagnostic interventions. He considers psychiatric evaluation inadequate to diagnose psychogenic pain, because psychopathology does not confirm it and the absence of detected psychopathology does not rule it out. Instead, he advocates a detailed neurological and neurophysiological assessment (Ochoa, in press). He holds that in most of these patients, weakness and sensory loss are not organically based. In a group of 270 patients with RSD/causalgia-like symptoms, which he prefers to label CPSMV (chronic pains associated with various sensory, motor, and vasomotor phenomena), he found neurological lesions sufficient to explain the complaints in 34%, lesions insufficient to explain complaints in 11%, and absence of neurological illness in 55%. Yet, he states that while motor and sensory assessments can accurately distinguish organic from nonorganic *weakness and sensory loss*, they can not distinguish organic from nonorganic *pains* (Ochoa 1995b). For example, profound sensory loss or weakness that disappears with placebo cannot be due to a structural lesion, yet pain that disappears with placebo may well be of nociceptive origin. Ochoa's emphasis on neurological findings recalls Shumacker and Abramson's 1949 report that 11 of 142 cases of "RSD" were judged to represent a psychiatric disorder, and that the best diagnostic sign was simultaneous contraction of agonist and antagonist muscles in response to a command, so that instead of movement there was only tremor or rigidity.

Ochoa (1994) proposed the following criteria for psychogenic neuromuscular symptoms:

1. Give-way weakness and EMG of full interference pattern alternating with intermissions in the absence of extrapyramidal disease (unclear whether this distinguishes conversion from malingering)
2. Placebo-induced normalization of weakness, and probably, placebo-induced normalization of dystonia
3. Placebo-induced normalization of hypoesthesia
4. Video surveillance
5. Reversal of all symptoms with psychiatric treatment

He notes pointedly that just as failure to detect pathology does not rule out organic disease, failure to detect psychopathology does not rule out psychiatric illness.

Ochoa's positions are controversial and perhaps somewhat extreme, yet they highlight the inability of psychiatric interview (and psychological testing) to reliably identify psychogenic pain. While it is reasonable to *suspect* this diagnosis when extreme dysfunction and somatic complaints are associated with a lack of dysphoria (the well-known "conversion V" on MMPI testing and "la belle indifference" of an earlier era), these findings cannot confirm it. Nor is the onset of symptomatology following a psychic trauma definitive (unless, of course, symptoms immediately follow the stress in the absence of injury). In a highly competitive, stressful culture with support for the infirm, virtually all disability has the potential for associated "secondary gain."

In contrast, a neurological deficit that reverses with suggestion is not a neurological deficit. A paralyzed hand that moves in sleep or that is calloused is not paralyzed. The lack of ambiguity and subjectivity in such observations supports Ochoa's belief that neurological findings should determine a diagnosis of psychogenicity. A caveat, however, is warranted. Neurologically "impossible" findings have subsequently found explanations. Many people demonstrate transient increases in strength in response to confidence or suggestion. Movement disorders commonly abate with relaxation and increase with anxiety. Finally, is the well-known but often forgotten concurrence of psychogenic symptoms with organic ones. Thus, pseudoseizures do not preclude epilepsy. Similarly, confirmation of psychogenic paralysis, dystonia, and such does not disprove organic pain and weakness.

FACTITIOUS ILLNESS AND MALINGERING

Most authorities have declared that malingering, while difficult to distinguish from conversion, is quite uncommon. Yet, there appear to be no data to support conclusions regarding its frequency. There are, however, hints from other fields. In 54 patients with unexplained intractable diarrhea, 47 had stool examinations for laxatives, of which seven were positive (14%). All had denied use of laxatives (Bytzer et al. 1989). Weintraub (1995b) cites two industry studies showing that 20–46% of persons surveyed considered purposeful misrepresentation of compensation claims to be acceptable. These studies suggest that factitious illness and malingering may not be rare, but do not provide information as to how often they present as pain or, more specifically, RSD. These studies suggest keeping an open mind as to the possibility of the diagnosis.

Factitious lymphedema has been noted in several cases (Smith 1975; Carlson et al. 1977). Jarventausta et al. (1987) reported a case of factitious pain and swelling of the upper arm. In a similar case, thought to represent Munchausen's syndrome, Rodriguez-Moreno et al. (1990) noted that the edema, demineralization, and bone scan were "indistinguishable from reflex sympathetic dystrophy." Another, apparently inadvertently self-inflicted case, was attributed to pathological grief (Dopson 1979). We have seen similar cases, in which it appeared that a tourniquet had been used to compress the arm or leg, and other cases in which extremities were chronically positioned so as to compromise circulation. Ochoa and Verdugo (1993) comment that this "ligature sign" has been considered evidence for RSD as well as for factitious illness. In most of these cases, neither conscious nor unconscious symptom production could be proved, yet such seems likely. These patients may show edema, trophic changes, and "allodynia," leading to the misdiagnosis of reflex sympathetic dystrophy. Ochoa (1994) also described cases of clear malingering that resembled RSD.

It was noted long ago that "pain can be evaluated only by the individual experiencing it" (Livingston 1943), and we are urged to view pain as just what the patient says it is. Yet, Weintraub (1995a) cautions, ". . . it becomes necessary for physicians confronted by bizarre and intractable symptoms, especially in litigation, to resist the urge to believe the patient and develop a healthy skepticism and cautious approach." Often, discussions become emotionally charged, as some clinicians criticize physicians who "slander" patients with the determination of malingering, while others decry the naiveté of accepting without question patients' reports of symptoms that lack objective corroboration, either from examination or collateral sources.

Faust (1995) reviews studies demonstrating that clinicians are not skillful at detecting deception, even when they are confident of their judgments. He hypothesizes that several factors impede detection: (1) The hazards of missing a medical condition usually outweigh those of overdiagnosis. (2) Physicians are taught to believe their patients and to sympathize with them. (3) It is usually in the patient's best interests to present factual information. (4) The physician's obligation is normally to the patient and his or her interests.

Scientific objectivity seems the appropriate route between suspicious disbelief and gullible naiveté. Such objectivity is difficult to achieve because we only know that deception occurs, but not how often, and we have few objective tools to distinguish it from psychogenic pain. Our need to identify and ally ourselves with patients in the therapeutic situation conflicts with the need for scientific objectivity in litigation and determinations of entitlement. Perhaps a "trust but verify" posture is best, or even separation of the roles of "treater" from "certifier."

TREATMENT IMPLICATIONS

While the treatment of RSD is beyond the scope of this chapter, the following section presents some therapeutic strategies whose benefit may be inferred from the material reviewed.

PSYCHOPHYSIOLOGIC INTERVENTIONS

The pronounced ability of psychophysiological factors to exacerbate RSD suggests that interventions that target psychophysiologic reactivity and increase volitional control would be useful. Unfortunately, reports are sparse and often only anecdotal descriptions of single cases.

Grunert et al. (1990) reported that thermal biofeedback training provided good success in a series of 20 refractory patients, 14 of whom had returned to work at one year follow-up. Blacker (1980), Barowsky et al. (1987), Alioto (1981), and Blanchard (1979) also reported efficacy in single-case studies.

Hypnosis has been tried as well. Gainer (1992) reported three cases of RSD that had benefited only transiently from sympathetic blocks. With hypnosis, all patients were able to achieve warming of the extremity and long-term relief of symptoms, including dystonia in one case. Finer and Graf (1968) described changes in pain and circulation in causalgia in response to hypnosis. Shumacker and Abramson (1949) successfully treated psychiatric cases with suggestion after administering amobarbital.

DRUG CONSIDERATIONS

The common occurrence of pain on sympathetic stimulation suggests that drugs with this property might best be avoided. The short-acting benzodiazepines and opioids are associated with pronounced catecholamine release as trough levels are approached in those accustomed to their use (rebound). It is possible that the use of sedating antidepressants or antihistamines as anxiolytics can circumvent this difficulty.

INTERDISCIPLINARY TREATMENT

Interdisciplinary treatment may be optimal, given the likelihood that a preponderance of patients will have both neurological and psychological pathology. In addition to treatments for the primary condition, it may be essential to eliminate barriers to use of the involved extremity—whether fear, hopelessness, or disincentives to recovery—to prevent irreversible changes.

CONCLUSIONS

1. There is no good evidence that true RSD is a psychogenic condition.
2. It is highly likely that anxiety, stress, and chemical dependence increase nociception in RSD. Appropriate treatment with relaxation and antidepressants should help.
3. The severe pain of causalgia is the cause of psychiatric suffering and not the converse.
4. Pathologic signs and symptoms in RSD may be worsened by volitional or inadvertent behaviors, such as immobilization and disuse. These behaviors may be motivated by fear, misinformation, or regressive urges. Thus, although maladaptive, they may not indicate psychopathology.
5. Patients with conversion disorder and factitious illness may be erroneously diagnosed with RSD and thus receive inappropriate treatment. Their failure to respond may mislead professionals into the belief that RSD is a psychiatric condition.
6. Conversion/factitious mechanisms may be more likely to mimic RSD than other pain syndromes. If true, such cases should be relatively rare in the primary care setting and increasingly common in tertiary care and beyond.
7. We lack definitive information as to whether aberrant behavior following a trivial injury can produce RSD that otherwise would not occur. We also do not know whether high levels of state or trait anxiety can do so.

In a given patient with symptoms suggestive of reflex sympathetic dystrophy, the diagnostic goal is not to determine whether the psyche causes RSD, but to determine whether the patient has psychogenic pain, RSD, or RSD made worse by behavioral and psychological factors.

A caveat is warranted. Self-fulfilling prophecies are a risk in patients with RSD, such that evaluators create that which they perceive. Much disability in injured workers may be generated by "the system" that challenges the validity of patient complaints and introduces harmful delays in treatment. Some patients with RSD are initially undiagnosed or suspected of having functional symptoms, which leads to exaggerated efforts to convince physicians of the severity of illness. These efforts may backfire by appearing insincere. Those who fear a psychiatric diagnosis may so deny and minimize psychological problems and stresses that they create the impression of somatization. Teasell and Shapiro (1995) describe the preoccupation with proving the legitimacy of their complaints, once labeled as psychogenic. Thus, ironically, the physician's misdiagnosis of psychogenicity could interact with the patient's fear of this diagnosis to create the signs that support the diagnosis.

Our understanding of the physiology and treatment of reflex sympathetic dystrophy will be facilitated by developing homogeneous populations for study. This effort may be fostered by establishing exclusion criteria, such that RSD could not be diagnosed in the presence of nonphysiologic neurological findings, abatement of deficit symptoms (as opposed to pain) with placebo, or evidence of self-inflicted injury.

Investigation of psychological factors in RSD is needed. Prospective studies of injured and operated persons are necessary to identify the factors that facilitate development of the syndrome. Alternatively, early case identification may permit prospective treatment studies to determine factors associated with outcome.

SUMMARY

The widely acknowledged "RSD personality" is clearly unsubstantiated. Evidence is good that RSD is strongly altered by behavioral and affective disturbances and may at times promote such disturbances. Conversely, appropriate behaviors and interventions that stabilize affects are likely to be beneficial. Conversion and dissimulation may masquerade as RSD or may co-exist with it in the form of conscious or unconscious exaggeration. Diagnosis in such cases is difficult and current criteria are often more suggestive than definitive.

REFERENCES

Affleck, G., Urrows, S., Tennen, H. and Higgins, P., Daily coping with pain from rheumatoid arthritis: patterns and correlates, Pain, 51 (1992) 221–229.

Alioto, J.T., Behavioural treatment of reflex sympathetic dystrophy, Psychosomatics, 22 (1981) 539–540.

American Psychiatric Association, Diagnostic and Statistical Manual of Mental Disorders: DSM III-R, American Psychiatric Association, Washington, D.C., 1987.

American Psychiatric Association staff, Diagnostic and Statistical Manual of Mental Disorders: DSM-IV, American Psychiatric Association, Washington, D.C., 1994.

Barowsky, E.I., Zweig, J.B. and Moskowitz, J., Thermal biofeedback in the treatment of symptoms associated with reflex sympathetic dystrophy, J. Child Neurol., 2 (1987) 229–232.

Bernstein, B.H., Singsen, B.H., Kent, J.T., Kornreich, H., King, K., Hicks, R. and Hanson, V., Reflex neurovascular dystrophy in childhood, J. Pediatr., 93 (1978) 211–215.

Bhatia, K.P., Bhatt, M.H. and Marsden, C.D., The causalgia-dystonia syndrome, Brain, 116 (1993) 843–851.

Bigos, S.J., Battié, M.C., Spengler, D.M., Fisher, L.D., Fordyce, W.E., Hansson, T.H., Nachemson, A.L. and Wortley, M.D., A prospective study of work perceptions and psychosocial factors affecting the report of back injury, Spine, 16 (1991) 1–6.

Blacker, H.M., Volitional sympathetic control, Anesth. Analg., 59 (1980) 785–788.

Blanchard, E.B., The use of temperature biofeedback in the treatment of chronic pain due to causalgia, Biofeedback Self Regul., 4 (1979) 183–188.

Bonica, J.J., Causalgia and other reflex sympathetic dystrophies. In: J.J. Bonica, J.C. Liebeskind and D.G. Albe-Fessard (Eds.), Proceedings of the Second World Congress on Pain, Advances in Pain Research and Therapy, Vol. 3, Raven Press, New York, 1979, pp. 141–166.

Bruehl, S. and Carlson, C.R., Predisposing psychological factors in the development of reflex sympathetic dystrophy, Clin. J. Pain, 8 (1992) 287–299.

Bytzer, P., Stokholm, M., Andersen, I., Klitgaard, N.A. and Schaffalitzky de Muckadell, O.B., Prevalence of surreptitious laxative abuse in patients with diarrhea of uncertain origin: a cost benefit analysis of a screening procedure, Gut, 30 (1989) 1379–1384.

Carlson, M.J., Linscheid, R.L. and Lucas, A.R., Recognition of factitial hand injuries, Clin. Orthop., 122 (1977) 222–227.

Cassileth, B.R., Lusk, E.J., Strouse, T.B., Miller, D.S., Brown, L.L., Cross, P.A. and Tenaglia, A.N., Psychosocial status in chronic illness: a comparative analysis of six diagnostic groups, N. Engl. J. Med., S311 (1984) 506–511.

Ciccone, D.S. and Grzesiak, R.C., Cognitive dimensions of chronic pain, Soc. Sci. Med., 19 (1984) 1339–1345.

Contrada, R.J. and Drants, D.S., Stress, reactivity, and type A behavior: current status and future directions, Annals of Behavioral Medicine, 10 (1988) 64–70.

Cooke, E.D. and Ward, C., Vicious circles in reflex sympathetic dystrophy, a hypothesis: discussion paper, J. R. Soc. Med., 83 (1990) 96–99.

Crisson, J.E. and Keefe, F.J., The relationship of locus of control to pain coping strategies and psychological distress in chronic pain patients, Pain, 35 (1988) 147–154.

Crook, J. and Tunks, E., Defining the "chronic pain syndrome": an epidemiological method. In: H.L. Fields, R. Dubner and F. Cervero (Eds.), Proceedings of the Fourth World Congress on Pain, Advances in Pain Research and Therapy, Vol. 9, Raven Press, New York, 1985, pp. 871–877.

DeGood, D.E., Cundiff, G.W., Adams, L.E. and Shutty, M.S., Jr., A psychosocial and behavioral comparison of reflex sympathetic dystrophy, low back pain, and headache patients, Pain, 54 (1993) 317–322.

DeLeo, D., Magni, G., Rossi, F. and Rosetto, F., Psychologische Faktoren beim Sudeck syndrom, Deutsche Medizinsche Wollenschrift, 108 (1983) 7199.

De Takats, G., Sympathetic reflex dystrophy, Med. Clin. North Am., 49 (1965) 117–129.
De Takats, G. and Miller, D.S., Post-traumatic dystrophy of the extremities: a chronic vasodilator mechamsm, Arch. Surg., 46 (1943) 469–479.
Dopson, C., Unresolved grief presenting as chronic lymphedema of the hand, Am. J. Psychiatry, 136 (1979) 1333–1334.
Doupe, J., Cullen, C.H. and Chance, G.Q., Post-traumatic pain and the causalgic syndrome, J. Neurol. Neurosurg. Psychiatry, 7 (1944) 33–48.
Drucker, W.R., Hubay, C.A., Holden, W.D. and Bukovnic, J.A., Pathogenesis of posttraumatic sympathetic dystrophy, Am. J. Surg., 97 (1959) 454–464.
Ecker, A., Norepinephrine in reflex sympathetic dystrophy: a hypothesis, Clin. J. Pain, 5 (1989) 313–315.
Egle, U.T. and Hoffmann, S.O., Psychosomatic aspects of reflex sympathetic dystrophy. In: M. Stanton-Hicks, W. Janig and R.A. Boas (Eds.), Reflex Sympathetic Dystrophy, Kluwer Academic Publishers, Boston, 1990, pp. 29–36.
Faust, D., The detection of deception, Neurol. Clin., 13 (1995) 255–265.
Finer, B. and Graf, K., Circulatory changes accompanying hypnotic imagination of hyperalgesia and hypoalgesia in causalgic limbs, Zeitschrift für die Gesamte Experimentelle Medizin, 146 (1968) 97–114.
Fishbain, D.A., Goldberg, M., Meagher, B.R., Steele, R. and Rosomoff, H., Male and female chronic pain patients categorized by DSM-III psychiatric diagnostic criteria, Pain, 26 (1986) 181–197.
Fishbain, D.A., Goldberg, M., Labbe, E., Steele, R. and Rosomoff, H., Compensation and non-compensation chronic pain patients compared for DSM-III operational diagnoses, Pain, 32 (1988) 197–206.
Fishbain, D.A., Rosomoff, H.L. and Rosomoff, R.S., Drug abuse, dependence and addiction in chronic pain patients, Clin. J. Pain, 8 (1992) 77–85.
Fordyce, W.E., Behavioral methods for chronic pain and illness, C.V. Mosby, St. Louis, 1976.
Fordyce, W.E., Fowler, R.S., Lehman, J.F., Delateur, B.J., Sand, P.L. and Trieschmann, R.B., Operant conditioning in the treatment of chronic pain, Arch. Phys. Med. Rehabil., 54 (1973) 399–408.
Gainer, M.J., Hypnotherapy for reflex sympathetic dystrophy, Am. J. Clin. Hypn., 34 (1992) 227–232.
Gamsa, A., The role of psychological factors in chronic pain. I. A half century of study, Pain, 57 (1994a) 5–15.
Gamsa, A., The role of psychological factors in chronic pain. II. A critical appraisal, Pain, 57 (1994b) 17–29.
Grunert, B.K., Devine, C.A., Sanger, J.R., Matloub, H.S. and Green, D., Thermal self-regulation for pain control in reflex sympathetic dystrophy syndrome, J. Hand Surg., 15 (1990) 615–618.
Guze, S.B., The validity and significance of the clinical diagnosis of hysteria (Briquet's syndrome), Am. J. Psychiatry, 132 (1975) 138–141.
Haddox, J.D., Psychologic support of the patient with reflex sympathetic dystrophy. In: M. Stanton-Hicks, W. Jänig and R.A. Boas (Eds.), Reflex Sympathetic Dystrophy, Kluwer Academic Publishers, Boston, 1990a, pp. 143–150.
Haddox, J.D., Psychological aspects of reflex sympathetic dystrophy. In: M. Stanton Hicks (Ed.), Pain and the Sympathetic Nervous System, Kluwer Academic Publishers, Boston, 1990b.
Haddox, J.D., Abram, S.E. and Hopwood, M.H., Comparison of psychometric data in RSD and radiculopathy, Reg. Anesth., 13 (1S) (1988) 27.
Harkapaa, K., Jarvikoski, A., Mellin, G., Hurri, H. and Luoma, J., Health locus of control beliefs and psychological distress as predictors for treatment outcome in low-back pain patients: results of a 3-month follow-up of a controlled intervention study, Pain, 46 (1991) 35–41.
Hemler, D.E., McAuley, R.A. and Belandres, P.V., Common clinical presentations among active duty personnel with traumatically induced reflex sympathetic dystrophy, Mil. Med., 153 (1988) 493–495.
Holden, W.D., Sympathetic dystrophy, Arch. Surg., 57 (1948) 373–384.

Horowitz, S.H., Iatrogenic causalgia: classification, clinical findings, and legal ramifications, Arch. Neurol., 41 (1984) 821–824.
Jarventausta, T.H. and Telaranta, T.K., Factitious pain and swelling of the upper arm: case report, Acta. Chir. Scand., 153 (1987) 71–72.
Jensen, M.P., Turner, J.A. and Romano, J.M., Self-efficacy and outcome expectancies: relationship to chronic pain coping strategies and adjustment, Pain, 44 (1991a) 263–269.
Jensen, M.P., Turner, J.A., Romano, J.M. and Karoly, P., Coping with chronic pain: a critical review of the literature, Pain, 47 (1991b) 249–283.
Katon, W., Egan, K. and Miller, D., Chronic pain: lifetime psychiatric diagnoses and family history, Am. J. Psychiatry, 142 (1985) 1156–1160.
Kori, S.H., Miller, R.P. and Todd, D.D., Kinisophobia: a new view of chronic pain behavior, Pain Management, 3 (1990) 35–43.
Kramlinger, K.G., Swanson, D.W. and Maruta, T., Are patients with chronic pain depressed? Am. J. Psychiatry, 140 (1983) 747–749.
Lankford, L.L., Reflex sympathetic dystrophy. In: J.M. Hunter, L.H. Schneider, E.J. Macklin and J.A. Bell (Eds.), Rehabilitation of the Hand, C.V. Mosby, St. Louis, 1978, pp. 763–786.
Lankford, L.L., Reflex sympathetic dystrophy of the upper extremity. In: J.E. Flynn (Ed.), Hand Surgery, 3rd ed., Williams & Wilkins, Baltimore, 1982, pp. 656–670.
Lidz, T. and Payne, R.L., Causalgia: report of recovery following relief of emotional stress, Archives of Neurology and Psychiatry, 53 (1945) 222–225.
Livingston, W.K., Pain mechanisms: a physiologic interpretation of causalgia and its related states, MacMillan, New York, 1943.
Lynch, M.E., Psychological aspects of reflex sympathetic dystrophy: a review of the adult and paediatric literature, Pain, 49 (1992a) 337–347
Lynch, M.E., Psychological aspects of reflex sympathetic dystrophy, IASP Newsletter, Oct./Sept. (1992b) 2–3.
Mailis, A. and Wade, J., Profile of caucasian women with possible genetic predisposition to reflex sympathetic dystrophy: a pilot study, Clin. J. Pain, 10 (1994) 210–217.
Mayfield, F.H. and Devine, J.W., Causalgia, Surgery, Gynecology and Obstetrics, 80 (1945) 631–635.
Merskey, H., Psychiatry and pain. In: R.A. Sternbach (Ed.), The Psychology of Pain, 2nd ed., Raven Press, New York, 1986.
Merskey, H., Regional pain is rarely hysterical, Arch. Neurol., 45 (1988) 915–918.
Merskey, H. and Bogduk, N. (Eds.), Classification of Chronic Pain, Descriptions of Chronic Pain Syndromes and Definition of Terms, 2nd ed., IASP Press, Seattle, 1994, pp. 40–43.
Miller, E., Defining hysterical symptoms (Editorial), Psychol. Med., 18 (1988) 275–277.
Miller, D.S. and De Takats, G., Post-traumatic dystrophy of the extremities: Sudeck's atrophy, Surgery, Gynecology and Obstetrics, 75 (1942) 558–582.
Mitchell, S.W., Moorehouse, G.R. and Keen, W.W., Gunshot Wounds and Other Injuries of Nerves, Lippincott, Philadelphia, 1864.
Moberg, E., The shoulder-hand-finger syndrome, Surg. Clin. North Am., 40 (1960) 367–373.
Ochoa, J.L., Reflex sympathetic dystrophy: a disease of medical understanding, Clin. J. Pain, 8 (1992) 363–366.
Ochoa, J.L., CPSMV: Chronic Pains Associated with Positive and Negative Sensory, Motor, and Vasomotor Manifestations. Description of Heterogeneous Clinical Entities and Differential Diagnosis of their Sociopathological and Psychopathological Substrates. Presented at: Controversies in Neuroscience V: Persistent Pain, August 19–21, 1994, Neurological Sciences Institute, Portland, OR.
Ochoa, J.L., Reflex sympathetic dystrophy: a common clinical avenue for somatoform expression, Neurol. Clin., 13 (1995a) 351–363.
Ochoa, J.L., Letter to editor, Muscle Nerve, 4 (1995b) 458–462.
Ochoa, J.L. and Verdugo, R.J., The mythology of reflex sympathetic dystrophy and sympathetically maintained pains, Physical Medicine Rehabilitation Clinics of North America, 4 (1993) 151–162.
Ochoa, J.L., Verdugo, R.J. and Campero, M., Pathophysiological spectrum of organic and

psychogenic disorders in neuropathic pain patients fitting the description of causalgia or RSD. In: G.F. Gebhart, D.L. Hammond and T.S. Jensen (Eds.), Proceedings of the 7th World Congress on Pain, Progress in Pain Research and Management, Vol. 2, IASP Press, Seattle, 1994, pp. 483–494.

Osterweis, M., Kleinman, A. and Mechanic, E. (Eds.), Pain and Disability: Clinical, Behavioral, and Public Policy Perspectives, Institute of Medicine, Committee on Pain, Disability, and Chronic Illness Behavior, National Academy Press, Washington, D.C., 1987.

Pak, T.J., Martin, G.M., Magness, J.L. and Kavanaugh, G.J., Reflex sympathetic dystrophy: review of 140 cases, Minn. Med., 53 (1970) 507–512.

Pilowsky, I., Abnormal illness behavior, Br. J. Med. Psychol., 42 (1960) 347–351.

Pilowsky, I., Pain and illness behaviour: assessment and management. In: P. Wall and R. Melzack (Eds.), Textbook of Pain, Churchill Livingstone, New York, 1984, 765–775.

Poulsen, D.L., Hansen, H.J., Langemark, M., Olesen, J. and Bech, P., Discomfort or disability in patients with chronic pain syndrome, Psychother. Psychosom., 48 (1987) 60–62.

Purtell, J.J., Robins, E. and Cohen, M.E., Observations on clinical aspects of hysteria: a quantitative study of 50 hysteria patients and 156 control subjects, JAMA, 146 (1951) 902.

Rizzi, R., Visentin, M. and Mazzetti, G., Reflex Sympathetic dystrophy. In: C. Benedetti, C.R. Chapman and G. Moricca, (Eds.), Advances in Pain Research and Therapy, Vol. 7, Raven Press, New York, 1984.

Rodriguez-Moreno, J., Ruiz-Martin, J.M., Mateo-Soria, L., Rozadilla, A. and Roig-Escofet, D., Munchausen's syndrome simulating reflex sympathetic dystrophy, Ann. Rheum. Dis., 49 (1990) 1010–1012.

Roe, S., Mailis, A. and Umana, M., Effect of intravenous sodium amytal on sympathetic skin responses, limb temperatures and pain (poster), Annual Meeting of the American Pain Society, November 10, 1994a, Orlando, Florida.

Roe, S., Mailis, A. and Umana, M., Effect of intravenous sodium amytal on cutaneous hyperalgesia and bone pressure thresholds in patients with pain. Poster, Annual Meeting of the American Pain Society, November 10, 1994b, Orlando, Florida.

Rudy, T.E., Kerns, R.D. and Turk, D.C., Chronic pain and depression: toward a cognitive-behavioral mediation model, Pain, 35 (1988) 129–140.

Schott, G.D., An unsympathetic view of pain, Lancet, 345 (1995) 634–636.

Schwartzman, R.J. and McLellan, T.L., Reflex sympathetic dystrophy: a review, Arch. Neurol., 44 (1987) 555–561.

Sherry, D.D. and Weisman, R., Psychological aspects of childhood reflex neurovascular dystrophy, Pediatrics, 81 (1988) 572–578.

Shumacker, H.B. and Abramson, D.I., Posttraumatic vasomotor disorders, Surgery, Gynecology and Obstetrics, 88 (1949) 417–434.

Smith, R.J., Factitious lymphedema of the hand, J. Bone Joint Surg. Am., 57 (1975) 89–94.

Stanton-Hicks, M., Jänig, W., Hassenbusch, S., Haddox, J.D., Boas, R. and Wilson, P., Reflex sympathetic dystrophy: changing concepts and taxonomy, Pain, 65 (1995) 127–133.

Steinert, H., Nickel, O. and Hahn, K., Three-phase bone scanning in reflex sympathetic dystrophy. In: M. Stanton-Hicks, W. Janig and R.A. Boas (Eds.), Reflex Sympathetic Dystrophy, Kluwer Academic Publishers, Boston, 1990, 177–185.

Sternbach, R.A. and Timmermans, G., Personality changes associated with the reduction of pain, Pain, 1 (1975) 177–181.

Subbarao, J. and Stillwell, G.K., Reflex sympathetic dystrophy syndrome of the upper extremity: analysis of total outcome of management of 125 cases, Arch. Phys. Med. Rehabil., 62 (1981) 549–554.

Tamoush, A.J., Causalgia: redefinition as a clinical pain syndrome, Pain, 10 (1981) 187–197.

Teasell, R.W. and Shapiro, A.P., Letter to editor, Muscle and Nerve, 4 (1995) 456–457.

Turk, D.C., Meichenbaum, D. and Genest, M., Pain and Behavioral Medicine: A Cognitive-Behavioral Perspective, Guilford Press, New York, 1983.

U.S. Commission on the Evaluation of Pain, Report of the Commission on the Evaluation of Pain,

Appendix C: Summary of the National Study of Chronic Pain Syndrome, U.S. Department of Health and Human Services, Social Security Admistration, Office of Disability, Government Printing Office, Washington, D.C., 1987.

Van Houdenhove, B., Algoneurodystrophy: a psychiatrist's view, Clin. Rheum., 5 (1986) 399–406.

Van Houdenhove, B., Vasquez, G., Onghena, P., Stans, L., Vandeput, C., Vermaut, G., Vervaeke, G., Igodt, P. and Vertommen, H., Etiopathogenesis of reflex sympathetic dystrophy: a review and biopsychosocial hypothesis, Clin. J. Pain, 8 (1992) 300–306.

Van Spaendonck, K.P.M., Van Heusden, H.A., The, R., Kampen, C. and Goris, R.J.A., Posttraumatische dystrofie en persoonlijkheidstype. In: R.J.A. Goris (Ed.), Posttraumatische dystrofie, PAOG, Nijmegen, 1992, pp. 39–43.

Waylett-Rendall, J., Therapist's management of reflex sympathetic dystrophy. In: J.M. Hunter, L.H. Schneider, E.J. Macklin and J.A. Bell (Eds.), Rehabilitation of the Hand, C.V. Mosby, St. Louis, 1978, pp. 787–792.

Weintraub, M.I., Regional pain is usually hysterical, Arch. Neurol., 45 (1988) 914–915.

Weintraub, M.I., Malingering and conversion reactions (preface), Neurol. Clin. 13 (1995a) xi–xii.

Weintraub, M.I., Chronic pain in litigation: what is the relationship? Neurol. Clin., 13 (1995b) 341–349.

Weiss, W.U., Psychological aspects of RSD syndrome, American Journal of Pain Management., 4 (1994) 67–72.

White, J.C. and Sweet, W.H., Pain and the Neurosurgeon: A Forty-year Experience, C.C. Thomas, Springfield, IL, 1969.

Wilson, R.L., Management of pain following peripheral nerve injuries, Orthop. Clin. North Am., 12 (1981) 343–359.

Zachariae, L., Incidence and course of posttraumatic dystrophy following operation for Dupuytren's contracture, Acta Chir. Scand. Suppl., 336 (1964) 6–51.

Correspondence to: Edward C. Covington, MD, Director, Chronic Pain Rehabilitation Program, The Cleveland Clinic Foundation, 1995 Euclid Ave, Cleveland, OH 44195, USA. Tel: 216-444-5964; Fax: 216-444-9248.

12

Use of Regional Anesthetics for Diagnosis of Reflex Sympathetic Dystrophy and Sympathetically Maintained Pain: A Critical Evaluation

Michael Stanton-Hicks,[a] P. Prithvi Raj,[b] and Gabor B. Racz[c]

*[a]Pain Management Center, Cleveland Clinic Foundation, Cleveland, Ohio,
[b]Pain Medicine Center, Los Angeles, California, and [c]Department of
Anesthesiology, Texas Tech University Health Science Center,
Lubbock, Texas, USA*

The value of regional anesthesia as an aid to the diagnosis of complex regional pain syndrome (CRPS) type I (reflex sympathetic dystrophy; RSD) can probably be attributed to Doupe and colleages (1944), who were considerably influenced by the efficacy of sympathetic blocks that were performed on injured servicemen during World War II. Others including Kwan (1935), Ross (1932) and Livingston (1943), all contemporaries, contributed to the idea that the relief of pain following sympatholysis is fundamental to a diagnosis of causalgia and reflex sympathetic dystrophy. However, association of the sympathetic nervous system in sensibility and even motor function has its roots in the writings of Claude Bernard, that great physiologist who was probably the first scientist to emphasize the importance of experimental technique in obtaining valid clinical observations (Bernard 1852). In a classical experiment, he removed the superior cervical ganglion in the cat and described the effects on skin sensation and blood flow in the affected organ (Bernard 1851).

Leriche (1916), a surgeon, wrote extensively about the effects of sympathetic activity on pain sensation, a fact that empirically led him to strip the sympathetic plexus from blood vessels in causalgic states of the lower extremities. While this procedure of course makes little physiological sense, it helped to cement further the idea of sympathetic dysfunction with these dysautonomias. Leriche was also the first to use procaine to block sympathetic ganglia for many conditions, including causalgia and angina (Leriche 1949). Bonica (1953, 1973, Bonica et al. 1979), in his many writings, consistently related the relief of burning dysesthesia, hyperalgesia to mechanical and cold stimuli, and hyperpathia by sympathetic blockade to be commensurate with a diagnosis of reflex sympathetic dystrophy or causalgia. Because of the technical difficulties inherent in the application of paravertebral sympathetic blockade, Bonica emphasized that if such techniques are to be reliable as diagnostic or prognostic tests, certain rigorous rules should be followed. He emphasized, for example, the need to block the cervicothoracic chain from the middle cervical ganglia to the fourth thoracic ganglion to ensure that sympathetic fibers (Kuntz's nerves; Kuntz 1953) not ascending from the thorax within the thoracic sympathetic trunk would be interrupted. While most clinicians employ the anterior paratracheal technique, a posterior paravertebral approach may be necessary to achieve the additional blockade of the upper four thoracic sympathetic ganglia.

In addition to assessing the subjective response of pain relief, it is important to determine the completeness of sympatholysis by some objective method such as surface temperature in the distal extremities and peripheral autonomic surface potential ([PAPS] reflex response) (Knezevic et al. 1985). Quantitative sweat testing (QSART; Low et al. 1983) is a valuable test of sudomotor function, but because it is an *axon reflex,* it can not be used to test the effect of sympatholysis. Quantitative sensory testing (QST) is a negative test (Kissen et al. 1987). In a similar manner, Bonica (1979) emphasized that for complete interruption of the lower sympathetic trunk, it is necessary to include the last thoracic sympathetic ganglion with all of the lumbar ganglia. While acknowledging the potential for misinterpretation resulting from barriers to diffusion, placebo effect, and technical competence, Bonica emphasized that diagnostic and prognostic integrity can only be sustained if these procedures are performed at least three times. To determine whether a patient is a "placebo responder," some investigators suggest that saline should replace the local anesthetic for at least one block (Ochoa et al. 1994). However, saline, either at room temperature or warmed to body temperature, may itself produce *measurable* evidence of a sympathetic block, together with the relief of burning dysesthetic symptoms or other nociceptive pain (Chapter 10, this volume). Other physical factors such as osmolality can affect nerve excitability; an example is the experiment by Fink et al. (1979), who used hyposmolar saline-sucrose to induce conduction block in vitro. A frequent misconception is the apparent paradox associated with the relief of burning dysesthesia and cold mechanical allodynia after sympatholysis in the presence of a hyperemic, dry, hot extremity. The idea of a hyperactive sympathetic nervous system has prevailed and has made it easier to accept the relief of such symptoms by sympatholysis in a clinically cold, ischemic, and sweaty extremity.

While this latter clinical picture of SMP fits the hypothesis of Roberts (1986), remaining unanswered is the question at what point does norepinephrine induce nociception? It would appear that this might occur when the background sympathetic tone is low or at least if the system is not hyperactive.

That norepinephrine can induce pain in certain states (e.g., SMP) is well established (Walker and Nulsen 1948; Wallin et al. 1976). Also, recent research seems to indicate that both the alpha-1 adrenoceptor (Davis et al. 1991; Campbell et al. 1992) and the alpha-2 adrenoceptor (Sato and Perl 1991; Jänig and McLachlan 1994) are implicated in nociception.

Do local humoral factors override postganglionic sympathetic influence in this acute stage of CRPS type I (RSD), thus presenting the clinically hot, pink, dry (but sometimes sweaty) picture? Or is there a fundamental change in the reactivity "of the adrenoceptor" such that it now reacts either directly or indirectly to the influence of norepinephrine?

Proper interpretation of any alpha-adrenergic challenge, be it by interference with the postganglionic sympathetic fiber or a pharmacologic attack at the alpha-adrenergic receptor, requires that the foregoing unexplained factors be kept in mind. In SMP (Fig. 1), it is postulated that peripheral tissues express alpha-1 adrenoceptors (Campbell et al. 1992; Meyer et al. 1992). Activation of nociceptors by the release of norepinephrine on previously inactive alpha-1 receptors is a source of pain. Nociceptor activity leads to a sensitization of central pain-signaling neurons such that input from low-threshold mechanoreceptors now has the capacity to evoke pain. Persisting activity in these nociceptors also maintains the central-signaling neurons in a

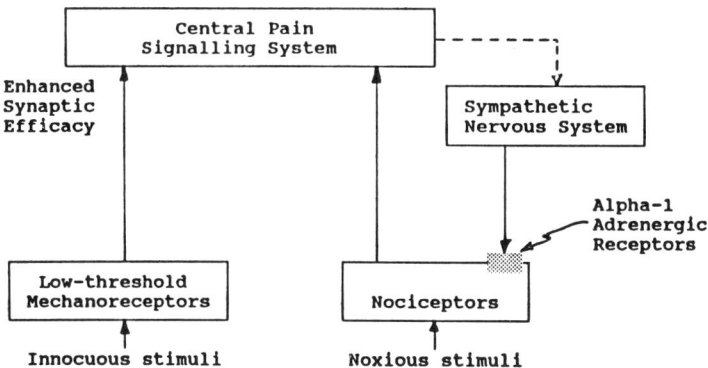

Fig. 1. Mechanism of sympathetically mediated pain. (Raja et al. 1991)

sensitized state. Although the original injury may heal, the sympathetically associated mechanism persists via the action of norepinephrine on nociceptor-related adrenoceptors. If a sympathetic block is performed at this stage, the sympathetically maintained activation of nociceptors is eliminated. Removal of the tonic nociceptor input to the CNS terminates the sensitization of central pain-signaling neurons and results in disappearance of the touch-evoked pain.

The above model differs from that proposed by Roberts (1986), who postulated that the central sensitization was maintained by sympathetically driven activity and low-threshold mechanoreceptors. However, vigorous tactile stimulation during a sympathetic block does not produce pain (Treede et al. 1992). This observation would suggest that activity in low-threshold mechanoreceptors does not appear to be the critical factor sustaining central sensitization.

The paradox may be more difficult to explain by a simple or single mechanism if we consider the results of Price and colleagues. In their study, a group of patients who had various somatosensory abnormalities including burning dysesthesia, touch-evoked allodynia, numbness, dysesthesia, and paroxysmal pain, responded to sympatholysis with relief of symptoms (Price et al. 1989). The investigators asked, "Why should blocking of any kind of peripheral sympathetic interaction eliminate the ability of naturally and electrically evoked A-beta volleys to evoke pain?" Furthermore, why should the central effect of A-beta input be rapidly normalized by block of a peripheral sympathetic effect?

In sympathetically independent pain, the factors that maintain the central state of hyperexcitability may be diverse. These factors may include sustained nociceptor input in normal nociceptive afferent fibers due to traction on periosteum, muscle, blood vessels, and epineurium, which may result from trauma or surgery. Another source of ongoing nociceptor input may be regenerating nerve sprouts in an end-bulb neuroma or a neuroma-in-continuity (Wall and Gutnick 1974; Jänig 1988).

Clinical evidence indicates that successful management of patients with SMP is dependent on early diagnosis and appropriate therapy aimed at interrupting the sympathetic innervation to the affected region. SMP should be suspected when pain and hyperalgesia are disproportionate to the injury and persist well beyond the healing period. The diagnosis should be confirmed by a random series of blocks with careful assessment of their effects on each occasion; failing this, it is then appropriate to administer one or more placebo-controlled blocks.

Pharmacologic end-organ blockade by alpha-adrenoceptor agonists is also used to diagnose RSD and causalgia. Hannington-Kiff (1977) introduced the technique with quanethidine as an alternative method of preventing the action of noradrenaline on its effector organs. While many different substances such as bretylium have been used, quanethidine is particularly advantageous, not only because it displaces noradrenaline stores, but also because it prevents its reuptake and has a strong affinity for local tissues, thereby preventing its rapid elimination. Although the block is nonselective, it is simple to perform, does not require technical expertise, and may be employed in the presence of systemic anticoagulation. The principal disadvantages of intravenous regional sympathetic blockade are that it can only be used in the extremities, and widespread systemic effects may attend the release of guanethidine into the circulation and cause severe hypotension, which in some cases can be delayed for several hours after tourniquet release.

Also important is the relationship between local anesthetic sympathetic blockade and intravenous alpha-adrenoceptor blockade with phentolamine, which Arnér (1991) and Raja et al. (1991) suggest is equally helpful to the diagnosis of sympathetically maintained pain. Although its proponents claim that the technique is more effective in detecting the placebo responder, its interpretation is similarly fraught with the difficulty of differentiating between a placebo responder and a normal physiologic placebo response (Chapter 10, this volume).

The ensuing physical changes that characterize RSD are merely components in the multifactorial breakdown of physiologic function. Under such circumstances, a somatosensory block will be necessary to establish a diagnosis that is consistent with nociceptive pain but without a requirement for a concomitant sympathetic component. Therefore, all the other clinical features relating to a diagnosis of RSD, or causalgia in the presence of a known nerve lesion, must be present to establish a diagnosis. The temporal changes in the pathophysiology of these conditions not only test the clinical acumen of the clinician, but also the ability to interpret the results of regional anesthetic procedures that are employed in diagnosis.

REGIONAL ANESTHETIC TECHNIQUES OF SYMPATHOLYSIS

UPPER EXTREMITY: STELLATE GANGLION BLOCK

Although several approaches to the cervical sympathetic chain have been described, Leriche and Fontain (1934) were the first to describe the anterior approach. Two techniques are commonly employed. The most common uses the transverse process of C6 (Chaussignac's tubercle); the other is a more medial approach at the C7 level with the anterolateral aspect of the vertebral body as the target (Stanton-Hicks et al. 1986; Moore 1954).

In brief, the procedure is carried out as follows. The patient is placed supine with a roll beneath the shoulders to promote hyperextension of the neck. Chaussignac's tubercle is plapated medial to the sternocleidomastoid muscle. While using the palpating fingers to protect the carotid artery in its sheath, the clinician introduces a needle to the C6 tubercle and injects the local anesthetic (Fig. 2). Attention must be paid to several anatomical features to ensure a successful response. While the depth of the C6 tubercle from the skin may vary, the tubercle itself lies more anterior than the junction of the transverse process and the vertebral body. Regardless of the specific location encountered at C6, if the palpating fingers properly displace the skin posteriorly, the depth tends to be between 2 and 2.5 cm. The important difference between the medial and lateral location on the transverse process at C6 relates to the presence of the longus colli muscle. It is located over the lateral aspect of the vertebral body and medial portion of the transverse process. It does not cover the C6 tubercle; only the prevertebral fascia that invests the longus colli muscle also covers the C6 tubercle. Therefore, if the needle contacts the medial aspect of the transverse processes at a depth somewhat greater than expected, the clinician should be prepared to withdraw the needle 0.5 cm to avoid injection into the longus colli muscle. Injection into the muscle belly

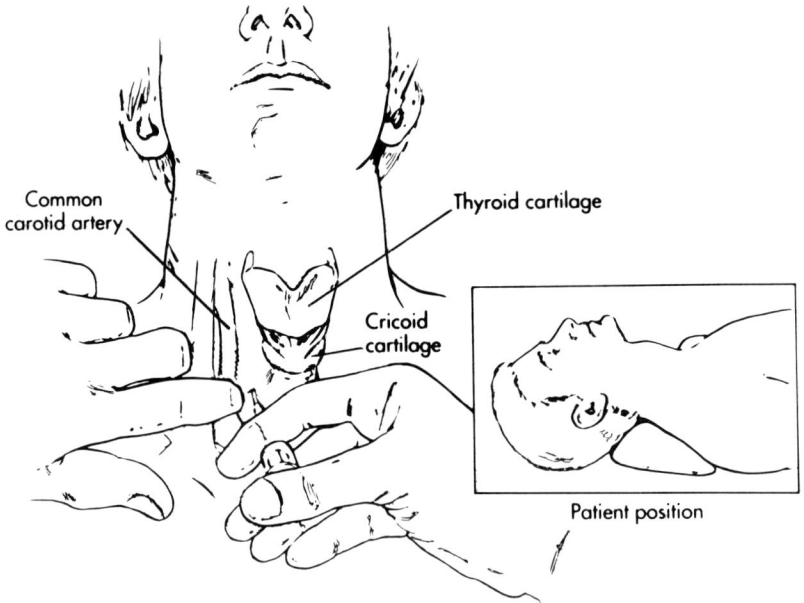

Fig. 2. Stellate ganglion block. C6 anterior tubercle is directly beneath the operator's index finger. The carotid artery is retracted laterally when necessary. The needle is perpendicular to all skin planes and is inserted directly posterior. Inset: patient positioned for stellate ganglion block. Pillow or roll should be between the shoulders to extend the neck, bring the esophagus midline, and facilitate palpation of Chaussignac's tubercle. (Raj 1992)

will limit caudad diffusion of the local anesthetic in the correct tissue plane and, by lateral diffusion behind the overlying fascia, may in turn induce a somatosensory block.

Block of the stellate ganglion at the body of C7 obviates several potential hazards including vertebral artery injection, injection into the dural sheath, and injection behind the longus colli muscle. Introduction of a needle at the anterolateral aspect of the vertebral body of C7 allows the injectate to be deposited on the periosteum of the vertebral body and its extension as fascia over the longus colli muscle and facilitates movement of the solution not only over the stellate ganglion but also retropleural into the thorax to bathe the upper thoracic sympathetic ganglia. As before, the patient is placed supine with the head hyperextended and C7 is identified 2 cm or two fingerbreadths below the C6 vertebra. The needle is introduced between the palpating fingers and the trachea, which allows the needle to contact the anterolateral aspect of the vertebral body. A particular advantage of the lower anterior approach to the stellate ganglion is block of the upper three to four thoracic ganglia, a point already emphasized by Bonica to achieve adequate sympatholysis for the upper extremity (Bonica et al. 1979).

The local anesthetic must be injected in a routine and systematic fashion. An initial test dose must be injected in all cases. Less than a milliliter of solution injected intravascularly can result in the loss of consciousness or seizures. Prior to any injection, careful aspiration must be performed, either for blood or CSF. If aspiration is negative, the test dose of .5–1 ml is administered and verbal contact is maintained with the patient. Generally, the injection of 10–15 ml will reliably block most of the sympathetic influence to the upper extremity.

EVIDENCE OF SYMPATHOLYSIS

Interruption of the sympathetic supply to the head by blockade of conduction in preganglionic axons that pass through the stellate ganglion is demonstrated by the presence of a Horner's syndrome: myosis (pinpoint pupil), ptosis (drooping of the upper eyelid), and enophthalmos (sinking of the eyeball). Associated findings are conjunctival injection, nasal congestion, and facial anhidrosis. These signs may occur without complete interruption of the postganglionic sympathetic supply to the upper extremity. Evidence of sympathetic block to the upper extremity, with an increase of temperature $\geq 35°C$ at the fingertip, includes visible engorgement of veins on the back of the hand and forearm, dryness of the skin, and the subjective feeling of warmth.

It is important that, in addition to the usual clinical signs of Horner's syndrome, dilatation of skin veins, dryness of the skin, and changes in color, the clinician use at least one of the supportive objective measurements to verify the efficacy of sympatholysis. It can not be overemphasized that routine sympathetic blocks performed in the clinic are associated with a less than complete sympathetic block. While technical considerations may play a large part in the failure to achieve complete sympatholysis, pathophysiology will also affect the success of these procedures. Even in the hands of an experienced anesthesiologist, it is probably not possible to achieve more than 70–75% interruption of the postganglionic sympathetic axons in an extremity with routine simple stellate ganglion or lumbar sympathetic blocks. A rise in skin temperature $\geq 35°C$ at the fingertip indicates a $\geq 90\%$ sympathetic block. Appropriate objective measures are plethesmography, thermographic imaging, or one of the other measurements decribed above.

SIDE EFFECTS AND COMPLICATIONS

Side effects of stellate ganglion block should be distinguished from its complications. In addition to the signs described above, block of the recurrent laryngeal nerve with complaints of hoarseness, a feeling of fullness in the throat, and occasionally shortness of breath may occur. An uncommon complication is block of the phrenic nerve, which will result in paralysis of the hemidiaphragm but will cause respiratory embarrassment only in those patients whose respiratory reserve is already compromised. Partial brachial plexus block can also result if the local anesthetic has been deposited behind the prevertebral fascia (Carron and Litwiller 1975).

Intravascular injection is most likely to occur into the vertebral artery because of its proximity to the injection site. If unrecognized, this problem will usually result in immediate loss of consciousness, seizures, and occasionally severe arterial hypotension (Moore 1954). Cerebral air embolism has been reported during this procedure (Moore 1954; Adelman 1948).

The risk of pneumothorax can occur, although a rare event if the C6 approach is used. While injection at the C7 vertebral body should never be associated with a pneumothorax, if the needle is allowed to deflect laterally, then it should be remembered that the pleura over the apex of the lung could certainly be penetrated.

LUMBAR SYMPATHETIC BLOCK

Lumbar sympathetic blocks are used extensively for the diagnosis and treatment of reflex sympathetic dystrophy, causalgia, and SMP. While regional anesthetic block of the sympathetic nerves can also be performed by spinal, epidural, and in part by peripheral nerve block (see below), the relief of pain after lumbar sympathetic block will most clearly delineate SMP from other types of pain. While the preganglionic sympathetic neurons have their cell bodies in the anterolateral horn of the spinal cord at the T10, T11, T12, L1, L2, and sometimes L3 spinal cord segments, their preganglionic fibers that project through white rami and descend in the sympathetic trunk to the lower three lumbar and upper three sacral sympathetic ganglia. While a small percentage of these postganglionic fibers pass directly to the aortic and hypogastric plexuses, most axons pass to the sympathetic trunk as rami communicantes to join the L1–5 and upper three sacral nerves. Because the last thoracic and upper two lumbar spinal nerves receive two sets of rami, one ascending from the sympathetic trunk to the spinal nerves and representing white rami, the other traveling in the sympathetic trunk to spinal nerves, as gray rami in a descending course, these nerves would not be blocked during standard lumbar sympathetic blockade. It is for this reason that, as has been mentioned, Bonica advocated blocking at the T12 and L1 levels to achieve total interruption of the sympathetic outflow to the lower limb.

TECHNIQUE

Two techniques are in common use: a lateral approach first described by Braun and Läwen (1951) and later reemphasized by Reid et al. (1970), and the classical paravertebral approach described by Mandl (1926).

Lateral approach

With the patient positioned prone, this technique has some advantages over the classical approach in that it is a more direct path to the sympathetic trunk and its ganglia, it causes less discomfort for the patient, and it is unnecessary to use the transverse process as a depth marker. The entry site is made opposite the spinous processes of L2, L3, and sometimes L4, depending upon whether one or more needles are used for the procedure. Entry is made 7–8 cm from the midline, and the direction for insertion and its depth may be corroborated by fluoroscopic imaging in two planes (Stanton-Hicks 1990) (Fig. 3).

Each needle is introduced slowly until it comes in contact with the anterolateral aspect of the vertebral body. Ideally, this position is verified by fluoroscopic imaging and represents that area of the retroperitoneal space where the psoas fascia becomes continuous with the periosteum over the ventral portion of the vertebral body (analogous to the longus colli muscle and the cervical vertebral bodies). Exact placement of the needle may be determined by using a water-soluble nonionic contrast material. Dispersion of the local anesthetic can be tracked with this contrast marker. Generally, a volume of 15–20 ml is necessary to ensure adequate spread over at least three vertebral bodies.

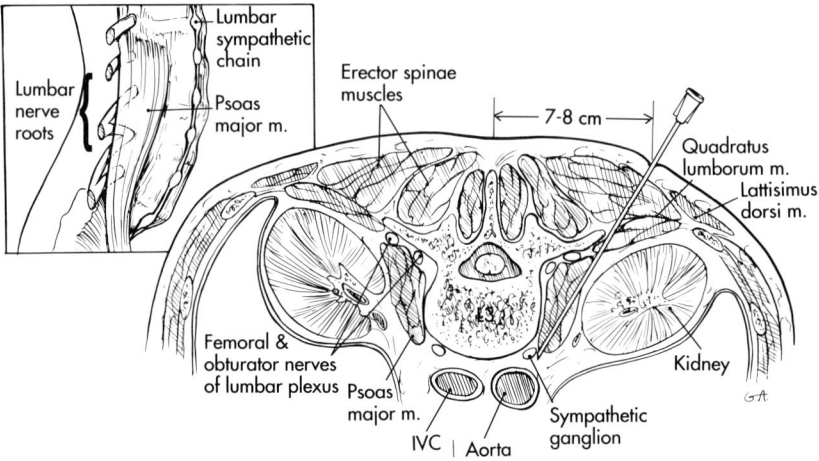

Fig. 3. Anatomy of the lumbar sympathetic chain. The sympathetic chain has migrated to the anterolateral border of the vertebral bodies. The chain is separated from the somatic nerve roots by the large psoas muscle. (Raj 1992)

Classic (paramedian) approach (Walker et al. 1978; Kappis and Gerlach 1932)

As with the lateral approach, the patient is placed prone and the spinous processes of L2–4 are identified. Needle insertion is placed much closer to the midline at about 4–5 cm. The needle is advanced at a steep (70–80°) angle to reach the transverse process at a depth of approximately 4–6 cm. The needle is then repositioned inferiorly to pass caudad to the transverse process and continue adjacent to but touching the vertebral body. Its position and depth can be controlled by fluoroscopy; as before, the use of a water-soluble nonionized contrast material will identify the correct tissue plane. Injection of the local anesthetic may be observed by watching its dispersion under fluoroscopy (see above); it should, for optimal sympatholysis, spread over at least three vertebral bodies.

EVIDENCE OF SYMPATHOLYSIS

Evidence of sympathetic block in the ipsilateral extremity will be demonstrated by dilatation of the superficial veins in the foot, an increase in temperature of the toes (34–35°C), a dryness of the skin, and a subjective feeling of warmth. See Table I for tests of autonomic function.

Table I
Tests for efficacy of sympathetic block

Sympathetic Function

Skin Plethysmography and "Ice Response"

Skin Conductance Response (SCR)
Previously referred to as sympathogalvanic response (SGR), this is a simple measure of activity in sudomotor neurons. It is dependent on changes in skin conductance but is also subject to habituation.

Skin Potential Response (SPR) (PASP)
SRP reflects activity in sudomotor neurons and changes in sodium flux of the sweat glands. Measurement requires a modified ECG, and has the advantage that no external signal source is required.

The Cobalt Blue Test
Filter papers soaked in cobalt blue are applied to corresponding areas of the upper extremity. A color range from blue to pink indicates sweating.

Cold Pressor Test
In conjunction with telethermography, this test enables the sympathetic response to be monitored after a nonaffected extremity is placed in ice-cold water. The cutaneous response demonstrated by surface cooling, which under normal physiologic conditions should be followed by rewarming of the skin after 20–25 minutes, will be delayed for 45 minutes or longer in cases of dysautonomia.

Blood Flow Measurements

Occlusion Skin Plethysmography

Temperature Measurement
Contact thermistors or noncontact, passive infrared measurement on corresponding areas (fingertips) of the ipsilateral and contralateral extremities on at least three sites should register $\geq 34°C$ with adequate sympatholysis. Complete sympatholysis under normal physiological circumstances should achieve a temperature measurement at the fingertips of $\geq 35°C$. Noncontact telethermography has the advantage of allowing regional temperature differences of $0.1°C$ to be measured over the total area.

Laser Doppler Flowmetry (Fluxmetry)
This technique offers an excellent, noninvasive measurement of changes in skin blood flow.

SIDE EFFECTS AND COMPLICATIONS

The most common side effect of lumbar sympathetic blockade is backache, which results from placement of the needles through the paravertebral muscles of the back. This side effect should be carefully explained to patients beforehand, because a heating pad or ice packs along with rest and occasional muscle relaxants may be necessary.

Intravascular injections of large volumes of local anesthetics can produce serious, systemic, toxic reactions. This result is obviated by the use of dynamic imaging during injection (Stanton-Hicks 1990; Moore 1975).

Trauma to the kidney or ureter may occur if a proper technique is not followed (Reed, personal communication, 1985). Block of the genitofemoral nerve, occurs in between 10–15% of cases and because of its frequency, should be explained to patients beforehand (Hatangdi and Boas 1985). Not infrequently in this instance, patients may experience a burning dysesthesia in the dermatome of the genitofemoral nerve.

EFFICACY

Recent studies have indicated that the adequacy of sympathetic blockade in SMP does not consistently correlate with the degree of pain relief obtained (Treede et al. 1992). Not withstanding the variables introduced by the widely differing technical skills, lack of uniform protocols, and as emphasized by Bonica, the need for obsessive attention to detail when performing these sympatholytic regional anesthetic procedures, there are several other possible reasons for the relief of pain in the absence of successful sympathetic block. One is that a placebo response is elicited, already referred to earlier (Roberts 1986, Verdugo and Ochoa 1993). A second reason is that the pain relief is due to the regional spread of local anesthetic to nearby somatic afferent nerves and their dorsal root ganglia (tracking of the solution alongside the rami communicantes, which can be avoided by the use of dynamic fluoroscopic imaging) (Stanton-Hicks 1990). This regional spread may also occur with stellate ganglion injections and is of course inevitable when using epidural and intrathecal injections (Löfström et al. 1980). A third possibility is the systemic absorption of locally injected lidocaine, which produces analgesia through an action distant from the injection site (e.g., dorsal root entry zone) (Rowbotham and Fields 1989). Fourth, in the case of pharmacologic adrenoceptor blockade, drugs like phentolamine have many other effects such as blocking ATP-regulated potassium ion channels so their site of action is not specifically on alpha-adrenergic receptors (McPherson and Angus 1989; Dunne 1991). Given that none of the commonly used methods of reversible sympathetic block are truly specific, a false-positive diagnosis of SMP may be made whenever pain relief is achieved by any methods in common use. The evaluation of pain is subjective. A linear scale such as the Visual Analog Scale (VAS), with units of either 1–10 (or 10–100) where zero is no pain and 10 equals excruciating (unbearable) pain, is used most commonly. As an example, a shift of 75% from a patient's baseline pain on the VAS would be consistent with a diagnosis of SMP, e.g., from 10 to 3, or 7 to 0. Obviously, because pain is subjective and continually variable, a smaller percentage reduction in a patient's pain symptoms, e.g., from 7 to 4, would still represent a significant component of SMP. It also would represent some residual pain, which under the circumstances, can be termed sympathetically independent pain (SIP) (Campbell et al. 1992b), i.e., it is not affected by sympatholysis. This situation, however, presupposes that *complete* sympatholysis in this respect has been achieved.

In a study that compared the effects of stellate ganglion block and intravenous phentolamine in patients with a presumptive diagnosis of sympathetically maintained, Dellemijn et al. (1994) found that both procedures provide information that is complementary to, and may be necessary, to substantiate a clinical diagnosis (Fig. 4). In fact, each procedure supplies different information. For example, the change in skin temperature after sympatholysis had no bearing on the relief of pain. In the case of phentolamine, usually associated with minimal skin temperature change, pain relief may correlate with the magnitude of systolic blood pressure fall. Interestingly, changes in the quantitative sensory testing (QST) over the thenar eminence following stellate ganglion block suggested that pain relief was, in this instance, correlated with a partial deficit in thermal discrimination. To explain the greater relief of pain that was associated with stellate ganglion block, the authors provided at least two possibilities, neither of which is related to the degree of sympathetic blockade: systemic uptake of the local anesthetic and the potential spread to adjacent somatosensory nerves (Fig. 5). The foregoing

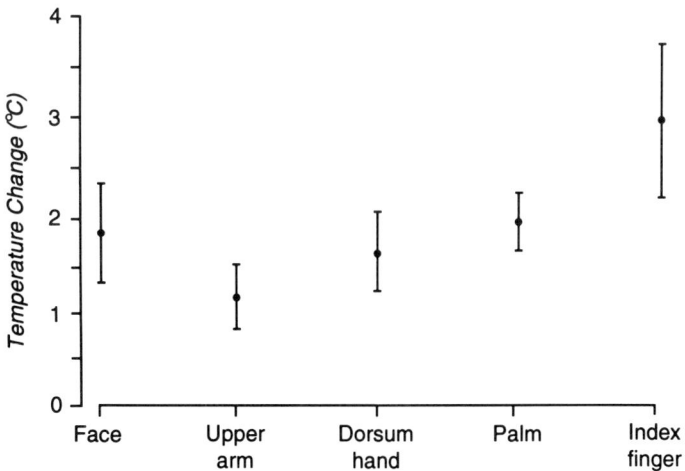

Fig. 4. Ipsilateral temperature change following stellate ganglion block. Absolute change in skin temperature of the ipsilateral arm was greater the more distal in the limb it was measured. Absolute temperature changes in the face were comparable to the palm. Error bars are ± 1 SEM. (Dellemijn et al. 1994)

aspect of this study corroborates the results of Treede et al., who also found that pain relief from stellate ganglion and lumbar sympathetic conduction blocks are not related to the degree of sympathetic block (Treede et al. 1992). From the foregoing results, it is clear that supplemental testing of patients with a presumptive diagnosis of RSD/SMP requires the utmost care when monitoring the outcome of sympathetic blockade by either method. Because of its ability to document the effect of local anesthetic action on small-diameter axons, QST is useful in cases where doubt as to the diagnosis remains. Not only should local anesthetic sympatholysis be undertaken in conjunction with the phentolamine test, but it also may be necessary to use intravenous lidocaine, when, for example, pain relief has been realized with stellate ganglion block but not phentolamine. Such an approach would help to exclude the possibility of diffusion by the local anesthetic to nearby spinal nerves.

Lack of pain relief with effective sympathetic blockade can also occur. Obviously, if the pain is truly independent of activity within the sympathetic nervous system, no pain relief is expected. A more difficult problem is the determination of whether sympatholysis in the area of interest has occurred. Obviously, only objective tests in the ipsilateral territory and not subjective observations will substantiate whether interruption of the postganglionic sympathetic outflow has occurred (Moore 1975; Hardy and Wells 1989).

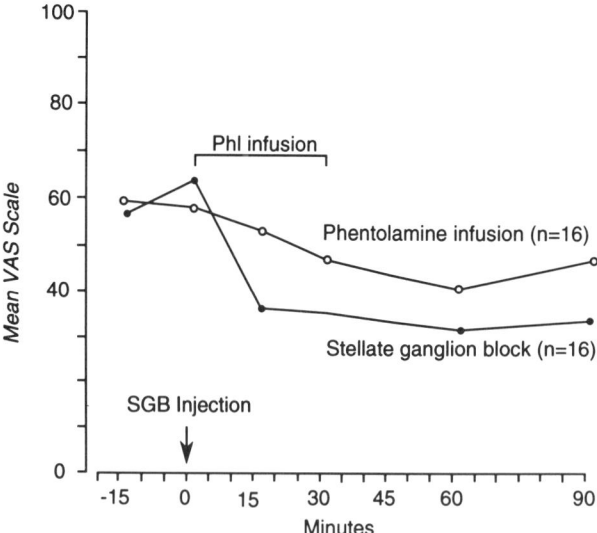

Fig. 5. Mean pain intensity visual analog scale (VAS) scores during stellate ganglion block and phentolamine. Open circles represent phentolamine infusion and filled circles represent stellate ganglion block. Phentolamine was administered at a constant rate during the 30-minute infusion period. (Dellemijn et al. 1994)

Quantitative thermal sensory testing is a useful tool for documenting blockade of small-caliber afferent axons from local anesthetic spread. With the stellate ganglion block, careful monitoring of the temperature changes on both hands may provide a better index of which patients achieve adequate blockade of sympathetic outflow than available by simply measuring the temperature in the ipsilateral hand. Sympathetic block with intravenous phentolamine does not produce a sensory deficit and elicits minimal changes in skin temperature or none at all. Thus, although less potent in relieving pain at the 35-mg dose (recommended by Raja et al. 1991), phentolamine appears to be more specific in its action than is stellate ganglion block.

The differentiation of SMP from SIP depends on the sensitivity and specificity of the sympatholytic techniques. Unfortunately, no single technique now available is adequate to make this distinction. With this circumstance in mind, we can redefine SMP in the upper extremity as: (1) pain that is relieved by both phentolamine infusion and stellate ganglion block, and (2) that sympathetic blockade by stellate ganglion injection does not produce weakness or sensory deficit to either warm or cold stimuli, and (3) the poststellate ganglion block temperature in the hand and face is greater ipsilateral to the block.

DIFFERENTIAL NERVE BLOCK

Although differential nerve block resulting from the use local anesthetics has been studied for many years, considerable controversy concerning the differential susceptibility of nerve fibers to local anesthetic conduction block remains. Some of the controversy stems from different approaches to the problem and different definitions of what constitutes "differential block." Gasser and Erlanger (1929) studied the effect of cocaine on the dog saphenous nerve. Although they found that the compound action potential (CAP) of small nerve fibers disappeared before the CAP of large fibers, some of the large fibers had been blocked before all of the small fibers. This phenomenon is called a relative differential block or differential rate of block. Nathan and Sears (1961) applied local anesthetics to cat spinal nerve roots. They found critical local anesthetic concentrations that would completely block small myelinated fibers without blocking large myelinated fibers. They referred to this phenomenon as an "absolute differential block" and required that equilibrium be established between the nerve and local anesthetic solution. Between small myelinated fibers and C (GR IV) fibers, they found a relative differential block; A-delta (GR III) fibers were blocked first. Franz and Perry (1974) obtained single-unit recordings from the cat saphenous nerve and were able to produce an absolute differential block only when the local anesthetic was applied to less than 4 mm of nerve. When greater than 4 mm of nerve were bathed in a procaine solution, a differential rate of block was obtained, with A-delta (GR III) and C (GR IV) fibers being blocked before A-alpha. Gissen et al. (1980, 1982) used desheathed rabbit vagus and sciatic nerve preparations and initially found a differential rate of block, with C (GR IV) fibers being blocked before A-alpha fibers. However, when equilibrium was established between the nerve and local anesthetic solution, the A-alpha fibers were blocked more extensively than were the C (GR IV) fibers.

INTERPRETATION

While the technique of differential spinal block is not important to this discussion, it should be understood that two approaches, an anterograde and retrograde administration, are used. The latter is simpler and only requires the use of one concentration sufficient to block all modalities, whereas the anterograde injection requires sequential use of three concentrations of local anesthetic after the saline placebo is first injected.

If the patient's pain is relieved following the first injection, the mechanism underlying the patient's pain is regarded as psychogenic. It is well established that 30–35% of all patients who have true organic pain will obtain relief from an inactive agent, so relief following the injection of normal saline may simply represent a *normal* placebo (physiologic) reaction. However, this response can usually be differentiated clinically from true psychogenic pain, because the placebo reaction is usually of rather short duration and is generally self-limiting. The possibility that pain is entirely psychogenic is substantiated or refuted by the findings of a psychological evaluation and, when in doubt, repeated provocative tests of sympatholysis. If the patient does not obtain relief from the placebo injection; and if he or she does obtain relief following the injection 0.25% procaine, a sympathetic mechanism is implicated as a basis of the patient's symptoms. This conclusion is reinforced when there are no signs of testable sensory blockade.

If the 0.25% procaine solution does not provide pain relief, but it is achieved by the 0.5% procaine dose, pain relief must be a factor of sensory block, i.e., blockade of the A-delta (GR III) or C (GR IV) fibers, which suggests a somatic or organic basis for the patient's pain. However, if the patient does not obtain relief with either 0.25% or 0.5% procaine, then 1% procaine (and sometimes when necessary 5% procaine) should be injected to produce blockade of all modalities. Should this concentration relieve the pain, the mechanism is still regarded as somatic, the presumption being that the patient has an elevated critical sensory blocking threshold. If the patient fails

to obtain relief despite a complete sympathetic, sensory, and motor blockade, then a central nervous mechanism is implicated. Central mechanisms include:
- a lesion higher in the central nervous system than the level of the spinal anesthesia
- psychogenic pain
- the phenomena known as *encephalization*
- malingering

Although this technique of differential spinal blockade has proved to be extremely effective, it does have several drawbacks: (1) The technique is quite time-consuming because the physician must wait for an adequate time after each injection to allow the various responses to become evident. In cases where the 1% concentration of procaine does not provide a complete blockade of all modalities, an additional injection of 5% procaine is necessary; (2) Each injection deposits an increasing amount of procaine in the subarachnoid space, so that following blockade of all modalities, considerable time is necessary for full recovery; (3) The anterograde administration requires the needle to remain in place throughout the procedure, which forces the patient to remain in the lateral position.

DIFFERENTIAL EPIDURAL BLOCK

Because of its complexity and imposition on time, differential spinal block is now rarely used. It has been replaced by the epidural route, which can be applied at any segmental level. While an anterograde sequence of placebo solution and blocking concentrations of local anesthetics similar to the technique of differential spinal can be used, some consider the retrograde approach to have an advantage in cases where there is a high functional or psychogenic overlay. Usually normal saline followed by one of the short-acting local anesthetics including 2-chloroprocaine, lidocaine, or mepivacaine in a motor-blocking concentration is used. Interpretation of the results follows the same sequence as that for a spinal differential block.

EFFICACY OF LOCAL ANESTHETICS FOR DIFFERENTIAL BLOCKING

Ford et al. (1984) examined differential rate of blocking by local anesthetic of peripheral nerves in an in vivo model. The model was constructed to be reasonably similar to the human clinical state (Fig. 6).

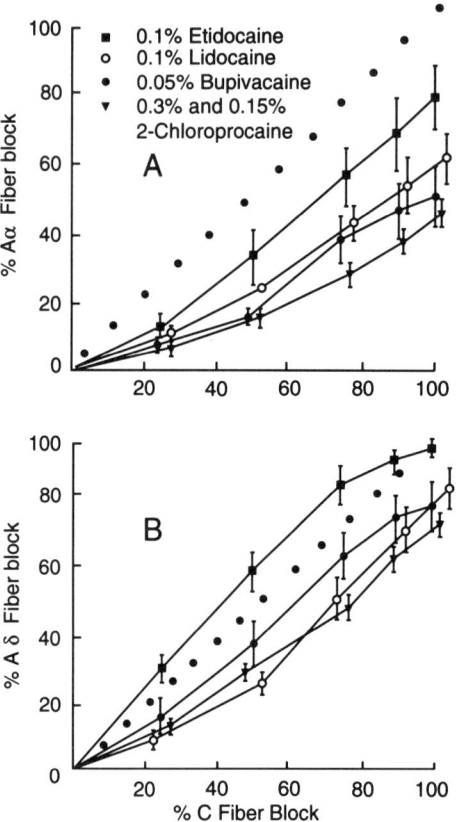

Fig. 6. Relation of C-fiber block to A-alpha-fiber block **(A)** and A-delta-fiber block **(B)**. Each point is the average ± SEM of at least five blocks. The dotted line is the reference line for no differential block. (Ford et al. 1984)

SUMMARY

In the final analysis it is clear that none of the methods that are directed toward interrupting the alpha-adrenoceptor, either pharmacologically, or by conduction block, are entirely reliable, reproducible, easy to interpret, or have a high degree of specificity. In fact, differential blocks by any route have the least specificity and at best can only be considered screening tests of sympathetic function. The problem of placebo, false-positive results, and the possibility that a nonadrenoceptor-dependent mechanism, albeit indirect, might indeed lower the specificity of the different methods still remains. Certainly the disparity between the relief of pain after conduction sympathetic block and the phentolamine test may merely reflect the failure in each case of an appropriate dose response. In support of sympatholysis by whichever method, are compelling data that would still seem to implicate the alpha-1 adrenoceptor in nociception. What is clear, however, is that interpretation of the response to sympatholysis must be taken in context with the total clinical picture. Because the diagnosis of RSD is essentially one of exclusion, any contributory tests of clinical features that are reproducibly unique to these conditions must remain a part of the standard diagnostic protocol. Sympatholysis, whether pharmacologic or by conduction block, is one such test. Until new knowledge regarding a mechanism on pathophysiology should suggest otherwise, regional anesthetic with the limitations already discussed in this test is a centerpiece in the diagnosis of RSD/SMP.

REFERENCES

Adelman, M.H., Cerebral air embolism complicating stellate ganglion block, Journal of Mt. Sinai Hospital, 15 (1948) 28–30.
Arnér, S., Intravenous phentolamine test: diagnostic and prognostic use in reflex sympathetic dystrophy, Pain, 46 (1991) 7–22.
Bernard, C.L., Influence du grand sympathique sur la sensitibilité et sur la calorification, C.R. Soc. Biol. (Paris) 3 (1851) 163–164.
Bernard, C.L., Sur les nerfs vasculaires et caloriques du grand sympathique, C.R. Acad. Sci. III, XXXIV (1852).
Bonica, J.J., The Management of Pain, Lea & Febiger, Philadelphia, 1953.
Bonica, J.J., Causalgia and other reflex sympathetic dystrophies, Postgrad. Med., 53 (1973) 143.
Bonica, J.J. and Buckley, F.P., Regional analgesia with local anesthetics. In: J.J. Bonica (Ed.), The Management of Pain, 2nd ed., Lea & Febiger, Philadelphia, 1990, pp. 883–966.
Bonica, J.J., Liebeskind, J.C. and Albe-Fessard, L.B. (Eds.), Advances in Pain Research and Therapy, Vol. 3, Raven Press, New York, 1979, pp. 141–166.
Braun, H.K. and Läwen, A., Die örtliche Betäugung, 9 Aufl., Barth, Leipzig, 1951.
Campbell, J.N., Meyer, R.A. and Raja, S.N., Is nociceptor activation by alpha-1 adrenoceptors the culprit in sympathetically maintained pain? APS Journal, 1 (1992a) 3–11.
Campbell, J.N., Meyer, R.A., Davis, K.D. and Raja, S.H., Sympathetically maintained pain: a unifying hypothesis. In: W.D. Willis (Ed.), Hyperalgesia, Raven Press, New York, 1992b, pp. 141–149.
Carron, H. and Litwiller, R., Stellate ganglion block, Anesth. Analg., 54 (1975) 567–570.
Davis, E., Treede, R-D., Raja, S.N., Meyer, R.A. and Campbell, J.N., Topical application of clonidine relieves hyperalgesia in patients with sympathetically maintained pain, Pain, 47 (1991) 309–317.
Dellemijn, H.L., Fields, R.R., Allen, W.R., McKay, W.R. and Rowbotham, M.C., The interpretation of pain relief and sensory changes following sympathetic blockade, Brain, 117 (1994) 1475–1487.
Doupe, J., Cullen, C.H. and Chance, G.O., Post-traumatic pain and the causalgia syndrome, J. Neurol. Psychiatry, 7 (1944) 33–48.
Dunne, M.J., Block of ATP-regulated potassium channels by phentolamine and other alpha-adrenoreceptor antagonists, Br. J. Pharmacol., 103 (1991) 1847–1850.
Fink, B.R., Barsa, J. and Calkins, D.F., Osmotic swelling effects on neural conduction, Anesthesiology, 51 (1979) 418–423.
Ford, D.J., Raj, P.P., Singh, P., Regan, K.M. and Ohlweiler, D., Differential peripheral nerve block by local anesthetics in the cat, Anesthesiology, 60 (1984) 28–33.

Franz, D.N. and Perry, R.S., Mechanisms for differential block among single myelinated and nonmyelinated axons by procaine, J. Physiol. (Lond), 236 (1974) 193–210.

Gasser, H.S. and Erlanger, J., The role of fiber size in the establishment of a nerve block by pressure or cocaine, Am. J. Physiol., 88 (1929) 581–591.

Gissen, A.J., Covino, B.G. and Gregus, J., Differential sensitivities of mammalian nerve fibers to local anesthetic agents, Anesthesiology, 53 (1980) 467–474.

Gissen, A.J., Covino, B.G. and Gregus, J., Differential sensitivity of fast and slow fibers in mammalian nerve. III. Effect of etidocaine and bupivacaine in fast/slow fibers, Anesth. Analg., 61 (1982) 570–575.

Hannington-Kiff, J.G, Relief of Sudeck's atrophy by regional intravenous guanethidine, Lancet, 1 (1977) 1132–1133.

Hardy, P.A.J. and Wells, J.C.D., Extent of sympathetic blockade after stellate ganglion block with bupivacaine, Pain, 36 (1989) 193–196.

Hatangdi, V.S. and Boas, R.A., Lumbar sympathectomy: a single needle technique, Br. J. Anaesth., 57 (1985) 285–289.

Jänig, W., Pathophysiology of nerve following mechanical injury. In: R. Dubner, G.F. Gebhart and M.R. Bond (Eds.), Proceedings of the Vth World Congress on Pain, Pain Research and Clinical Management, Vol. 3., Elsevier, Amsterdam, 1988, pp. 89–108.

Jänig, W. and McLachlan, E.M., The role of modifications in noradrenergic peripheral pathways after nerve lesions in the generation of pain. In: H.L. Fields and J.C. Liebeskind (Eds.), Pharmacological Approaches to the Treatment of Chronic Pain: New Concepts and Critical Issues, Progress in Pain Research and Management, Vol. 1, IASP Press, Seattle, 1994, pp. 101–128.

Kappis, M. and Gerlach, F., Paravertebal injection of procain in diagnosis, Med. Klin., 19 (1932) 1184–1187.

Kissin, I., McDanal, J., Brown, P.T., Xavier, A.V. and Bradley, E.L., Jr., Sympathetic blockade increases tactile sensitivity. Anesth. Analg., 66 (1987) 1251–1255.

Knezevic, W. and Bajada, S., Peripheral autonomic surface potential: quantitative technique for recording autonomic neural function in man, Clin. Exper. Neurol., 21 (1985) 201–210.

Kuntz, A., Autonomic Nervous System, 4th ed., Lea & Febiger, Philadelphia, 1953.

Kwan, S.T., The treatment of causalgia by thoracic sympathetic ganglionectomy, Ann. Surg., 101 (1935) 222–227.

Leriche, R., De la causalgie envisagée comme une nevrite du sympathique et des son traitement par la dénudation et l'excision des plexus nerveux périartériels, Presse Med., 24 (1916) 178–180.

Leriche, R., La Chirurgie de la Douleur, Masson, Paris, 1949.

Leriche, R. and Fontain, R.L., Anaesthésie isolée du ganglion étoile: sa technique, se indications, ses resultas, Presse Med., 42 (1934) 846.

Livingston, W.K., Pain Mechanisms: A Physiologic Interpretation of Causalgia and its Related States, MacMillan, New York, 1943.

Löfström, J.B., Lloyd, J.W. and Cousins, M.J., Sympathetic neural blockade of upper and lower extremity. In: M.J. Cousins and P.O. Bridenbaugh (Eds.), Neural Blockage in Clinical Anesthesia and Management of Pain, J.B. Lippincott, Philadelphia, 1980, pp. 355–382.

Low, P.A., Caskey, P.E., Tuck, R.R., Fealey, R.D. and Dyck, P.J., Quantitative sudomotor axon reflex test in normal and neuropathic subjects, Ann. Neurol., 14 (1983) 573–580.

Mandl, F., Die Paravertebral Injection, Springer Verlag, Vienna, 1926.

McPherson, G.A. and Angus, J.A., Phentolamine and structurally related compounds selectively antagonize the vascular actions of the K+ channel opener, cromakalim, Br. J. Pharmacol., 97 (1989) 941–949.

Meyer, R.A., Raja, S.N., Treede, R-D., Davis, K.D. and Campbell, J.N., Neural mechanisms of sympathetically maintained pain. In R.F. Schmidt and W. Jänig (Eds.), Reflex Sympathetic Dystrophy: Pathophysiological Mechanisms and Clinical Implications, VCH, Weinheim, 1992.

Moore, D.C., Stellate Ganglion Block, Charles C. Thomas, Springfield, IL, 1954.

Moore, D.C., Anterior (paratracheal) approach for block of the stellate ganglion. In: Regional

Block: A Handbook for Use in the Clinical Practice of Medicine and Surgery, 4th ed., Charles C. Thomas, Springfield, 1975, pp. 123–137.

Nathan, P.N. and Sears, T.A., Some factors concerned in differential nerve block by local anesthetics, J. Physiol. (Lond.), 157 (1961) 565–585.

Ochoa, J.L., Verdugo, R.J. and Campero, M., Pathophysical spectrum of organic and psychogenic disorders in neuropathic patients fitting the description of causalgia or reflex sympathetic dystrophy. In: G.F. Gebhardt, D.L. Hammond and T.S. Jensen (Eds.), Proceedings of the 7th World Congress on Pain, Progress in Pain Research and Management, Vol. 2, IASP Press, Seattle, 1994, pp. 483–494.

Price, D.D., Bennett, G.J. and Rafii, A., Psycho-physical observations on patients with neuropathic pain relieved by a sympathetic block, Pain, 36 (1989) 273–288.

Raj, P.P. (Ed.), Practical Management of Pain, 2nd ed., Mosby–Year Book, St. Louis, 1992, p. 784.

Raja, S.N., Reflex sympathetic dystrophy: pathophysiological basis for therapy, Pain Digest, 2 (1992) 278.

Raja, S.N., Treede, R.D., Davis, K.D. and Campbell, J.N., Systemic alpha-adrenergic blockade with phentolamine: a diagnostic test for sympathetically maintained pain, Anesthesiology, 74 (1991) 691–698.

Reid, W., Watt, J.K. and Gray, T.G., Phenol injection of the sympathetic chain, Br. J. Surg., 57 (1970) 45–50.

Roberts, W.J., A hypothesis on the physiological basis for causalgia and related pains, Pain, 24 (1986) 297–311.

Ross, J.P., Causalgia, St. Bartholomew Hospital Reports, 65 (1932) 103.

Rowbotham, M.C. and Fields, H.L., Topical lidocaine reduces pain in postherpetic neuralgia, Pain, 38 (1989) 297–301.

Sato, J. and Perl, E.R., Adrenergic excitation of cutaneous pain receptors induced by peripheral nerve injury, Science, 251 (1991) 1608–1610.

Stanton-Hicks, M., Blocks of the sympathetic nervous system. In: M. Stanton-Hicks (Ed.), Pain and the Sympathetic Nervous System, Kluwer Academic Publishers, Boston, 1990, pp. 153–164.

Stanton-Hicks, M., Abram, S. and Nolte, H., Sympathetic blocks. In: P.P. Raj, (Ed.), Practical Management of Pain, Year Book Medical Publishers, Chicago, London, 1986, pp. 661–681.

Treede, R.-D., Davis, K.D., Campbell, J.N. and Raj, S.N., The plasticity of cutaneous hyperalgesia during sympathetic ganglionic blockade in patients with neuropathic pain, Brain, 115 (1992) 607–621.

Verdugo, R. and Ochoa, J.L., Placebo-controlled somatic and sympathetic blocks in patients with prior diagnosis of causalgia, RSD or SMP (abstract). In: G.F. Gebhardt, D.L. Hammond and T.S. Jensen (Eds.), Proceedings of the 7th World Congress on Pain, Progress in Pain Research and Management, Vol. 2, IASP Press, Seattle, 1993, pp. 560–561.

Walker, A.E. and Nulsen, F., Electrical stimulation of the upper thoracic portion of the sympathetic chain in man, Archives of Neurology and Psychiatry, 59 (1948) 559–560.

Walker, P.M., Key, J.A., McKay, I.M. and Johnston, K.W., Phenol sympathectomy for vascular occlusive disease, Surg. Gynecol. Obst. 146 (1978) 741–744.

Wall, P.D. and Gutnick, M., Properties of afferent nerve impulses originating from a neuroma, Nature, 248 (1974) 740–743.

Wallin, G., Torebjörk, E. and Hallin, R., Preliminary observations on the pathophysiology of hyperalgesia in the causalgic pain syndrome. In: Y. Zottiman (Ed.), Sensory Functions of the Skin in Primates, Pergammon, New York, 1976, pp. 489–502.

Correspondence to: Michael Stanton-Hicks, MB BS, Dr. med. FRCA, ABPM, Director, Pain Management Center, Cleveland Clinic Foundation, 9500 Euclid Ave., Cleveland, Ohio 44100, USA, Tel: 216-444-3736; Fax: 216-444-9248.

Epilogue

Although the topics of the chapters of this book were chosen at a 1993 conference in Orlando, Florida, USA, they do not represent a direct transcription of the proceedings but rather an amalgam of ideas that were synthesized from this conference. The conference sought to develop a broad consensus as to what constitutes "reflex sympathetic dystrophy" (RSD) and "complex regional pain syndrome" (CRPS). There was agreement:

- to change the taxonomy
- that numerous patients have RSD/CRPS, but exact epidemiology needs to be determined, i.e., the incidence and prevalence
- that these patients are readily recognized by certain universally accepted clinical criteria, but that these symptoms vary over time
- that the diagnostic criteria require further refinement and, if possible, quantification to provide a better subdivision of patient groups, to develop better inclusion and exclusion criteria, as well as to define differential diagnosis for disorders that mistakenly may be misdiagnosed as RSD/CRPS, and
- that further human and animal research is necessary to investigate the mechanisms that lead to the clinical phenomenology in these patients

The consensus statement acknowledged that it should be possible to develop a more consistent and rational approach to treatment of these patients, even though treatment itself was not discussed. After all, most patients with RSD/CRPS are not seen in academic hospitals, but are treated in community hospitals and in private clinics. In these settings patients frequently go from doctor to doctor, including many specialists (internal medicine, anesthesiology, orthopedics, neurology, surgery, emergency medicine, psychiatry/psychology, etc.) who either do not recognize what these patients have nor know how to treat them. In this way the ground is laid for inappropriate diagnosis and treatment; individual patients may, over the course of years, undergo many types of treatment, which in some cases may be extreme, leading to amputation of limbs, bilateral sympathectomy, long-lasting psychotherapy, long-lasting pharmacotherapy, and chronic invalidism. These disasters in private and professional life are legend, yet the therapeutic approaches in too many patients who suffer from RSD/CRPS frequently have little rational basis and may, in some hands, for example, consist of mindless numbers of sympathetic blocks having little if any therapeutic effect. In many patients, delay of adequate and appropriate treatments, including sympathetic blocks, leads to a situation in which treatments that may have been effective early in the course of the disease become completely ineffective. The reason for this failure of delayed treatment is poorly understood. Also, the place for and nature of exercise therapy is not appreciated in many quarters.

As might be expected, many controversies arose throughout the conference. In all cases they reflected the differing opinions and experiences, mostly from treatment of heterogeneous groups of patients in academic centers. These patients are not necessarily representative of those who are seen much earlier after the initiating event at community hospitals or private practices. These controversies are also reflected in several chapters in this volume (e.g., those by Baron et al., Boas, Low et al., and Wilson et al.). The editors had no intention of hiding these disagreements, and the authors were encouraged to express their opinions because they represent the chaotic nature and present state of the field. In this sense, neither editors nor authors would wish to imply that the articles in this book represent *all* aspects of RSD/CRPS.

A contemporary window on this medical syndrome can be gleaned from a literature search through the Medline System from 1966 to 1995. Two sets of key words were used as follows:

Group I—Conventional Key Words: reflex sympathetic dystrophy, sympathetically maintained pain, and sympathetic nervous system and pain. Papers dealing with these subjects were pooled together: 1,775 papers were published between 1966 and 1995.

Group II—Traditional Key Words: causalgia, algodystrophy, and Sudeck. These papers also were pooled together: 1,041 papers were published between 1966 and 1995. About 43% of the papers listed in this group also appeared under one of the key words of the first group, i.e., these papers are included in the first group.

The hypothetical question was asked: "How many papers of both groups are concerned with (or claim to be concerned with) pathophysiological aspects?"

Fig. 1 presents the results of this literature search. The data clearly show that the number of papers per year of the first group (RSD/SMP, sympathetic nervous system and pain) rose exponentially, by a factor of six to seven-fold between 1966–1974 and 1990–1995; extrapolations for the period 1995–1999 project a mean of about 200 papers per year. The mean number of papers in the second group (causalgia, algodystrophy, Sudeck) remained almost stagnant, increasing by a factor of 1.6 between 1966–1974 and 1990–1995. Finally, the inset in Fig. 1 shows that the fraction of all papers dealing with pathophysiological aspects rose from roughly 15% in 1966–1974 to 40% in the period 1990–1995.

This literature underscores the importance of material covered in this book and the attention that this disorder has attracted from the medical and scientific community since 1980. Undoubtedly, this attention will increase during the next five years. The tangible increase in experimental clinical and animal work addressing pathophysiological aspects holds considerable promise that ultimately an understanding of the different mechanisms that operate in RSD/CRPS will accrue from this activity. This is a fundamental message that, we hope, will trigger new and more original research than has been the case in the past.

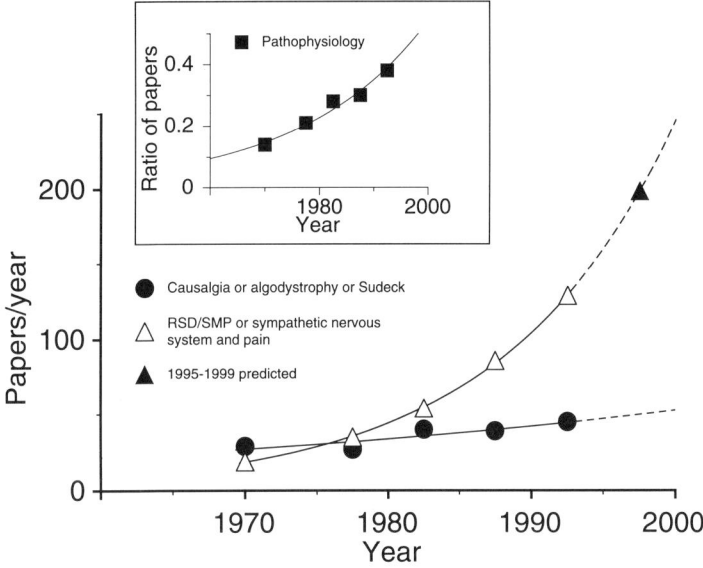

Fig. 1. Medline search for papers listing the key words reflex sympathetic dystrophy, sympathetically maintained pain, and sympathetic nervous system and pain (group 1, △), and the key words causalgia, algodystrophy, and Sudeck (group 2, ●). Ordinate scale, mean number of papers published per year during the respective periods (1966–74, 75–79, 80–84, 85–89, 90–mid-95). The predicted value spans the period 1995–1999. Inset: percentage of all papers (N=2384) concerned with pathophysiological aspects.

Index

A
Adolescence, reflex sympathetic dystrophy in, 67, 75
α-Adrenergic receptors, 219–220
Afferents
  affecting blood vessels, 13
  C fibers. *See* C fibers, afferent
  coupling with sympathetic neurons, 11–12
  mechanically insensitive, 138
  primary
    conduction velocity, 160
    in dynamic mechanical allodynia mediation, 159–162
    electrical stimulation, 159–160
    local anesthetic block, 162
    microneurography, 162
    nerve compression block, 161–162
    sensitivity and axon diameter, 159
  sensitization in trauma, 10–11
Afferents, nociceptive
  acute pain signaling, 124–125
  excitability in neuralgia, 124
  heat hyperalgesia mediation, 128–130
  stimulus-independent pain mediation, 126–127
  unmyelinated
    and brush-evoked pain, 134
    mechanically sensitive, 139, 141
    nonresponsiveness to mechanical stimulation, 138
    pressure hyperalgesia mediation, 137–138
    sensitization to catecholamines, 130–133
Alcoholism, 196
Allodynia
  central nervous system processing, 43
  cold, 167–168, 170
  in CRPS diagnosis, 85
  definition, 154
  dynamic mechanical
    afferent mediation, 159–162
    evoked sensations, 156–158
    patient description of, 156
    physiopathology, 159–162
    sensory evaluation, 156–158, 170
    temporal summation, 163
  dynamic *vs.* static, 154–155
  heat, 163–167, 170
  mechanoreceptor function, 134, 220
  in reflex sympathetic dystrophy, 28–29, 56
  sensory evaluation
    electrical skin stimulation, 159
    methods, 98, 156–158, 170
    nerve compression block, 161–162
    thermal stimulation, 163, 167
    threshold assessment, 157–158
  spinal substrates, 14
  static mechanical, 158–159, 170
Amitriptyline, 73
Analgesia
  nonopioid, endogenous, 3
  opioid, endogenous, 3
  placebo. *See* Placebo effect
  sympathetic nerve block efficacy, 228–231
Anesthetics, local
  in differential blocking, 233–234
  pharmacodynamics, 186
  in sympathetic nerve block, 34–35
    diagnostic use, 217–237
    history, 217–218
    regional spread, 228
Animal experimentation, 107. *See also* Models, animal
Antidepressants, tricyclic, 73
Anti-inflammatory drugs, nonsteroidal, 73
Anxiety, 89, 177–179
Autonomic nerve block. *See* Sympathetic nerve block
Autonomic testing, 100–101
Autotomy, in transection neuroma, 112–113
Axons
  reflex sweat response, 51, 99, 218
  sensitivity, 159

B

Behavior therapy, 72
Behavioral responses, 195–196
Biofeedback, 72
Blood vessels, afferent control, 13
Bone changes, 30, 69
Bone scan, three-phase, 30, 69
Bradykinin, in hyperalgesia, 130
Brush-evoked pain, 134–136
Bupivacaine, 112

C

Catecholamines
 physiopathology, 131–132
 and postganglionic terminals, 132
 and stump neuromas, 131
Causalgia
 in children, 67
 classification, 81–82
 definition, 6, 101
 diagnosis
  criteria, 101–102
  differential, 28
  with guanethidine, 220–221
 epidemiology, 33
 motor function impairment, 33
 peripheral nerve injuries, 33, 36
 and personality, 197
 as regional pain syndrome, 110
 skin temperature, 36–37
 and sympathectomy failure, 117–118
 symptoms, 33, 44, 102
Central nervous system
 allodynia processing, 43
 injuries in CRPS, 89, 111
 physiopathology, 113
 in reflex sympathetic dystrophy, 42–43
 sympathetic function in, 1
C fibers, afferent
 conduction velocity, 160
 heat-pain threshold, 125, 129
 warmth perception assessment, 167
Children
 causalgia in, 67
 reflex sympathetic dystrophy
  diagnosis, 69–70
  differences from adults, 68
  disability, 71
  drug therapy, 72–73
  occurrence, 67
  psychological aspects, 70–72
  and sympathetic nerve block, 73–74
  symptoms, 68
  treatment, 72–75
Circulation, skin, 29

Cognition, 175, 201–202
Cold
 hyperalgesia, 142, 167–169
 hypoalgesia, 167–169
 probe testing, 168–169
Complex regional pain syndrom (CRPS)
 age factors, 27
 behavioral changes, 84
 central nervous system
  injuries, 89, 111
  physiopathology, 42–43
 classification, 6, 81–84, 91
 clinical questions, 18–19
 diagnosis
  criteria, 88–89, 96–97, 102–104
  differential, 28, 90
  tests for, 34–36
 epidemiology, 27
 and extremity disuse, 89
 genetic predisposition, 89
 movement disorders in, 87
 neural pathways to target organs, 14
 as neurological disease, 15–19
 nomenclature, 6, 79–81
 physiopathology, 8–9, 25–26, 44
 psychological aspects, 7, 89
 and repetitive noxious stimulation, 89–90
 sensory testing
  in differential diagnosis, 151–152
  in management, 152
  methods, 170
 somatosensory changes, 86
 sympathetic activity in, 14, 26, 87
 sympathetic efferent system in, 173
 symptoms, 7–9, 25, 85–88
 and thermoregulation, 42, 87
 tissue changes, 13
 trophic changes in, 88
 type I. *See* Reflex sympathetic dystrophy
 type II. *See* Causalgia
 type III, 81–82
 types combined in same patient, 34
 vasomotor response, 87
Conditioning, classical, 175
Conditioning, operant, 202
Confrontational defense, 3
Constriction injury, chronic
 animal models, 108
 characteristics of pain, 116
 drug therapy, 114–115
 pain mapping in, 110
 sympathectomy in, 116
 and sympathetic vasoconstriction, 116

CRPS. *See* Complex regional pain syndrome (CRPS)
Cuff block, 161–162

D
Defense behavior, 3
Depression, 89
Desipramine, 73
Differential nerve block
  epidural, 233
  with local anesthetics, 233–234
  neurophysiology, 231–232
  in psychogenic pain, 232
  spinal, 232–233
  therapeutic use, 232–233
Double-blind studies, 181–182
Drug dependence, 196
Dysalgia, 81
Dysesthesia, 155

E
Edema, 29, 98
Efferents
  pathways to target organs, 1–2
  physiopathology, 8
  role in complex regional pain syndrome, 173
Electrical stimulation, transcutaneous. *See* Transcutaneous electrical nerve stimulation (TENS)
Epinephrine, 5
Erythromelalgia, 141–142
Expectation, in placebo effect, 176–178

F
Factitious illness, 207–208
Fear, 89, 202
Flight reaction, 3

G
Genetic predisposition, 89
Guanethidine, 5, 35, 220–221

H
Heat
  hyperalgesia
    nociceptor mediation, 128–130
    and skin temperature, 135
    tests for, 163–165, 167
  hypoalgesia, 163–165
  probe testing, 167
Hidden infusion, 181, 182–183
HLA antigens, 89
Homeostasis, 1

Hyperalgesia
  afferent mechanisms, 123–150
  chemical, 130
  cold
    mechanisms, 142
    tests for, 167–169, 170
  in CRPS diagnosis, 85
  in deep tissues, 143
  definition, 154
  drug therapy, 112, 118
  dynamic *vs.* static, 154–155
  evaluation of, 98
  heat
    nociceptor mediation, 128–130
    sensory evaluation, 170
    and skin temperature, 135
  mechanical
    blunt pressure, 137–141
    brush-evoked pain, 134–136
    impact stimuli, 141–142
    pinprick, 136–137
    sensory evaluation, 158, 170
    subtypes, 127
  norepinephrine stimulation, 118–119
  physiopathology, 4
  primary, 127
  secondary, 127
  with spontaneous pain, 4
  static mechanical, 158–159
  stimulus-induced, 127
  tissue damage in extremities, 4
  tissue inflammation, 4, 128
Hyperhidrosis, 42
Hyperpathia
  definition, 154
  sensory evaluation, 164–165
Hypoalgesia
  cold, 167–169
  definition, 154
  heat, 163–165
Hypoesthesia, 154

I
Impact stimuli, 141–142
Inflammation
  and chemical sensitivity, 138–139, 141
  pain control mechanisms, 126
  in reflex sympathetic dystrophy, 30
Ischemia test, 36, 100

L
Learning, 175–176
Lidocaine
  in sympathetic nerve block, 184, 186
  systemic absorption, 228

Lumbar sympathetic block
  complications, 227–228
  evidence of sympatholysis, 226, 227
  lateral approach, 225–226
  paramedian approach, 226
  utilization, 224–225

M

Malingering, 203, 207–208
Mechanoreceptors
  receptive field size, 138
  in touch-evoked pain, 134, 159, 220
Mental disorders, 196–197, 200
Mesencephalon, 3
Models, animal. *See also* Animal experimentation
  chronic constriction injury, 108
  pain
    mapping, 110–111
    sympathetically maintained, 108–109
    time factors in, 109
  partial nerve transection, 108
  spinal nerve transection, 108
Mononeuropathy, 37
Motivation, in placebo response, 177
Motoneurons, 13
Movement disorders
  in CRPS diagnosis, 87
  in reflex sympathetic dystrophy, 98, 99
Musculoskeletal system, 29–30

N

Nerve constriction, chronic, 37
Nerve transection, 108
Nervous system disorders, 153–154
Neural pathways, 14
Neuralgia
  pressure hyperalgesia in, 138
  stimulus-independent pain, 126–127
  symptom-oriented approach, 124
Neurons
  afferent. *See* Afferents, nociceptive
  efferent. *See* Efferents
  sympathetic
    coupling with afferent neurons, 11–12
    discharge patterns, 12
    physiopathology, 12–13
    vasoconstrictor, 42
Neuropathic pain, 153–154
N-methyl-D-aspartate (NMDA) receptor blockers
  in long-term pain relief, 112
  in peripheral neuropathy therapy, 111–112
Nociception
  α-adrenergic receptors in, 219–220

definition, 153
norepinephrine-induced, 219–220
pain in, 153
Nociceptors
  acute pain signaling, 124–125
  continuous discharge in neuropathy, 126
  in glabrous skin, 130
  in heat hyperalgesia, 135–136
  norepinephrine responsiveness, 118–119
  norepinephrine stimulation, 117
  sensitization, 10–11, 118–119
  stimulation in autotomy, 112
  in touch-evoked pain, 134–136, 159
Norepinephrine
  in hyperalgesia, 118–119
  in nociception, 219–220
  sympathectomy and responsiveness, 117
Nortriptyline, 73

O

Operant conditioning, 202
Osteoporosis, 30, 100

P

Pain
  adrenoceptor-mediated, 117
  affective-motivational dimension, 178–179
  animal models, 108–109
  characteristics, 56, 60, 81, 97
  classification, 123
  clinical probability scale, 56, 58
  cold-evoked, 167–169
  in deep tissues, 143
  discomfort evaluation, 166–167
  evoked, 153
  extraterritorial, 110–111
  heat-evoked
    probe tests, 167
    temporal characteristics, 166–167
    thermal stimulation, 163–165
  intensity, 164–166
  nervous system adaptation, 123
  nociceptive *vs.* neuropathic, 153
  orthostatic, 28
  psychogenic. *See* Psychogenic pain
  psychological factors, 178–179, 201–202
  sensory-discriminative dimension, 178
  spontaneous, 4, 85, 152–153
  stimulus-independent, 123
  and sympathetic nervous system
    afferent physiopathology, 11–12
    generalized reactions, 3
    localized and selective reactions, 4
    mechanisms, 9–13
    physiopathology, 4

target organs, 12–13
tissue damage in extremities, 4
threshold stimulation, 153
visceral, 4
Paresthesia, 155
Pediatrics. *See* Children
Phentolamine, 5, 69–70
Peripheral autonomous pain syndrome, 80
Peripheral edema vascular abnormality, 80–81
Peripheral nerve injuries
  animal models, 108–109
  in causalgia, 33, 36
  drug therapy, 112, 114
  pain control in, 115–116
  physiopathology, 114–115
  and sympathetic system, 115–116
Peripheral nervous system, sympathetic function in, 1
Personality
  in causalgia, 197
  in reflex sympathetic dystrophy, 197–199
  and response to pain, 201
  retrospective assessment, 199
Phantom pain, 112
Phentolamine
  in diagnostic studies, 69–70
  in pain relief, 5
  in SMP assessment, 186–187, 221, 228
  vs. stellate ganglion block, 229
Physical therapy, 72
Pinprick hyperalgesia, 136–137
Placebo effect
  and anxiety, 177–179
  assessment of
    control methods, 181–183
    natural history of pain intensity, 179–180
    observational problems, 180–181
  cognitive factors, 175, 178–179
  and desire for relief, 177–178
  environmental factors, 174
  expectation in, 176–178
  learning in, 175–176
  motivation in, 177
  multiple dimensions of pain, 178–179
  and saline, 184, 186, 218
  situational factors, 174
  in sympathetic nerve block, 6–7, 218
  in sympathetically maintained pain, 183–188, 228
Polyneuropathy, 37
Pressure hyperalgesia
  and chemical sensitivity, 138–139, 141

  in neuralgia, 138
  nociceptive afferent mediation, 137
Procaine, 218
Protopathia, 56
Psychogenic pain, 202–206, 232–233
Psychological aspects
  family factors, 70–72
  instruments, 99
  locus of control, 201
Psychophysiology, 194–195

Q

Quantitative sensory testing (QST), 218
Quantitative sweat evaluation
  abnormal indices, 53–54
  as axon reflex, 218
  in sudomotor evaluation, 50-51, 53–54, 98–99
  utilization, 52
Quantitative sudomotor axon reflex test (QSART), 50
  abnormalities, 54–55, 62–65
  in diagnosis, 57–60
  recordings, 52–53
Quiescence, 3

R

Radionuclide imaging, children *vs.* adults, 69
Reaction time, 160–161
Reflex sympathetic dystrophy (RSD)
  bone metabolism, 30
  central nervous system, physiopathology, 42–43
  in children and adolescents, 67–77
  classification, 81–82
  and deep tissue injuries, 113
  definition, 5–6, 93
  diagnosis
    autonomic testing, 100–101
    in children, 69–70
    clinical scales, 58–65, 94–96
    correlation of clinical and laboratory indices, 62–65
    criteria, 57, 94–97, 103
    differential, 28
      vs. factitious illness, 207–208
      vs. malingering, 207–208
      vs. psychogenic pain, 203–206
    physical examination, 98–99
    miscellaneous testing, 100
    radiography, 100
  drug therapy, 72–73
  edema in, 29, 98
  inflammation in, 30

Reflex sympathetic dystrophy *(cont.)*
  laboratory diagnosis
    bone scans, three-phase, 69, 100
    criteria for abnormality, 53–54
    pain probability scale, 56, 58
    patient characteristics, 50, 51
    scales for, 58–60, 62–65, 94–96
    skin vasomotor response, 52–53, 99
    sudomotor evaluation, 50–52, 99
    validity of, 57
  musculoskeletal function in, 29–30
  neurological function, 15–19, 61
  osteoporosis in, 30
  pain
    characteristics, 56, 60–61, 97
    orthostatic, 28
    somatosensory functions, 27–28
  physiopathology, 4, 44
  psychological aspects
    absence of reaction, 193
    alcoholism, 196
    behavior, 195–196
    in children, 70–72, 200–201
    comparison with other pain
      syndromes, 199–200
    drug dependence, 196
    mental disorders, 196–197
    and outcome, 200–201
    overview, 191–193
    personality, 197–199
    psychiatric complications, 193
    psychophysiology, 194–195
    stress, 194–195
    therapy, 208–209
  as regional pain syndrome, 110
  skin
    blood flow, 29, 39–41
    temperature, 38
  spontaneous remission, 32, 44
  staging, 32
  sweating in, 29, 50–51, 61
  swelling in, 98
  sympathetic functions in, 37–38, 61–64, 93–94, 97–98
  sympathetic nerve block
    diagnostic use, 57, 94–95, 100, 217–218
    placebo effects, 6–7, 184–186
    therapeutic use, 5, 73–75
  symptoms
    autonomic changes, 61, 93
    clinical characteristics, 27, 37, 43–44, 49–66, 97–98
    combination and variability, 31
    external stimuli affecting, 31
    sensory changes, 8–9, 28–29, 97
    trophic changes, 30, 44, 61, 98, 99
    vasomotor changes, 61
  time factors, 31
Regional sensitization disorder, 80
Remission, spontaneous, 32, 44
RSD. *See* Reflex sympathetic dystrophy (RSD)
RSD/SMP. *See* Reflex sympathetic dystrophy (RSD)
RSO, resting sweat output. *See* Sudomotor evaluation; Sweating

S
Saline, 184, 186, 218
Sciatic nerve diseases, 112–113
Sciatic nerve injury in rats, 113
Scintigraphy. *See* Radionuclide imaging
Sensation disorders
  in CRPS diagnosis, 86
  and disease confirmation, 151–152
  nomenclature, 155
  stimulus-defined *vs.* mechanistic-defined, 155–156
  testing, 98, 151–152
SIP (Sympathetically independent pain). *See* Sympathetically maintained pain (SMP)
Skin
  blood flow, 29, 36–37, 39–41
  trophic changes, 30, 88
Skin temperature
  in causalgia, 36–37
  in chronic nerve constriction, 37
  criteria for abnormality, 54
  in CRPS diagnosis, 87
  and heat hyperalgesia, 135
  in reflex sympathetic dystrophy, 38, 99
  resting conditions, 38, 40
  under thermal load, 39
SMP. *See* Sympathetically maintained pain (SMP)
Stellate ganglion block
  advantages of, 223
  complications, 224
  evidence of sympatholysis, 223–224
  technique, 221–223
  vs. phentolamine in SMP diagnosis, 229
Stress, psychological, 194–195
Sudeck's atrophy, 100
Sudomotor evaluation. *See also* Sweating
  criteria for abnormality, 53–54
  evoked response, 52, 99
  methods, 50–51, 98, 218
  resting output, 52, 99

Sweating. *See also* Sudomotor evaluation
  in CRPS diagnosis, 87
  laboratory evaluation, 50–55
  in reflex sympathetic dystrophy, 29, 99
Swelling, 86, 98
Sympathectomy
  and neuralgia, 118
  and norepinephrine responsiveness, 117
  and pain recurrence, 117–118
  in peripheral pain relief, 115–116
Sympathetic nerve block
  in children, 73–75
  diagnostic use, 6–7, 34–35, 57, 94–95, 100, 183–184
  efficacy, 228–231
  evaluation of completeness, 218–219
  failure of, 230
  methods
    α-adrenergic receptor agonists, 220–221
    local anesthetics, 34–35, 217–237
    lumbar sympathetic block, 224–228
    saline, 184, 186, 218
    stellate ganglion block, 221–224
  in pain relief, 5, 73–75
  and placebo response, 6–7, 183–186, 218
Sympathetic nervous system
  anatomy, 1–3
  and central nervous system function, 1
  chronic pain maintenance, 131
  efferents, 1, 8
  neural pathways to target organs, 1–2, 14
  pain
    afferent and sympathetic neuron coupling, 11–12
    mechanisms, 9–13
    spontaneous, with hyperalgesia, 4
    target organs, 12–13
    and tissue damage in extremities, 4
    and tissue inflammation, 4
    visceral, 4
  and skin temperature, 36–37
Sympathetically independent pain (SIP). *See* Sympathetically maintained pain (SMP)
Sympathetically maintained pain (SMP)
  animal models, 108–109
  assessment
    phentolamine test, 186–187, 221
    placebo response, 183–188
    sympathetic nerve block, 183–186
  central processing of, 219–220
  chemical hyperalgesia in, 130–131
  and chronic compression syndrome, 116
  classification, 81–83
  definition, 4
  diagnosis
    differential, 7, 231
    false-positive, 228
    phentolamine *vs.* stellate ganglion block, 229
  hyperexcitability factors, 220
  management of, 220
  in peripheral neuropathy
    animal models, 115–116
    in humans, 116
  sympathectomy induction, 117
  as symptom, 6, 26
  and unmyelinated afferent fibers, 131–132
  without nerve injury, 118–119
Sympatholysis. *See* Sympathetic nerve block

T

Temperature, skin. *See* Skin temperature
TENS. *See* Transcutaneous electrical nerve stimulation (TENS)
Tests, diagnostic
  complex regional pain syndrome
    guanethidine, 35
    ischemia, 36, 100
    phentolamine, 35–36
    sympathetic nerve block, 34–35
  dynamic mechanical allodynia, 156–158
  heat-evoked pain, 163–167
  mechanical hyperalgesia, 158
  static mechanical allodynia, 158–159
  static mechanical hyperalgesia, 158–159
Thermal stimulation, 163–169
Threshold stimulation
  cold, 167–168
  definition, 153
  electrical, 159–160
  heat, 163–165
Touch-evoked pain. *See* Allodynia
Transcutaneous electrical nerve stimulation (TENS), 72, 159–160
Transection neuroma, 112–113
Trazodone, 73
Tremor, 29–30

V

Vasoconstriction
  in chronic constriction injury, 116
  physiopathology, 41–42
  and skin blood flow, 39–41
Vasomotor response
  in CRPS diagnosis, 87
  indices, 50–51
  measurement, 52–53, 98
Visceral pain, 4